Smart Fertilizers and Innovative Organic Amendments for Sustainable Agricultural Systems

Smart Fertilizers and Innovative Organic Amendments for Sustainable Agricultural Systems

Editors

Maria de la Luz Mora
Cornelia Rumpel
Marcela Calabi-Floody

MDPI • Basel • Beijing • Wuhan • Barcelona • Belgrade • Manchester • Tokyo • Cluj • Tianjin

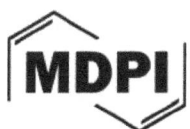

Editors

Maria de la Luz Mora
Center of Plant-Soil Interaction and Natural Resources Biotechnology, Scientific and Biotechnological Bioresource Nucleus, Universidad de la Frontera
Chile

Cornelia Rumpel
CNRS, Institute of Ecology and Environmental Sciences, UMR 7618 (CNRS, Sorbonne U, UPEC, INRAE, IRD)
France

Marcela Calabi-Floody
Center of Plant-Soil Interaction and Natural Resources Biotechnology, Scientific and Biotechnological Bioresource Nucleus, Universidad de la Frontera
Chile

Editorial Office
MDPI
St. Alban-Anlage 66
4052 Basel, Switzerland

This is a reprint of articles from the Special Issue published online in the open access journal *Agronomy* (ISSN 2073-4395) (available at: https://www.mdpi.com/journal/agronomy/special_issues/smart_fertilizers_sustainable-agricultural).

For citation purposes, cite each article independently as indicated on the article page online and as indicated below:

LastName, A.A.; LastName, B.B.; LastName, C.C. Article Title. *Journal Name* **Year**, *Volume Number*, Page Range.

ISBN 978-3-0365-2762-8 (Hbk)
ISBN 978-3-0365-2763-5 (PDF)

Cover image courtesy of Cornelia Rumpel

© 2021 by the authors. Articles in this book are Open Access and distributed under the Creative Commons Attribution (CC BY) license, which allows users to download, copy and build upon published articles, as long as the author and publisher are properly credited, which ensures maximum dissemination and a wider impact of our publications.

The book as a whole is distributed by MDPI under the terms and conditions of the Creative Commons license CC BY-NC-ND.

Contents

About the Editors vii

Preface to "Smart Fertilizers and Innovative Organic Amendments for Sustainable Agricultural Systems" ix

María de la Luz Mora, Marcela Calabi-Floody and Cornelia Rumpel
Closing Biogeochemical Cycles and Meeting Plant Requirements by Smart Fertilizers and Innovative Organic Amendments
Reprinted from: *Agronomy*, 11, 1158, doi:10.3390/agronomy11061158 1

Luca Incrocci, Rita Maggini, Tommaso Cei, Giulia Carmassi, Luca Botrini, Ferruccio Filippi, Ronald Clemens, Cristian Terrones and Alberto Pardossi
Innovative Controlled-Release Polyurethane-Coated Urea Could Reduce N Leaching in Tomato Crop in Comparison to Conventional and Stabilized Fertilizers
Reprinted from: *Agronomy* 2020, 10, 1827, doi:10.3390/agronomy10111827 7

Muhammad Izhar Shafi, Muhammad Adnan, Shah Fahad, Fazli Wahid, Ahsan Khan, Zhen Yue, Subhan Danish, Muhammad Zafar-ul-Hye, Martin Brtnicky and Rahul Datta
Application of Single Superphosphate with Humic Acid Improves the Growth, Yield and Phosphorus Uptake of Wheat (*Triticum aestivum* L.) in Calcareous Soil
Reprinted from: *Agronomy* 2020, 10, 1224, doi:10.3390/agronomy10091224 27

Ana Paula Bettoni Teles, Marcos Rodrigues and Paulo Sergio Pavinato
Solubility and Efficiency of Rock Phosphate Fertilizers Partially Acidulated with Zeolite and Pillared Clay as Additives
Reprinted from: *Agronomy* 2020, 10, 918, doi:10.3390/agronomy10070918 43

Isis Vega, Cornelia Rumpel, Antonieta Ruíz, María de la Luz Mora, Daniel F. Calderini and Paula Cartes
Silicon Modulates the Production and Composition of Phenols in Barley under Aluminum Stress
Reprinted from: *Agronomy* 2020, 10, 1138, doi:10.3390/agronomy10081138 67

Ahmed Fathy Yousef, Mohamed Ahmed Youssef, Muhammad Moaaz Ali, Muhammed Mustapha Ibrahim, Yong Xu and Rosario Paolo Mauro
Improved Growth and Yield Response of Jew's Mallow (*Corchorus olitorius* L.) Plants through Biofertilization under Semi-Arid Climate Conditions in Egypt
Reprinted from: *Agronomy* 2020, 10, 1801, doi:10.3390/agronomy10111801 85

Iraj Emadodin, Thorsten Reinsch, Raffaele-Romeo Ockens and Friedhelm Taube
Assessing the Potential of Jellyfish as an Organic Soil Amendment to Enhance Seed Germination and Seedling Establishment in Sand Dune Restoration
Reprinted from: *Agronomy* 2020, 10, 863, doi:10.3390/agronomy10060863 99

Thomas Klammsteiner, Veysel Turan, Marina Fernández-Delgado Juárez, Simon Oberegger and Heribert Insam
Suitability of Black Soldier Fly Frass as Soil Amendment and Implication for Organic Waste Hygienization
Reprinted from: *Agronomy* 2020, 10, 1578, doi:10.3390/agronomy10101578 109

Anne-Maïmiti Dulaurent, Guillaume Daoulas, Michel-Pierre Faucon and David Houben
Earthworms (*Lumbricus terrestris* L.) Mediate the Fertilizing Effect of Frass
Reprinted from: *Agronomy* **2020**, *10*, 783, doi:10.3390/agronomy10060783 . . . . **121**

Marie-Liesse Aubertin, Cyril Girardin, Sabine Houot, Cécile Nobile, David Houben, Sarah Bena, Yann Le Brech and Cornelia Rumpel
Biochar-Compost Interactions as Affected by Weathering: Effects on Biological Stability and Plant Growth
Reprinted from: *Agronomy* **2021**, *11*, 336, doi:10.3390/agronomy11020336 . . . . **129**

Verónica Berriel, Jorge Monza and Carlos H. Perdomo
Cover Crop Selection by Jointly Optimizing Biomass Productivity, Biological Nitrogen Fixation, and Transpiration Efficiency: Application to Two *Crotalaria* Species
Reprinted from: *Agronomy* **2020**, *10*, 1116, doi:10.3390/agronomy10081116 . . . . **143**

Chau Thi Da, Phan Anh Tu, John Livsey, Van Tai Tang, Håkan Berg and Stefano Manzoni
Improving Productivity in Integrated Fish-Vegetable Farming Systems with Recycled Fish Pond Sediments
Reprinted from: *Agronomy* **2020**, *10*, 1025, doi:10.3390/agronomy10071025 . . . . **155**

About the Editors

Maria de la Luz Mora leads an interdisciplinary research group (Plant–Soil Interaction and Plant Biotechnology) and contributes significantly to plant production, especially in the cereal, meat, and milk industries in southern Chile. Dr. Mora is the author and co-author of more than 190 scientific publications with contributions of international researchers, doctorate students, and post doctorates. In addition, she has lead and participated in several International Cooperation Programs with Research Centers of excellence. She has been the Director of the Scientific and Technological Bioresources Nucleus (Bioren-Ufro) since 2009. During her career, she has directed several National and Co-International projects. She was the creator of the Doctorate Program in Sciences of Natural Resources, and she also has advised about 20 PhD students. She has been working on projects that contribute to the knowledge to understand the coupled C-N-P cycles to contribute to food security and production.

Cornelia Rumpel is a soil biogeochemist working for the French National Research Center (CNRS) at the Institute of Ecology and Environment in Paris, France. Her work is concerned with the dynamics of organic matter at the molecular scale and the biogeochemical cycling of carbon, nitrogen, and phosphorus in natural and managed ecosystems. She focuses on temperate and tropical environments and has contributed to the change of several paradigms. Her recent work focuses on the development of innovative agroecological strategies to increase soil carbon sequestration. She has supervised 18 PhD students to successful completion of their thesis, has published more than 200 papers in international peer reviewed journals, and is listed as a highly cited researcher.

Marcela Calabi-Floody is an interdisciplinary researcher with a strong vision on development and innovation (R&D&i), with expertise in nanotechnology, soil–organic matter interactions, and smart biofertilizer generation. She works in La Frontera University at the Scientific and Technological Bioresource Nucleus (BIOREN) in the field of nanotechnology associated with C sequestration and smart fertilizer development. In addition, she has specialized in nanotechnological and the biotechnological management of agricultural wastes (development, revaluation, and reuse) in order to improve its utilization as C sequestration matrix in soils. Dr. Calabi-Floody has directed and co-directed more than 18 national and international research projects, generating a strong collaboration network. With this research network, she has generated more than 25 high-level scientific articles published in international journals, and disseminated the results at national and international conferences.

Preface to "Smart Fertilizers and Innovative Organic Amendments for Sustainable Agricultural Systems"

Sustainable agricultural practices are needed to provide food security for a growing global population. Food production is usually associated with high nutrient inputs in the form of mineral fertilisers. Since the beginning of agriculture, such practices have led to soil degradation and the release of environmental contaminants. This book focuses on innovations in organic and inorganic fertiliser production. We have compiled studies presenting smart fertilization strategies. The idea for this book originated from the Chilean–French collaboration of the three guest editors during the MEC fellowship of Dr. Cornelia Rumpel at the Universidad de la Frontera in Temuco (Chile). The editors thank all authors for their excellent contributions

Maria de la Luz Mora, Cornelia Rumpel, Marcela Calabi-Floody
Editors

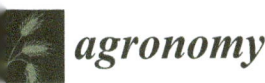

Editorial

Closing Biogeochemical Cycles and Meeting Plant Requirements by Smart Fertilizers and Innovative Organic Amendments

María de la Luz Mora [1], Marcela Calabi-Floody [1,2,*] and Cornelia Rumpel [1,3,*]

1. Center of Plant, Soil Interaction and Natural Resources Biotechnology, Scientific and Biotechnological Bioresource Nucleus, Universidad de La Frontera, BIOREN-UFRO, Av. Francisco Salazar, Temuco 01145, Chile; mariluz.mora@ufrontera.cl
2. Nano-Biotechnology Laboratory, Universidad de La Frontera, Temuco 4811230, Chile
3. Institute of Ecology and Environmental Sciences, UMR 7618 (CNRS, Sorbonne U, UPEC, INRAE, IRD), 75005 Paris, France
* Correspondence: marcela.calabi@ufrontera.cl (M.C.-F.); cornelia.rumpel@inrae.fr (C.R.)

1. Meeting the Growing Food Demand of the Global Population: Challenges for Sustainable Agriculture

Expansion of farmland with food production as a major service has been largely associated with conversion of natural ecosystems like the Amazon and Savanna into new agricultural land [1]. It has resulted in the large scale modification of natural landscapes and ecosystems, altering important climate interactions, such as surface moisture and microbial diversity, and strongly impacting greenhouse gas (GHG) emissions [2]. Indeed, current agricultural activities are the main contributors to GHG emissions, representing globally 20% of the annual atmospheric emissions [3]. They are largely driven by land use change and decoupling of biogeochemical cycles leading to land degradation, and soil organic matter loss since the introduction of agriculture [2,4]. Agriculture contributes to GHG emissions by releasing CO_2, N_2O and CH_4. The agricultural sector is the main contributor to N_2O and CH_4 emissions, which have 260 and 40 times greater global warming potential than CO_2. In particular, N fertilizers are important N_2O sources. Nowadays, it has become clear that agriculture is not only causing climate change by GHG emission, but that it is also highly vulnerable to climate change, which is threatening crop yields in many parts of the world [5]. Moreover, the green revolution in the 1960s, which strongly reformed and increased agricultural production, also had many adverse effects on the environment [6], including soil acidification and pollution of waterways through export of mineral fertilizers not taken up by plants [7,8]. The use of agrochemicals to fight weeds and pests led to biodiversity loss, and highlighted the need for an agroecological transition and a second green revolution. An additional challenge is the necessity to achieve food security of a growing global population [9].

As the earth surface covered by agricultural land (more than 40% of the total Earth surface) cannot be expended anymore [2], sustainable intensification of production on the existing area, while reducing mineral agrochemical use and adapting to climate change, is a great challenge for landowners, scientists and politicians. Recently, it has been suggested that increasing carbon storage in soils could be a solution to mitigate and to adapt to climate change while at the same time supporting agricultural production to increase food security [10,11]. Such a solution can only be brought to scale if region specific solutions adapted to pedoclimatic and socioeconomic conditions are employed [12]. One aspect of sustainable solutions is the replacement of mineral fertilizers by innovative strategies to enhance plant growth. In the light of circular economy, it was suggested that smart fertilization strategies could be based on the transformation of organic wastes from agricultural systems into innovative organic amendments [13,14] and/or carrier materials for beneficial microorganisms and/or enzymes [15]. While improving nutrient availability, fertilization strategies based on organic materials may be an avenue towards sustainable intensification.

Therefore, it is imperative to concentrate efforts to develop innovative fertilizers through biotechnological approaches with or without use of beneficial microorganisms that allow their viability in the soil in the face of an established microbiome. Innovative organic amendments with low GHG emission potential should be designed to foster terrestrial C sequestration and stabilization, capable of mitigating the environmental impact caused by the agricultural sector, while at the same time increasing soil health and adapting to climate change. For this Special Issue, we invited contributions dealing with innovations in organic and inorganic fertilization strategies in order to improve agricultural yields, while at the same time reducing negative externalities and increasing the soils' organic matter contents. It contains 11 articles reporting (1) the effects of new fertilization strategies on soils and plants, (2) characteristics of innovative organic amendments and (3) system innovations based on organic fertilization and waste recycling.

2. Smart Fertilizer Development and Their Effect on Soils and Plants

As the main limiting factor for food production is N and P availability, huge amounts of conventional N and P-fertilizer are applied per year, which often lead to environmental damage [16]. Especially N-fertilizer application at levels exceeding plant requirements leads to significant environmental consequences due to N losses, such as: nitrate (NO_3^-) leaching, ammonia (NH_3) volatilization, and nitrous oxide (N_2O) emission [8,17–19]. The N losses by urea application is one of the main problems in agricultural systems, where leaching of NO_3^- is one of the most important loss pathways due to its high mobility [20]. Incrocci et al. [21] used a (bio)technological approach to develop an innovative controlled-release polyurethane-coated urea fertilizer, which could considerably reduce the N leaching in tomato cultivations. Unlike N, phosphorus (P) is mainly fixed in the soil systems. Therefore, the efforts to improve P use efficiency are focusing on favoring slow release and preventing P fixation in the soil. In this context, Shafi et al. [22] reported that the incorporation of humic acid in combination with chemical P fertilizer can prevent the P fixation in calcareous soil, thus improving crop yield and wheat (*Triticum aestivum* L.) plants' P uptake. Teles et al. [23] developed a new P fertilizer with slow solubility through the partial acidification of rock phosphates, incorporating zeolite and pillared clay into partially acidulated phosphates with high adsorption characteristics. The mechanism of P release is based on the saturation the acidic sites of the clay materials before adsorption. These saturated sites may act as a vehicle for slow and gradual dissolution into soil solution. This strategy seems to be highly promising as it was able to compete with conventional fertilizers.

Mineral fertilization may also lead to soil acidification thereby increasing aluminum (Al^{3+}) toxicity [7,24,25]. In this context, Vega et al. [26] studied the beneficial effects of silicon application for mitigating Al^{3+} toxicity in sensitive barley cultivars. Their findings revealed that silicon fertilization could increase the resistance of barley to Al^{3+} toxicity by regulating the metabolism of phenolic compounds with antioxidant and structural functions.

A liquid biofertilizer combined with a microbial consortium was evaluated by Yousef et al. [27]. These authors used a bacteria and fungi consortium containing *Bacillus circulans*, *B. poylmyxa*, *B. megatherium*, *Candida* spp., and *Trichoderma* spp. and studied its combined effect with liquid biofertilizer on Jew's mallow plant production. They concluded that combined application of inorganic NPK plus biofertilizer is most beneficial to increase growth, yield, and nutrient accumulation of Jew's mallow plants.

3. Innovative Organic Amendments

In order to move to carbon neutrality in agricultural production in agreement with sustainable development goals and global governmental treaties to minimize climate change, different initiatives were launched, such as "4 per Thousand (4p1000)" at the COP21 in Paris, or the Agenda 2030 of the United Nations [28]. Recently, FAO and the Global Soil Partnership (GSP) established "RECSOIL: Recarbonization of global soils" as an initiative to implement the soil organic carbon (SOC) agenda by using the best tools and technologies available [29]. Organic amendments may be a keystone to increase SOC sequestration and provide food security through soil quality improvement. Reuse of organic waste and their transformation into organic amendments is a sustainable strategy that farmers need to apply and scientists have the challenge to innovate. In this context, Emadodin et al. [30] proposed jellyfish application as an organic soil amendment able to allow enhanced seedling growth and establishment of ryegrass on sand dune soil even under water scarcity conditions.

Under a circular economy approach, black soldier flies have the capacity to transform anthropogenic organic wastes into nutritious insect biomass (frass). The fertilizer potential of frass was studied by Klammsteiner et al. [31], who reported that it may serve as a valuable alternative to mineral fertilizers with beneficial effects on plant growth and not impairing the hygienic properties of soils. In addition, Dulaurent et al. [32] investigated the effect of earthworms (*Lumbricus terrestris* L.) on nutrient uptake and crop growth in the presence of frass from mealworm (*Tenebrio molitor* L.). Their study showed a synergistic effect between earthworms and frass on soil fertility and that earthworms thus may improve the efficiency of frass as an organic fertilizer.

Composting, vermicomposting and biochar production using organic wastes are known sustainable practices, which convert these raw materials into valuable organic amendments. Organic amendments may be used individually or in mixture to improve soil carbon sequestration and fertility at the same time [13,33,34]. Aubertin et al. [35] addressed the effect of weathering on biochar-compost mixture properties, their biological stability and their effect on plant growth after soil addition. They were able to show that weathering changed synergistic effects of biochar compost mixtures in terms of carbon sequestration potential and biomass production.

4. System Innovations Based on Organic Fertilization and Waste Recycling

Finally, in order to integrate sustainable agricultural practices, system innovations based on agroecological approaches and waste recycling must be employed. In this context, use of legumes as cover crops in agricultural rotations may reduce the production costs associated with the use of mineral N fertilizers, and also result in environmental benefits. In order to optimize biomass productivity, biological nitrogen fixation, and transpiration efficiency, Berriel et al. [36] evaluated the application of two *Crotalaria* species, specifically *C. juncea* and *C. spectabilis* grown under extreme environmental conditions with the finality to maximize their beneficial attributes, while minimizing water consumption through high transpiration. Their results showed that the *C. spectabilis* has advantages as legumes cover crop over *C. juncea*, in terms of transpiration as indicated by a ^{13}C isotopic analyses.

On the other hand, the chemical fertilizers dependence and/or its coming shortage is a global concern and a huge challenge in terms of food security [15,37]. Thus, the circular economy approach suggests that agricultural systems must become more efficient and favor reuse of their waste as fertilizers in order to reduce external inputs. In this context, recycling of fishpond sediments may be an alternative to reduce the reliance on synthetic fertilizers, due to its high nutritional value [38]. Da et al. [39] studied organic fertilizers based on a composted mixture of 30% of the Pangasius catfish pond sediment and 70% of agricultural waste in cucumber vegetable production. With this strategy, they reduced mineral fertilizer use by up to 75%. Therefore, their results provide evidence that system-inherent organic amendments can be integrated in fish–vegetable farming to provide a more diversified production system with tangible environmental benefits and potentially improved farm income.

The papers presented in this Special Issue indicate that there are multiple ways to increase the production efficiency of agriculture and to reduce external inputs using smart fertizers and innovative organic amendments. We suggest that such strategies should be scaled up to achieve sustainability in agriculture through waste recycling aiming a circular approach to close biogeochemical cycles.

Funding: The authors thank the Chilean government for providing a MEC grant N° MEC80180025 M.C.F. acknowledges funding from Chilean CONICYT (National foundation for Science and Technology) for the financial support under CONICYT-FONDECYT Regural project N° 1201375, and M.L.M thanks FONDECYT Regular N° 1181050. We also acknowledge ECOSSUD-CONICYT C13U02 for their financial support to encourage collaboration between French and Chilean research groups.

Data Availability Statement: Not applicable.

Acknowledgments: This Special Issue was launched during the sabbatical of C.R. at the Universidad de la Frontera (Temuco, Chile).

Conflicts of Interest: The authors declare no conflict of interest.

References

1. Campbell, B.M.; Beare, D.J.; Bennett, E.M.; Hall-Spencer, J.M.; Ingram, J.S.I.; Jaramillo, F.; Ortiz, R.; Ramankutty, N.; Sayer, J.A.; Shindell, D. Agriculture production as a major driver of the Earth system exceeding planetary boundaries. *Ecol. Soc.* **2017**, *22*. [CrossRef]
2. McDermid, S.S.; Mearns, L.O.; Ruane, A.C. Representing agriculture in Earth System Models: Approaches and priorities for development. *J. Adv. Model. Earth Syst.* **2017**, *9*, 2230–2265. [CrossRef] [PubMed]
3. IPCC. Global Warming of 1.5 C. 2018. Available online: https://ipcc.ch/report/sr15/ (accessed on 22 May 2021).
4. Sanderman, J.; Hengl, T.; Fiske, G.J. Soil carbon debt of 12,000 years of human land use. *Proc. Natl. Acad. Sci. USA* **2017**, *114*, 9575–9580. [CrossRef]
5. Ray, D.K.; Ramankutty, N.; Mueller, N.D.; West, P.C.; Foley, J.A. Recent patterns of crop yield growth and stagnation. *Nat. Commun.* **2012**, *3*, 1293. [CrossRef]
6. Pingali, P.L. Green revolution: Impacts, limits, and the path ahead. *Proc. Natl. Acad. Sci. USA* **2012**, *109*, 12–302. [CrossRef] [PubMed]
7. Mora, M.D.L.L.; Cartes, P.; Núñez, P.; Salazar, M.; Demanet, R. Movement of n0(3)-n and nh4-n in an andisol and its influence on ryegrass production in a short term study. *Rev. Cienc. Suelo Y Nutr. Veg.* **2007**, *7*, 46–64. [CrossRef]
8. Good, A.G.; Beatty, P.H. Fertilizing Nature: A Tragedy of Excess in the Commons. *PLoS Biol.* **2011**, *9*, e1001124. [CrossRef]
9. Poppy, G.M.; Jepson, P.C.; Pickett, J.A.; Birkett, M.A. Achieving food and environmental security: New approaches to close the gap. *Phil. Trans. R. Soc. B* **2014**, *369*, 20120272. [CrossRef] [PubMed]
10. Chabbi, A.; Lehmann, J.; Ciais, P.; Loescher, H.W.; Cotrufo, M.F.; Don, A.; SanClements, M.; Schipper, L.; Six, J.; Smith, P.; et al. Aligning agriculture and climate policy. *Nat. Clim. Chang.* **2017**, *7*, 307–309. [CrossRef]
11. Rumpel, C.; Amiraslani, F.; Chenu, C.; Cardenas, M.G.; Kaonga, M.; Koutika, L.-S.; Ladha, J.; Madari, B.; Shirato, Y.; Smith, P.; et al. The 4p1000 Initiative: Opportunities, limitations and challenges for implementing soil organic carbon sequestration as a sustainable development strategy. *Ambio* **2020**, *49*, 350–360. [CrossRef] [PubMed]
12. Amelung, W.; Bossio, D.; de Vries, W.; Kögel-Knabner, I.; Lehmann, J.; Amundson, R.; Bol, R.; Collins, C.; Lal, R.; Leifeld, J.; et al. Towards a global-scale soil climate mitigation strategy. *Nat. Commun.* **2020**, *11*, 5427. [CrossRef]
13. Barthod, J.; Rumpel, C.; Dignac, M.-F. Composting with additives to improve organic amendments. A review. *Agron. Sustain. Dev.* **2018**, *38*, 17. [CrossRef]
14. Zhao, S.; Schmidt, S.; Qin, W.; Li, J.; Li, G.; Zhang, W. Towards the circular nitrogen economy—A global meta-analysis of composting technologies reveals much potential for mitigating nitrogen losses. *Sci. Total. Environ.* **2020**, *704*, 135401. [CrossRef]
15. Calabi-Floody, M.; Medina, J.; Rumpel, C.; Condron, L.M.; Hernandez, M.; Dumont, M.; Mora, M.L. Chapter Three - Smart fertilizers as a strategy for sustainable agriculture. In: Donald LS, editor. *Adv. Agron.* **2018**, *147*, 119–157. [CrossRef]
16. Roy, R.N.; Finck, A.; Blair, G.J.; Tandon, H.L.S. Plant nutrition for food security. In *A Guide for Integrated Nutrient Management*; FAO Fertilizer and Plant Nutrition Bulletin: Rome, Italy, 2006; Volume 16.
17. Muñoz, C.; Paulino, L.; Monreal, C.; Zagal, E. Greenhouse Gas (CO_2 AND N_2O) Emissions from Soils: A Review. *Chil. J. Agric. Res.* **2010**, *70*, 485–497. [CrossRef]
18. Núñez, P.A.; Demanet, R.; Misselbrook, T.H.; Alfaro, M.; Mora, M.D.L.L. Nitrogen Losses under Different Cattle Grazing Frequencies and Intensities in a Volcanic Soil of Southern Chile. *Chil. J. Agric. Res.* **2010**, *70*, 237–250. [CrossRef]
19. Saggar, S.; Jha, N.; Deslippe, J.; Bolan, N.; Luo, J.; Giltrap, D.; Kim, D.-G.; Zaman, M.; Tillman, R. Denitrification and $N_2O:N_2$ production in temperate grasslands: Processes, measurements, modelling and mitigating negative impacts. *Sci. Total. Environ.* **2013**, *465*, 173–195. [CrossRef] [PubMed]
20. Omar, L.; Ahmed, O.H.; Majid, N.M.A. Improving Ammonium and Nitrate Release from Urea Using Clinoptilolite Zeolite and Compost Produced from Agricultural Wastes. *Sci. World J.* **2015**, *2015*, 1–12. [CrossRef]

1. Incrocci, L.; Maggini, R.; Cei, T.; Carmassi, G.; Botrini, L.; Filippi, F.; Clemens, R.; Terrones, C.; Pardossi, A. Innovative Controlled-Release Polyurethane-Coated Urea Could Reduce N Leaching in Tomato Crop in Comparison to Conventional and Stabilized Fertilizers. *Agronomy* **2020**, *10*, 1827. [CrossRef]
2. Shafi, M.I.; Adnan, M.; Fahad, S.; Wahid, F.; Khan, A.; Yue, Z.; Danish, S.; Zafar-Ul-Hye, M.; Brtnicky, M.; Datta, R. Application of Single Superphosphate with Humic Acid Improves the Growth, Yield and Phosphorus Uptake of Wheat (*Triticum aestivum* L.) in Calcareous Soil. *Agronomy* **2020**, *10*, 1224. [CrossRef]
3. Teles, A.P.B.; Rodrigues, M.; Pavinato, P.S. Solubility and Efficiency of Rock Phosphate Fertilizers Partially Acidulated with Zeolite and Pillared Clay as Additives. *Agronomy* **2020**, *10*, 918. [CrossRef]
4. Haygarth, P.M.; Bardgett, R.D.; Condron, L.M. Phosphorus and nitrogen cycles and their management. In *Soil Conditions and Plant Growth*; Gregory, P.J., Nortcliff, S., Eds.; Wiley-Blackwell: Hoboken, NJ, USA, 2013; pp. 132–159.
5. Mora, M.L.; Demanet, R.; Vistoso, E.; Gallardo, F. Influence of Sulfate Concentration in Mineral Solution on Ryegrass Grown at different pH and aluminium levels. *J. Plant Nutr.* **2005**, *28*, 1–16. [CrossRef]
6. Vega, I.; Rumpel, C.; Ruíz, A.; Mora, M.D.L.L.; Calderini, D.F.; Cartes, P. Silicon Modulates the Production and Composition of Phenols in Barley under Aluminum Stress. *Agronomy* **2020**, *10*, 1138. [CrossRef]
7. Yousef, A.F.; Youssef, M.A.; Ali, M.M.; Ibrahim, M.M.; Xu, Y.; Mauro, R.P. Improved Growth and Yield Response of Jew's Mallow (*Corchorus olitorius* L.) Plants Through Biofertilization Under Semi-Arid Climate Conditions in Egypt. *Agronomy* **2020**, *10*, 1801. [CrossRef]
8. Lal, R. Food security impacts of the "4 per Thousand" initiative. *Geoderma* **2020**, *374*, 114427. [CrossRef]
9. FAO. "RECSOIL: Recarbonization of Global Soils" a Tool to Support the Implementation of the Koronivia Joint Work on Agriculture; FAO: Rome, Italy, 2019.
10. Emadodin, I.; Reinsch, T.; Ockens, R.-R.; Taube, F. Assessing the Potential of Jellyfish as an Organic Soil Amendment to Enhance Seed Germination and Seedling Establishment in Sand Dune Restoration. *Agronomy* **2020**, *10*, 863. [CrossRef]
11. Klammsteiner, T.; Turan, V.; Juárez, M.F.-D.; Oberegger, S.; Insam, H. Suitability of Black Soldier Fly Frass as Soil Amendment and Implication for Organic Waste Hygienization. *Agronomy* **2020**, *10*, 1578. [CrossRef]
12. Dulaurent, A.-M.; Daoulas, G.; Faucon, M.-P.; Houben, D. Earthworms (Lumbricus terrestris L.) Mediate the Fertilizing Effect of Frass. *Agronomy* **2020**, *10*, 783. [CrossRef]
13. Agegnehu, G.; Bird, M.I.; Nelson, P.; Bass, A.M. The ameliorating effects of biochar and compost on soil quality and plant growth on a Ferralsol. *Soil Res.* **2015**, *53*, 1–12. [CrossRef]
14. Scotti, R.; Conte, P.; Berns, A.; Alonzo, G.; Rao, M.A. Effect of Organic Amendments on the Evolution of Soil Organic Matter in Soils Stressed by Intensive Agricultural Practices. *Curr. Org. Chem.* **2013**, *17*, 2998–3005. [CrossRef]
15. Aubertin, M.-L.; Girardin, C.; Houot, S.; Nobile, C.; Houben, D.; Bena, S.; Brech, Y.; Rumpel, C. Biochar-Compost Interactions as Affected by Weathering: Effects on Biological Stability and Plant Growth. *Agronomy* **2021**, *11*, 336. [CrossRef]
16. Berriel, V.; Monza, J.; Perdomo, C. Cover Crop Selection by Jointly Optimizing Biomass Productivity, Biological Nitrogen Fixation, and Transpiration Efficiency: Application to Two *Crotalaria* Species. *Agronomy* **2020**, *10*, 1116. [CrossRef]
17. Cordell, D.; Drangert, J.-O.; White, S. The story of phosphorus: Global food security and food for thought. *Glob. Environ. Chang.* **2009**, *19*, 292–305. [CrossRef]
18. Muendo, P.N.; Verdegem, M.C.J.; Stoorvogel, J.J.; Milstein, A.; Gamal, E.; Duc, P.M.; Verreth, J.A.J. Sediment accumulation in fish ponds: Its potential for agricultural use. *Int. J. Fisher. Aquat. Stud.* **2014**, *1*, 228–241.
19. Da, C.T.; Tu, P.A.; Livsey, J.; Tang, V.T.; Berg, H.; Manzoni, S. Improving Productivity in Integrated Fish-Vegetable Farming Systems with Recycled Fish Pond Sediments. *Agronomy* **2020**, *10*, 1025. [CrossRef]

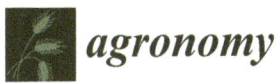

Article

Innovative Controlled-Release Polyurethane-Coated Urea Could Reduce N Leaching in Tomato Crop in Comparison to Conventional and Stabilized Fertilizers

Luca Incrocci [1], Rita Maggini [1,*], Tommaso Cei [1], Giulia Carmassi [1], Luca Botrini [1], Ferruccio Filippi [1], Ronald Clemens [2], Cristian Terrones [2] and Alberto Pardossi [1]

1. Department of Agriculture, Food and Environment, University of Pisa, 56124 Pisa, Italy; luca.incrocci@unipi.it (L.I.); tommaso.cei@gmail.com (T.C.); giulia.carmassi@unipi.it (G.C.); luca.botrini@unipi.it (L.B.); ferruccio.filippi@unipi.it (F.F.); alberto.pardossi@unipi.it (A.P.)
2. ICL Specialty Fertilizers, 6422 PD Heerlen, The Netherlands; ronald.clemens@icl-group.com (R.C.); cristian.terrones@icl-group.com (C.T.)
* Correspondence: rita.maggini@unipi.it

Received: 28 September 2020; Accepted: 17 November 2020; Published: 20 November 2020

Abstract: Large amounts of fertilizers are being used in agriculture to sustain growing demands for food, especially in vegetable production systems. Soluble fertilizers can generally ensure high crop yields, but excessive leaching of nutrients, mainly as nitrate, can be a major cause of water pollution. Controlled-release fertilizers improve the nutrient use efficiency and lower the environmental hazard, usually without affecting the production. In this study, an innovative controlled-release coated urea fertilizer was compared to conventional nitrogen (N) fertilizers and a soluble ammonium-based fertilizer containing a nitrification inhibitor, in a round table tomato cultivation. Both the water and N balance were evaluated for each treatment, along with the yield and quality of the production. The experiment was repeated in three different seasons (spring, autumn and summer-autumn) in a glasshouse to prevent the effect of uncontrolled rainfall. The results indicated that N leaching decreased by increasing the percentage of coated urea. The application of at least 50% total N as coated urea strongly reduced N leaching and improved N agronomic efficiency in comparison with traditional fertilizers, ensuring at the same time a similar fruit production. Due to reduced leaching, the total N amount commonly applied by growers could be lowered by 25% without detrimental effects on commercial production.

Keywords: nitrogen fertilizer; nitrification inhibitor; nitrogen leaching; nitrogen use efficiency; 3,4-dimethylpyrazole phosphate (DMPP)

1. Introduction

With the rapid increase of the global population, agriculture is required to satisfy the consequent boost in food demand worldwide. For example, in 2013 the production of primary foodstuffs such as wheat and maize reached 713 and 1018 millions of metric tons, respectively, and it has been estimated that in 2050 the world requirement will be 85% higher than in 2013 [1]. Along with water, considerable amounts of fertilizers have been thus far applied to raise the yield of agricultural crops. Nitrogen (N) is the main plant macronutrient and its concentration in natural soils is often deficient to ensure adequate plant growth and crop yield [2], eventually leading to high rates of N fertilization. Over a four-decade period from 1961 to 2013, the world consumption of N fertilizers has increased from 11.3 Tg N/year to 107.6 Tg N/year [3]. The use of fertilizers has especially increased in the intensive vegetable crop production system [4–6]. In China, N fertilization for the cultivation of vegetables exceeds 1000 and

3000 kg N/ha year in the open-field and greenhouse conditions, respectively. In the same country, in 2008, 17% of the national input of N fertilizers was devoted to the vegetable cropping system [7].

The conventional fertilizers that are commonly applied by growers are highly soluble salts and are liable up to 70% N losses due to volatilization and leaching [8]. These processes have two main undesirable effects: (1) a poor fertilization efficiency because the nutrient element is driven off the root zone, making it unavailable to the plant; (2) a harmful impact on the environment, due to either greenhouse gas emissions or surface water pollution by eutrophication. Nitrogen is commonly applied as nitrate ion, or it is quickly oxidized to this form through nitrification by soil microorganisms. The supply of different N forms or the nitrification process can cause hazardous volatilization losses as ammonia, N monoxide or other N oxides that could contribute to the greenhouse effect. In addition, nitrate ion is not retained by the soil and is easily leached [6,9].

Nitrogen leaching is generally more severe with intensive greenhouse cultures than with open-field crops, as plant growth is faster under controlled conditions and N fertilization represents an effective and low-cost practice to increase the production yield [6]. In fact, several authors drew attention to the occurrence of eutrophication and water pollution in the main European districts for protected vegetable crop production, such as Spain [10], Italy [11], The Netherlands [12], Poland [13] and Greece [14]. The environmental impact associated with nitrate leaching has become a major concern all over the world. In Europe, this has led to the introduction of the Nitrates Directive [15], to limit N pollution and improve water quality. According to the directive, the Nitrate Vulnerable Zones (NVZs) are land areas where drainage water from agricultural crops can cause contamination of larger water bodies by excess nitrate [16]. Hence, the limitation of fertilizers application in agriculture represents an effective measure to counteract nitrate pollution of surface water [17]. With N overfertilization, nitrate ion can also accumulate in the edible parts of several food crops [18]. Human intake of nitrate with the diet has been related to gastric cancer [19–21] and has directed the European Union toward a restriction to the nitrate content in food as a safety measure for the consumer [22].

Based on the above considerations, many efforts have been made to rationalize N fertilization. The application of enhanced efficiency fertilizers is a functional approach to achieve this purpose by limiting nutrient amounts in soils and at the same time reducing both N leaching and N volatilization losses. Enhanced efficiency fertilizers can be divided into three subgroups [23]: (i) slow-release fertilizers, (ii) stabilized fertilizers, (iii) controlled-release fertilizers. Slow-release fertilizers contain low solubility N compounds that become available to plants only after microbial degradation. Stabilized fertilizers contain chemical inhibitors, which slow down or stop biological processes. These include urease inhibitors that hinder the hydrolysis of urea by urease enzyme, or nitrification inhibitors such as dicyandiamide (DCD), or 3,4-dimethylpyrazole phosphate (DMPP), which prevent the oxidation of ammonium ion [24]. Controlled-release fertilizers are made of an inner core and an outer layer. The former is a water-soluble fertilizer such as urea, ammonium nitrate or potassium nitrate; the latter is a coating material such as sulfur, an alkyd- or polyurethane-like resin, a thermoplastic polymer or a mineral-based inorganic material [25]. Controlled-release fertilizers can also be made by the combination of sulfur-coated urea with an additional polymer or resin coating [26,27].

Two main limitations to the use of controlled-release fertilizers are their relatively high cost, and the difficulty to develop an adequate coating for irregularly shaped fertilizers or highly soluble compounds such as urea. The controlled-release fertilizer used in this study consisted of polyurethane-coated urea granules and was manufactured using an innovative polymer coating patented technology (E-MAX) that can be employed in combination with many types of fertilizers, including hygroscopic compounds or irregularly shaped materials. The release mechanism of coated fertilizers is based on the osmosis phenomenon produced by the diffusion of water through the coating, which leads to the solubilisation of the inner fertilizer. Water transfer through the coating layer is the rate determining step and depends on the chemical structure of the polymer, the thickness of the coating layer and the temperature. Therefore, for a given polymer with a fixed thickness, the release rate should be temperature-dependent and should be assessed through the temperature regime experienced by the coated fertilizer [28,29].

Thus, the release of nutrients into the soil could be predicted and controlled over time. With the E-MAX coating technology, the thickness of the polymer layer is well below 100 µm; the coating material is evenly spread and fixed on the whole surface of discrete 2- to 4-mm-diameter particles, degrades slowly and is essentially inert in the soil after the nutrient has been released. The work was aimed at evaluating: (i) the release curve and the effectiveness of the polyurethane-coated urea in relation to the plant N requirements in different climate growing conditions; (ii) the effect of this controlled-release fertilizer on N leaching and on the yield and quality of a soil greenhouse tomato cultivation in comparison with fertilization techniques that employ a nitrification inhibitor or soluble salts.

2. Materials and Methods

Although the controlled-release fertilizer used in this study was being developed and marketed mainly for open field application, three experiments were carried out in a glasshouse at the University of Pisa on round-table tomato plants (cultivar Hybrid F1 "OPTIMA"). The use of a greenhouse equipped with lysimeters allowed for the prevention of the negative effects of uncontrolled rainfall events and made possible to easily collect, measure and analyse water drainage and N leaching, thus enabling reliable computations of both water and N balance in the different treatments. The present study was focused on the time interval of N release by the coated urea (3–4 months) rather than to the long-term agronomical effects of the treatments. Therefore, the growing period lasted from the transplanting to the harvesting of the third or fourth truss and was shorter than that of a typical greenhouse cultivation of tomato, which is generally conducted until the ripening of the fifth or sixth truss. However, the growing conditions of the experiments closely resembled those of a real cropping system and enabled the evaluation of the yield and quality of the production.

2.1. Experimental Design

Three experiments were performed under different growing conditions: Experiment 1 (spring 2015), Experiment 2 (autumn 2015) and Experiment 3 (summer–autumn 2016). In all the experiments, either the stabilized or the controlled-release fertilizer were compared with a conventional treatment (CON). The distinct N treatments and fertilizer addition programs are detailed in Table 1. The same total N dose was applied in all the treatments using different N sources: (i) the inorganic salts potassium nitrate KNO_3, calcium nitrate $Ca(NO_3)_2$, ammonium nitrate NH_4NO_3 and ammonium sulphate $(NH_4)_2SO_4$; (ii) a stabilized fertilizer containing 26% total N (7.5% as nitrate and 18.5% as ammonium), with the addition of DMPP as a nitrification inhibitor (ENTEC® 26:0:0 Nitrogen-Phosphorus-Potassium, EuroChem Agro, Cesano Maderno, Italy); (iii) an innovative controlled-release fertilizer, manufactured using the E-MAX coating technology and consisting of granules of urea fertilizer coated by a permeable and very thin polyurethane layer (Agrocote® Max; ICL Specialty Fertilizers, Heerlen, The Netherlands; Patent EP 2672813 B1). The stabilized and controlled-release fertilizers will be hereafter indicated as DMPP and CU, respectively.

The total N dose was adapted to the different climate conditions of each experiment and, as plant growth is normally slower in autumn, N fertilization was necessarily lower in Experiment 2 than in Experiment 1 (300 kg/ha against 360 kg/ha) to prevent excess leaching. A reduced total N application in the cold season is consistent with the growers' common practice. For this reason, a similar absolute amount of CU or DMPP applied as base fertilization corresponded to a different percentage of total N. For example, Table 1 shows that the DMPP dose tested in Experiment 1 was 72 kg N/ha (20% of total N) and was comparable to the DMPP amount applied in Experiment 2 (75 kg N/ha; 25% of total N). Both the N dose and the N percentage are reported in Table 1 for each fertilizer.

Table 1. Description of the fertilization treatments applied in the three experiments and total cost of fertilizers.

Treatment	Short Description	Total N Dose	Base Fertilization	Top-Dressing (Fertigation)			Total Cost of Fertilizers	Total Cost of N Fertilizers
		kg N/ha	kg N/ha (% Total N)	kg N/ha (% total N)			€/ha	
				NH$_4$NO$_3$	Ca(NO$_3$)$_2$	KNO$_3$		
Experiment 1								
CON1	Growers' practice	360	72 (20) as (NH$_4$)$_2$SO$_4$	72 (20)	166 (46)	50 (14)	1887.04	1216.13
DMPP20	DMPP® 26.0.0	360	72 (20) as DMPP®	72 (20)	166 (46)	50 (14)	1874.51	1203.60
CU20	CU	360	72 (20) as CU	72 (20)	166 (46)	50 (14)	1875.47	1204.56
CU40	CU	360	144 (40) as CU	0	166 (46)	50 (14)	1898.95	1228.04
CU75-1	CU	360	270 (75) as CU	0	90 (25)	0	2002.21	1049.25
Experiment 2								
CON2	Growers' practice	300	75 (25) as (NH$_4$)$_2$SO$_4$	90 (30)	75 (25)	60 (20)	1624.54	1010.04
DMPP25	DMPP® 26.0.0	300	75 (25) as DMPP	90 (30)	75 (25)	60 (20)	1611.50	997.00
CU50	CU	300	150 (50) as CU	15 (5)	75 (25)	60 (20)	1636.95	1022.45
CU75-2	CU	300	225 (75) as CU	0	75 (25)	0	1606.69	653.73
Experiment 3								
CON3	Growers' practice	300	75 (25) as NH$_4$NO$_3$	90 (30)	75 (25)	60 (20)	1624.54	1010.04
CUred	CU reduced dose	225	150 (67) as CU	0	75 (33)	0	1475.88	522.92

The values between parentheses correspond to percentage of total N dose. CON: conventional treatment; DMPP: treatment with stabilized fertilizer; CU: treatment with coated urea. The total cost of N fertilizers and of all fertilizers were calculated using the following fertilizer prices: (NH$_4$)$_2$SO$_4$: N = 21%, 400 €/ton; NH$_4$NO$_3$ with DMPP (ENTEC 26): N = 26% 450 €/ton; coated urea (Agrocote®Max): N = 44%, 750 €/ton; KH$_2$PO$_4$: P$_2$O$_5$ = 52%, K$_2$O = 34%, 1760 €/ton; K$_2$SO$_4$: K$_2$O = 52%, 880 €/ton; Ca(NO$_3$)$_2$: N = 15.5%, Ca = 26%, 540 €/ton. The fertilizer prices are referred to an end-user located in Tuscany (Italy) in 2018.

For both conventional and stabilized fertilizers, the high solubility limited the amount that could be applied as base fertilization to 75 kg N/ha, to prevent detrimental salinity effects on the crop. In contrast, with the controlled-release CU fertilizer higher doses could be applied, up to 270 kg N/ha. The outcome of Experiment 1 was used to tune the conditions of the subsequent trial and, as in spring no significant effect was observed on the production with the CU20 treatment, higher CU doses were employed in autumn. In addition, at least 75 kg N/ha was applied in all the treatments as calcium nitrate. This amount was never decreased in the three experiments, to allow a sufficient calcium supply to the plants and ensure a correct calcium nutrition, preventing the occurrence of the blossom-end rot. For the CUred treatment, which employed a reduced N dose, the above amount of $Ca(NO_3)_2$ represented 33% of total N applied (Table 1).

In all the experiments, both N and water balance of the tomato culture were evaluated for each fertilization treatment. Inside the greenhouse, the plants were grown in lysimeters to enable reliable determination of water and N status in the growing system. Each lysimeter hosted four plants and consisted of a 200 L plastic tank (75 × 53 cm, height 50 cm), containing 20 L (5 cm) pumice layer at the bottom to ensure correct drainage. The pumice layer was topped off with 160 L sandy soil and peat (40 cm depth; 60:40 volume ratio; 1.2 kg/L specific weight). Along with the results of soil analyses, the main climatic parameters of the three experiments are reported in Table 2. The greenhouse heating guaranteed a minimum inner air temperature of 12.5 °C. Global radiation, air temperature, soil temperature at 15 cm depth and relative humidity (RH) were recorded every ten minutes by a climate station equipped with three different probes for soil temperature, connected to a database (Econorma, Treviso, Italy). The recorded values were used to calculate the cumulative radiation and the average daily values of RH, soil temperature and air temperature. The cumulative soil temperature was obtained by the sum of the values of daily average soil temperature recorded in each experimental period.

In each experiment, a zero-N fertilization treatment with the same levels of the other nutrients was also included for the assessment of N use efficiency. Although this is normally the control treatment in agronomic experiments, the main goal of the present study was to evaluate the effect of different fertilization strategies on the reduction of N leachate as compared with conventional fertilization. For this reason, the conventional treatment rather than the zero-N treatment was regarded as the control in our experiments.

After transplanting and until the end of the experimental period, each treatment was fertigated with nutrient solution to ensure a proper supply of all the macro- and micronutrients to the plants. Along with N, all the treatments of the three experiments received the same total amounts of phosphorus (P) and potassium (K), which were 1.4 and 12 g/plant, respectively (equivalent to 96 kg/ha P_2O_5 and 433 kg/ha K_2O). These P and K doses are commonly used by the greenhouse growers in Italy and were either applied as base fertilizers or supplied by fertigation. The total calcium supply ranged from 60 mg/L (that is the concentration in the irrigation water) to 150 mg/L. The latter value was reached only when calcium nitrate was used as a N source to prevent the occurrence of the blossom-end rot. The concentrations of the other elements in the nutrient solution were the following (mg/L): Mg 30; Na 230; Cl 320; Fe 2; B 0.27; Cu 0.24; Zn 0.29; Mn 0.55 and Mo 0.05. Depending on the treatment and on the phenological phase, different amounts of inorganic N fertilizers were added when necessary to the nutrient solution (Table 1) to achieve the same final N dose in each treatment. Specifically, NH_4NO_3 was supplied from transplanting until the blooming of the second truss, $Ca(NO_3)_2$ was employed until the ripening of the first truss and KNO_3 was added during the ripening stage, until the end of the experiment. The irrigation was generally applied twice a day, according to the climate conditions and the canopy development, in the same amount for all the treatments investigated.

The tomato plantlets were transplanted at the stage of six-seven true leaves, which in the three experiments corresponded to a different plant age (50–30 days), depending on the thermal growing conditions. Similarly, the end of the experimental period corresponded to the harvest of the fourth truss in Experiment 1 or to the harvest of the third truss otherwise.

Table 2. Climate and soil parameters measured in the three experiments. Temperature, humidity and radiation are reported as the average values inside the greenhouse during the whole experimental period. Soil parameters are reported as the initial values immediately before the beginning of each experiment.

Parameter	Experiment 1 Spring 2015	Experiment 2 Autumn 2015	Experiment 3 Summer/Autumn 2016
Growing period	20 March–7 July 2015	21 September 2015–28 January 2016	22 August–1 December 2016
Daily mean air temperature (°C)	22.7 ± 5.5	16.4 ± 3.9	20.4 ± 4.2
Daily mean soil temperature (°C)	22.4 ± 5.4	17.3 ± 3.9	20.7 ± 4.2
Air and soil temperature range (°C)	15–32	11–26	14–28
Cumulative average daily soil temperature (°C)	2459.9 ± 96.7	2245.8 ± 67.4	2079.1 ± 62.3
Relative humidity (%)	62.7 ± 7.7	79.6 ± 10.7	77.9 ± 11.4
Average daily global radiation (MJ/m^2·day)	10.5 ± 3.6	2.4 ± 0.7	5.0 ± 1.6
Cumulative global radiation (MJ/m^2)	1151.7 ± 43.8	299.9 ± 9.0	506.3 ± 15.2
pH	8.1 ± 0.1	6.8 ± 0.1	7.0 ± 0.1
Electrical Conductivity (mS/cm at 25 °C)	0.22 ± 0.08	0.29 ± 0.06	0.39 ± 0.08
Nitrate (mg NO$_3^-$/kg)	20 ± 2	28 ± 2	33 ± 4
Ammonium (mg NH$_4^+$/kg)	1.2 ± 0.2	7.0 ± 0.2	8.0 ± 0.3
Exchangeable Potassium (mg K$_2$O/kg)	140 ± 7	136 ± 5	129 ± 9
Exchangeable Calcium (mg Ca/kg)	2112 ± 11	2258 ± 13	2295 ± 13
Exchangeable Magnesium (mg Mg/kg)	80 ± 8	110 ± 8	91 ± 7
Assimilable Phosphorous (mg P$_2$O$_5$/kg)	76 ± 6	77 ± 6	70 ± 7
Assimilable Iron (mg Fe/kg)	388 ± 10	334 ± 16	388 ± 15
Assimilable Manganese (mg Mn/kg)	204 ± 8	215 ± 10	226 ± 11
Assimilable Zinc (mg Zn/kg)	6.0 ± 0.1	4.3 ± 0.5	6.2 ± 0.7
Assimilable Copper (mg Cu/kg)	5.9 ± 0.4	2.11 ± 0.02	3.20 ± 0.02
Soluble Boron (mg B/kg)	0.45 ± 0.04	0.21 ± 0.02	0.35 ± 0.04
Organic matter content (%)	2.31 ± 0.12	1.44 ± 0.10	4.15 ± 0.15
C/N	33.6 ± 0.6	14.0 ± 0.4	17.2 ± 0.2
Cationic Exchange Capacity (meq/100 g)	12.8 ± 1.0	11.6 ± 0.5	15.4 ± 1.1
Clay (%)	11.6 ± 0.9	6.2 ± 0.6	7.6 ± 0.8
Silt (%)	20.8 ± 1.2	20.5 ± 1.9	19.9 ± 1.1
Sand (%)	67.6 ± 2.1	73.3 ± 1.1	72.5 ± 2.2

Mean values ± standard deviation. n = 5 in Experiment 1; n = 3 in Experiment 2 and Experiment 3.

2.2. Analyses of Water, Soil, CU Granules and Plant Tissue Samples

The average values of the climate parameters (RH, air and soil temperature, cumulated global radiation) were recorded daily. Nitrogen was contained as urea in CU granules and in different chemical forms in water, soil and tissue samples. A summary of N determinations and analytical assays used can be found in Table 3.

Due to the autumn climate conditions, in both Experiments 2 and 3 the growing cycle was longer than in spring, while the crop evapotranspiration and the plant growth were strongly reduced. Therefore, an increase of the water collection period was necessary to maintain the same number of drainage samplings as Experiment 1. The cumulated drainage water was sampled from each container every 7–10 days in Experiment 1 and every 13–15 days in Experiment 2 and Experiment 3. The water samples were filtered on Whatman qualitative filter paper and analysed for the concentrations of nitrate (salicylic acid method) [30]; ammoniacal N (indophenol method) [31] and ureic N (enzymatic assay using a commercial kit; Megazyme International, Wicklow, Ireland). All the absorbance measurements were carried out using a Lambda35 UV-vis double beam spectrophotometer (Perkin Elmer, Waltham, MA, USA).

The soil samples were dehydrated at 40 °C in a ventilated oven and sieved to separate intact CU granules. The dried soil samples were extracted with water, 1 M KCl, 0.5 N NaHCO$_3$ at pH 8.5 or 1 N CH$_3$COONH$_4$ at pH 7.0, respectively, for the spectrophotometric determinations of nitrate [30], ammoniacal N [31] and available P [32] and for the assessment of exchangeable K by atomic absorption spectroscopy (AAS) [33]. In all cases, a 1:2 w/v extraction ratio was used. The total organic matter and the other soil parameters reported in Table 2 were assessed according to official methods the Italian Ministry of Agriculture and Forestry [34].

Table 3. Analytical assays used to determine nitrogen concentration in samples of water, soil, coated urea fertilizer and plant tissues in the three experiments.

Sample	Fraction of Total N	Determination	Chemical Form
	Ureic	Enzyme kit (urease)	Urea
Cumulated water drainage	Nitric	Spectrophotometric assay (nitrosalycilate method)	Nitrate
	Ammoniacal	Spectrophotometric assay (substituted indophenol method)	Ammonium + Ammonia
	Ureic	Enzyme kit (urease)	Urea
	Reduced	Kjeldahl method	Organic + Ammonium + Ammonia
Soil	Nitric	Spectrophotometric assay (nitrosalycilate method)	Nitrate
	Mineral	Nitrate + Ammoniacal N	Nitrate + Ammonium + Ammonia
	Total	Reduced + Nitrate	Organic + Nitrate + Ammonium + Ammonia
	Ureic	Enzyme kit (urease)	Urea
Coated urea fertilizer	Ammoniacal	Spectrophotometric assay (substituted indophenol method)	Ammonium + Ammonia
	Nitric	Spectrophotometric assay (nitrosalycilate method)	Nitrate
Plant tissues	Reduced	Kjeldahl method	Organic + Ammonium + Ammonia
	Organic	Reduced − Ammoniacal	N-containing organic compounds including urea
	Total	Reduced + Nitrate	Organic + Nitrate + Ammonium + Ammonia

The N amount retained by the coated urea granules was determined in all the CU treatments. At the beginning of each experiment, 2 g aliquots of the coated fertilizer were wrapped in net fabric before application to each lysimeter. Every 30 days during the cultivation period (for Experiments 1 and 2) and at the end of the cultivation period (for all three experiments), the wrappings were removed from the soil to collect the residual granules, which were gently washed with distilled water, oven-dried at 70 °C and powdered with mortar and pestle. The powder was dispersed into 200 mL distilled water and the filtered solution was analysed for the concentration of urea. For each cultivation period, the N release by the coated fertilizer was evaluated by the difference between the initial and final ureic-N amounts in the net-wrapped granules.

All the plant samples were dried in a ventilated oven at 70 °C till constant weight and ground in a mill to a fine powder. The crop yield was determined as the number and fresh weight of the fruits, which were picked weekly and divided into marketable and nonmarketable categories. To evaluate the quality of the production, four fruits from different plants were collected from each lysimeter in the middle of the harvesting period and were homogenized in a mixer. Part of each homogenized sample was oven-dried for dry matter determination; the remaining material was centrifuged, and the resulting juice was analysed for pH, EC, total soluble solids (determined by refractometry and expressed as °Brix) and total titratable acidity (determined by acid-base titration with 0.1 M sodium hydroxide and expressed as g citric acid in 100 mL juice). The shoot dry biomass production was determined at the end of each experiment. All the dry tissue samples were analysed for their contents of nitric, ammoniacal and reduced N, as described previously for soil samples.

2.3. Calculation of N and Water Balance Sheet and N Use Efficiency

A balance sheet for both water and N was computed for each treatment and experiment. Water evapotranspiration was calculated as the difference between water supply and water drainage (both measured); the leaching fraction was computed as the ratio between water drainage and water supply. The computation of N balance was based on the available amount during cultivation (initially contained in the soil or supplied through fertilization) and the amount that was actually removed (leached or absorbed by the plants) or remained in the soil at the end of the experiments. The amounts of fertilizers were weighed using a technical balance with 0.1 g precision and 1.0 kg/ha was cautiously assumed as the standard deviation for the total N applied. Soil mineral N was evaluated as the sum of nitric and ammoniacal N (Table 3) and was assessed both at the beginning (prior to base fertilization) and the end of each experiment. The total N amount of the system at the end of the experiment (N output) was evaluated as the sum of the N fractions that were absorbed by the plants, were lost by leaching, remained in the soil as mineral N or remained in the CU granules as residual urea. The final amount of urea in the soil was negligible (less than 0.1 mg/kg), due to both the controlled release by the CU fertilizer and to the fast leaching and mineralization processes that urea undergoes in soils [35]. The total N amount available during the growing period (N input) was calculated as the sum of the initial mineral amount in the soil and the amount applied with fertilizers, both as base fertilization and with fertigation (total N supplied). Based on the results of the zero-N treatments, some nitrogen use efficiency (NUE) indexes were calculated according to [36,37], using the following formulas:

$$\text{Agronomic Efficiency (AE)} = (Y - Y_0)/F$$

$$\text{Partial Factor Productivity (PFP)} = Y/F$$

$$\text{Apparent Recovery Efficiency by difference (REC)} = (U - U_0)/F$$

$$\text{Physiological Efficiency (PE)} = (Y - Y_0)/(U - U_0)$$

where Y and Y_0 (g/m^2 on a fresh weight basis) are the tomato yields with and without N fertilization, respectively; F is the total N supplied (g N/m^2) and U and U_0 (g N/m^2) are the N contents in fruits with and without N fertilization, respectively.

2.4. Statistical Analysis

A completely randomized design was adopted. As the statistical variability of the data was initially unknown, in Experiment 1 five replicates (lysimeters) were prudentially arranged. Based on the results of the first experiment, the number of replicates could be reasonably reduced to three in the subsequent trials to obtain an adequate statistical discrimination and limit the cost of data collection. Each replicate consisted of four tomato plants. The collected data were tested for normality and homoschedasticity by means of the Shapiro–Wilk's and Levene's test, respectively. The data were subjected to one-way ANOVA and the mean values were compared by Tukey test using the Statgraphics Plus 5.1 software (StatPoint, Inc., Herndon, VA, USA).

3. Results

For all the experiments, Table 4 reports the water balance, Table 5 shows the biomass and N distribution in different plant tissues and Table 6 reports the data concerning the yield and quality of the tomato production obtained with the different treatments. The N balance for the three experiments is reported in Table 7. Table 8 reports the NUE indexes that were calculated from the tomato yield (Y_0; kg/m^2 on a fresh weight basis) and the N content of fruits (U_0; g N/m^2) obtained without N fertilization (zero-N treatment).

In all the treatments, only negligible amounts of urea and ammonium (0–0.08 g N/m^2) were detected in the drainage water. Thus, N leached from the soil was almost completely in the form of nitrate ion.

In Experiment 1, the water balance was similar for the CON1, DMPP20 and CU20 treatments, while a higher water drainage and leaching fraction along with a lower evapotranspiration were observed for CU40 and CU75-1 treatments (Table 4). Both the dry biomass and the N concentration in the tissues were affected by N fertilization. Compared with CON1, all the treatments except CU20 increased the dry biomass of fruits. In addition, both CU40 and CU75-1 increased the fruit N concentration (Table 5). However, apart from slight differences in the number of fruits, the distinct treatments had no significant effect on the tomato yield or quality (Table 6).

Table 4. Effect of different fertilization strategies on the water balance.

Treatment	Water Supply (L/m^2)	Water Drainage (L/m^2)	Leaching Fraction (%)	Evapotranspiration (L/m^2)
		Experiment 1		
CON1	472.5 ± 19.2	67.5 ± 2.6 [b]	14.3 ± 2.2 [b]	405.0 ± 12.7 [a]
DMPP20	472.7 ± 19.4	61.3 ± 2.5 [b]	13.0 ± 2.9 [b]	411.4 ± 12.5 [a]
CU20	470.2 ± 20.1	66.6 ± 2.7 [b]	14.2 ± 2.5 [b]	403.5 ± 11.3 [a]
CU40	475.8 ± 19.1	94.6 ± 3.7 [a]	19.9 ± 3.4 [a]	381.2 ± 11.9 [b]
CU75-1	475.8 ± 17.7	97.8 ± 4.6 [a]	20.7 ±3.3 [a]	375,6 ± 11.0 [b]
		Experiment 2		
CON2	171.6 ± 9.3	38.4 ± 2.4 [b]	22.4 ± 1.8 [b]	133.3 ± 3.0 [a]
DMPP25	173.6 ± 7.2	39.8 ± 3.1 [b]	22.9 ± 2.1 [b]	133.8 ± 2.9 [a]
CU50	168.7 ± 6.9	41.7 ± 2.9 [b]	24.7 ± 1.9 [ab]	127.0 ± 3.2 [ab]
CU75-2	171.9 ± 8.2	46.7 ± 3.2 [a]	27.2 ± 2.1 [a]	125.2 ± 2.8 [b]
		Experiment 3		
CON3	321.4 ± 11.2	94.7 ± 4.7	29.5 ± 2.1	226.7 ± 6.5
Cured	326.3 ± 9.2	94.1 ± 5.6	28.8 ± 1.9	232.2 ± 5.8

Mean values ± standard deviation. In each experiment, different letters within the same column identify a significant difference ($p < 0.05$), according to Tukey test following one-way ANOVA. Mean values without any letters are not significantly different. CON: conventional treatment; DMPP: treatment with stabilized fertilizer; CU: treatment with coated urea.

Table 5. The influence of different fertilization strategies on the distribution of biomass and nitrogen in tomato tissues.

Treatment	Dry Biomass (g/m^2)			N Tissue Concentration (% Dry Biomass)		
	Leaves	Stems	Fruits	Leaves	Stems	Fruits
			Experiment 1			
CON1	179.4 ± 6.7 [b]	156.8 ± 10.1	717.0 ± 12.8 [c]	2.52 ± 0.03 [b]	2.25 ± 0.04 [ab]	2.95 ± 0.04 [b]
DMPP20	191.4 ± 9.4 [a]	155.9 ± 9.9	762.3 ± 12.5 [a]	2.60 ± 0.05 [a]	2.23 ± 0.02 [b]	3.04 ± 0.04 [ab]
CU20	194.5 ± 9.7 [a]	169.8 ± 9.7	714.7 ± 13.1	2.63 ± 0.04 [a]	2.28 ± 0.03 [ab]	3.00 ± 0.03 [b]
CU40	167.4 ± 5.3 [c]	155.3 ± 8.5	741.0 ± 15.1 [b]	2.62 ± 0.04 [a]	2.31 ± 0.03 [a]	3.10 ± 0.02 [a]
CU75-1	162,9 ± 5.5 [c]	154.8 ± 7.9	759.9 ± 13.2 [a]	2.68 ± 0.05 [a]	2.24 ± 0.03 [b]	3.12 ± 0.03 [a]
			Experiment 2			
CON2	206.6 ± 10.6 [a]	100.1 ± 6.7 [a]	195.8 ± 14.2 [b]	3.59 ± 0.03 [a]	3.00 ± 0.01 [ab]	3.44 ± 0.02 [ab]
DMPP25	189.5 ± 7.9 [b]	87.5 ± 6.5 [b]	189.9 ± 12.1 [b]	3.51 ± 0.02 [a]	3.16 ± 0.02 [a]	3.22 ± 0.01 [b]
CU50	198.4 ± 9.3 [ab]	85.9 ± 6.8 [b]	216.2 ± 14.6 [a]	3.46 ± 0.02 [ab]	2.83 ± 0.02 [bc]	3.49 ± 0.02 [a]
CU75-2	190.5 ± 8.4 [b]	101.0 ± 7.1 [a]	234.1 ± 15.2 [a]	3.22 ± 0.01 [b]	2.52 ± 0.02 [c]	3.60 ± 0.03 [a]
			Experiment 3			
CON3	191.9 ± 9.5	82.5 ± 6.1	197.6 ± 18.1	3.72 ± 0.03 [a]	2.61 ± 0.02	3.62 ± 0.02
Cured	184.0 ± 8.2	77.4 ± 5.8	214.4 ± 19.2	3.20 ± 0.02 [b]	2.72 ± 0.03	3.59 ± 0.02

Mean values ± standard deviation. For each column in each experiment, different letters identify a significant difference ($p < 0.05$), according to Tukey test following one-way ANOVA. Mean values without any letters are not significantly different. CON: conventional treatment; DMPP: treatment with stabilized fertilizer; CU: treatment with coated urea.

Table 6. The influence of different fertilization strategies on yield and quality of the tomato crop.

Treatment	Fruit Production						Fruit Quality				
	Fruit Yield (kg/m²)		Fruit Amount (n° Fruits/m²)		Average Fruit Weight (gFW/Fruit)	Fruit Dry Matter Content (%)	pH	EC (dS/m)	Total Soluble Solids (°Brix)	Titratable Acidity (g Citric Acid/100 mL)
	Total	Market Quality	Total	Market Quality						
Experiment 1										
CON1	12.8 ± 0.68	9.8 ± 0.9	59.0 ± 1.4 b	39.5 ± 1.6 ab	247.8 ± 22.1	5.60 ± 0.11	4.17 ± 0.04	5.23 ± 0.20	4.65 ± 0.20	0.57 ± 0.03
DMPP20	13.8 ± 0.79	10.4 ± 1.1	63.2 ± 2.2 ab	39.2 ± 1.5 ab	265.6 ± 28.2	5.52 ± 0.09	4.14 ± 0.03	5.14 ± 0.19	4.62 ± 0.23	0.58 ± 0.04
CU20	12.7 ± 0.71	9.8 ± 0.7	59.5 ± 1.8 ab	38.5 ± 1.6 b	255.3 ± 20.5	5.63 ± 0.15	4.14 ± 0.03	5.37 ± 0.24	4.45 ± 0.21	0.57 ± 0.04
CU40	13.4 ± 0.82	10.7 ± 0.8	65.7 ± 2.1 a	43.0 ± 2.9 a	248.8 ± 20.5	5.53 ± 0.10	4.16 ± 0.04	5.28 ± 0.21	4.57 ± 0.25	0.58 ± 0.05
CU75	13.5 ± 0.87	10.8 ± 0.9	64.6 ± 1.9 a	42.2 ± 3.1 a	254.7 ± 21.1	5.63 ± 0.14	4.15 ± 0.02	5.36 ± 0.25	4.63 ± 0.22	0.59 ± 0.06
Experiment 2										
CON2	4.21 ± 0.21 b	3.80 ± 0.31 b	33.5 ± 4.1	26.3 ± 2.4 b	144.8 ± 9.7 b	4.65 ± 0.08	4.42 ± 0.03 b	6.22 ± 0.34 b	4.10 ± 0.14 b	0.40 ± 0.03
DMPP25	4.04 ± 0.23 b	3.85 ± 0.41 b	33.8 ± 3.8	25.3 ± 2.5 b	152.5 ± 10.6 ab	4.70 ± 0.11	4.41 ± 0.03 b	6.87 ± 0.32 ab	4.40 ± 0.18 ab	0.45 ± 0.04
CU50	4.70 ± 0.31 ab	4.30 ± 0.35 ab	33.8 ± 3.9	27.3 ± 2.9 ab	155.0 ± 10.3 ab	4.60 ± 0.09	4.40 ± 0.04 b	6.65 ± 0.34 b	3.98 ± 0.14 b	0.42 ± 0.03
CU75	4.99 ± 0.33 a	4.70 ± 0.35 a	37.2 ± 4.2	30.0 ± 3.1 a	156.7 ± 10.1 a	4.69 ± 0.10	4.52 ± 0.04 a	7.54 ± 0.41 a	4.50 ± 0.15 a	0.41 ± 0.04
Experiment 3										
CON3	4.39 ± 0.19	3.77 ± 0.28	38.3 ± 3.9	26.3 ± 2.5	143.6 ± 10.9	4.50 ± 0.13	3.90 ± 0.04	5.23 ± 0.25	4.47 ± 0.09	0.73 ± 0.06
CUred	4.64 ± 0.18	4.08 ± 0.31	36.0 ± 3.7	28.8 ± 2.6	141.9 ± 11.2	4.62 ± 0.15	3.86 ± 0.05	5.14 ± 0.30	4.49 ± 0.07	0.65 ± 0.07

Mean values ± standard deviation. For each parameter in each experiment, different letters identify a significant difference ($p < 0.05$), according to Tukey test following one-way ANOVA. Mean values without any letters are not significantly different. CON: conventional treatment; DMPP: treatment with stabilized fertilizer; CU: treatment with coated urea. FW: fresh weight; EC: electrical conductivity.

Table 7. Nitrogen balance for different fertilization strategies in the three experiments.

N Distribution (kg/ha)					Treatments			
Experiment 1			CON1	DMPP20	CU20	CU40	CU75-1	
Input	Mineral soil content prior to fertilization (A)		39.2 ± 1.0	39.2 ± 1.0	39.2 ± 1.0	39.2 ± 1.0	39.2 ± 1.0	
	Supplied by base fertilization (B)	soluble salt	72.0 ± 1.0 [c]					
		DMPP		72.0 ± 1.0 [c]				
		CU			72.0 ± 1.0 [c]	144.0 ± 1.0 [b]	270.0 ± 1.0 [a]	
	Supplied by fertigation (C)		288.2 ± 2.5 [a]	287.5 ± 2.8 [a]	287.8 ± 3.1 [a]	216.3 ± 2.1 [b]	90.6 ± 1.1 [c]	
	Total N input (I)		399.4 ± 1.8	398.7 ± 2.0	399.0 ± 2.2	399.5 ± 1.3	399.8 ± 3.0	
Output	Mineral soil content after experiment (E)		40.6 ± 3.3 [c]	41.9 ± 4.3 [c]	47.3 ± 5.1 [c]	62.1 ± 5.8 [b]	72.9 ± 6.1 [a]	
	Residual in CU granules (F)				7.9 ± 1.5 [c]	15.8 ± 1.9 [b]	29.7 ± 2.5 [a]	
	Leached (G)		127.2 ± 8.1 [a]	97.8 ± 6.7 [b]	97.0 ± 7.1 [b]	57.2 ± 5.1 [c]	25.4 ± 3.1 [d]	
	Plant uptake (H)		272.4 ± 12.1 [b]	290.3 ± 13.5 [a]	290.2 ± 13.1 [a]	290.1 ± 12.7 [a]	296.5 ± 15.1 [a]	
	Total N output (O)		440.2 ± 14.1 [a]	430.0 ± 13.7 [a,b]	442.4 ± 15.1 [a]	425.2 ± 11.5 [b]	424.5 ± 12.5 [b]	
	N output − N input (Δ)		40.8	31.3	43.4	25.7	24.7	
	Relative error		9.27%	7.28%	9.81%	6.04%	5.82%	
Experiment 2			CON2	DMPP25	CU50		CU75-2	
Input	Mineral soil content prior to fertilization (A)		14.9 ± 1.0	14.9 ± 1.0	14.9 ± 1.0		14.9 ± 1.0	
	Supplied by base fertilization (B)	soluble salt	75.0 ± 1.0 [c]					
		DMPP		75.0 ± 1.0 [c]				
		CU			150.0 ± 1.0 [b]		225.0 ± 1.0 [a]	
	Supplied by fertigation (C)		224.5 ± 2.7 [a]	224.5 ± 2.9 [a]	144.1 ± 1.7 [b]		74.9 ± 0.3 [c]	
	Total N input (I)		314.4 ± 18.6	314.4 ± 18.7	309.0 ± 16.1		314.8 ± 14.5	
Output	Mineral soil content after experiment (E)		100.0 ± 9.1 [a]	110.8 ± 8.6 [a]	85.8 ± 7.1 [b]		89.8 ± 6.8 [b]	
	Residual in CU granules (F)				21.0 ± 2.2 [b]		31.5 ± 2.4 [a]	
	Leached (G)		46.0 ± 3.1 [a]	42.1 ± 2.9 [a]	28.4 ± 1.9 [b]		20.0 ± 2.1 [c]	
	Plant uptake (H)		171.4 ± 11.8 [a]	155.2 ± 12.4 [b]	168.5 ± 11.6 [a]		171.1 ± 12.1 [a]	
	Total N output (O)		317.4 ± 20.1	308.1 ± 17.2	303.7 ± 18.6		312.4 ± 21.2	
	N output − N input (Δ)		3.0	−6.3	−5.3		−2.4	
	Relative error		0.95%	−2.04%	−1.75%		−0.77%	

Table 7. Cont.

N Distribution (kg/ha)			Treatments	
Experiment 3			CON3	CUred
Input	Mineral soil content prior to fertilization (A)		20.3 ± 1.0	20.3 ± 1.0
	Supplied by base fertilization (B)	soluble salt	75.0 ± 1.0 [b]	
		CU		150.0 ± 1.0 [a]
	Supplied by fertigation (C)		229.0 ± 17.5 [a]	79.0 ± 8.1 [b]
	Total N input (I)		**324.3 ± 22.4 [a]**	**249.3 ± 23.1 [b]**
Output	Mineral soil content after experiment (E)		122.9 ± 12.4 [a]	87.8 ± 8.8 [b]
	Residual in CU granules (F)			16.5 ± 1.8
	Leached (G)		60.8 ± 6.1 [a]	21.0 ± 2.2 [b]
	Plant uptake (H)		164.6 ± 15.4 [a]	156.9 ± 11.2 [b]
	Total N output (O)		**348.3 ± 21.1 [a]**	**282.2 ± 17.5 [b]**
N output − N input (Δ)			24.0	32.9
Relative error			6.89%	11.66%

Mean values ± standard deviation. For each parameter, different letters identify a significant difference ($p < 0.05$), according to Tukey test following one-way ANOVA. CON: conventional treatment; DMPP: treatment with stabilized fertilizer; CU: treatment with coated urea. I = A + B + C; O = E + F + G + H; Δ = O − I; Relative error = Δ/O.

Table 8. Nitrogen use efficiency indexes calculated from the data collected in the three experiments.

Fertilization Treatment	AE (g FW/g N)	PFP (g FW/g N)	REC (g N/g N)	PE (g FW/g N)
		Experiment 1		
CON1	306.7 ± 15.4	355.0 ± 20.3	0.54 ± 0.05 [b]	568.5 ± 31.9
DMPP20	333.9 ± 20.1	382.2 ± 22.2	0.58 ± 0.04 [a,b]	576.9 ± 40.2
CU20	303.1 ± 15.1	351.4 ± 21.5	0.57 ± 0.03 [b]	534.1 ± 35.1
CU40	323.9 ± 16.2	372.2 ± 26.4	0.59 ± 0.04 [a]	548.9 ± 21.3
CU75-1	325.3 ± 18.3	373.6 ± 25.1	0.61 ± 0.05 [a]	532.8 ± 19.2
		Experiment 2		
CON2	102.39 ± 8.6 [b]	134.3 ± 10.2 [b,c]	0.19 ± 0.02 [b,c]	537.7 ± 23.5
DMPP25	96.97 ± 5.9 [b]	128.9 ± 12.3 [c]	0.17 ± 0.02 [c]	568.2 ± 27.2
CU50	120.09 ± 12.5 [a]	152.6 ± 14.1 [a,b]	0.22 ± 0.03 [a,b]	544.9 ± 21.1
CU75-2	125.84 ± 10.6 [a]	157.7 ± 12.0 [a]	0.24 ± 0.04 [a]	515.0 ± 20.9
		Experiment 3		
CON3	114.8 ± 10.4 [b]	144.4 ± 16.1 [b]	0.21 ± 0.03 [b]	536.9 ± 21.5
CUred	163.3 ± 12.6 [a]	202.6 ± 20.1 [a]	0.31 ± 0.04 [a]	530.5 ± 20.1

Mean values ± standard deviation. For each index and each experiment, a different letter indicates a significant difference, according to Tukey test following one-way ANOVA ($p < 0.05$). Mean values without any letters are not significantly different. Y0: tomato yield; U0: nitrogen content in fruits; AE: agronomic efficiency; PFP: partial factor productivity; REC: Apparent recovery efficiency by difference; PE: physiological efficiency; FW: fresh weight; CON: conventional treatment; DMPP: treatment with stabilized fertilizer; CU: treatment with coated urea. The values of Y0 (kg FW/m^2) and U0 (g N/m^2) used for the calculations were, respectively 1.74 ± 0.11 and 1.73 ± 0.15 in Experiment 1; 1.00 ± 0.09 and 0.76 ± 0.08 in Experiment 2; 0.90 ± 0.07, and 0.65 ± 0.05 in Experiment 3.

Concerning the N balance (Table 7), the total N plant uptake was lower in CON1 than the other treatments. The coated fertilizer (CU40 or CU75-1) was able to reduce N leaching by about 55% or 80% as compared to the control. The same effect was observed also for the DMPP20 and CU20 treatments, although to a lower extent (about 24% reduction). The soil contained always more mineral N at the end of the experiment than at the beginning, especially with the CU treatments that decreased N loss by leaching. However, in all the treatments the N output was higher than the N supplied. The REC index was significantly higher with the CU40 and CU75-1 treatments than with the control, while no significant difference was observed for AE and PFP (Table 8).

In Experiment 2, the water balance for the DMPP25 treatment was similar to that of the control. In contrast, both CU treatments exhibited the highest leaching fraction and the lowest evapotranspiration. Moreover, the CU75-2 produced the highest water drainage (Table 4). The different fertilizers affected the distribution of both dry matter and N content among plant organs, although the dry biomass of the whole plants remained generally unchanged (Table 5). The best results for yield and fruit quality were obtained with the CU75-2 treatment (Table 6). With the CU fertilizer, the total N plant uptake resulted similar to that of the control, but higher than that of the DMPP25 treatment. In addition, the coated fertilizer reduced N leaching, determined higher values of all the agronomical indexes and, in contrast with the outcome of Experiment 1, resulted in a lower final content of mineral N in the soil compared with the other treatments. At the end of Experiment 2, about 14% ureic N was still retained by the coated fertilizer (Tables 7 and 8).

The analysis of the CU granules during and at the end of the growing period gave similar results in both Experiments 1 and 2 (Figure 1). The N release into the soil by the CU fertilizer was temperature- rather than time-dependent and the whole set of data was fitted by an exponential-type function of the cumulative daily average soil temperature (thermal sum, X) with excellent correlation ($r^2 = 0.99$, n = 30). Nevertheless, for N release values below 80%, the relationship could be well described ($r^2 = 0.95$; n = 18) by the linear function (data not shown):

$$\% \text{ N release} = 3 + 0.05203 \times X$$

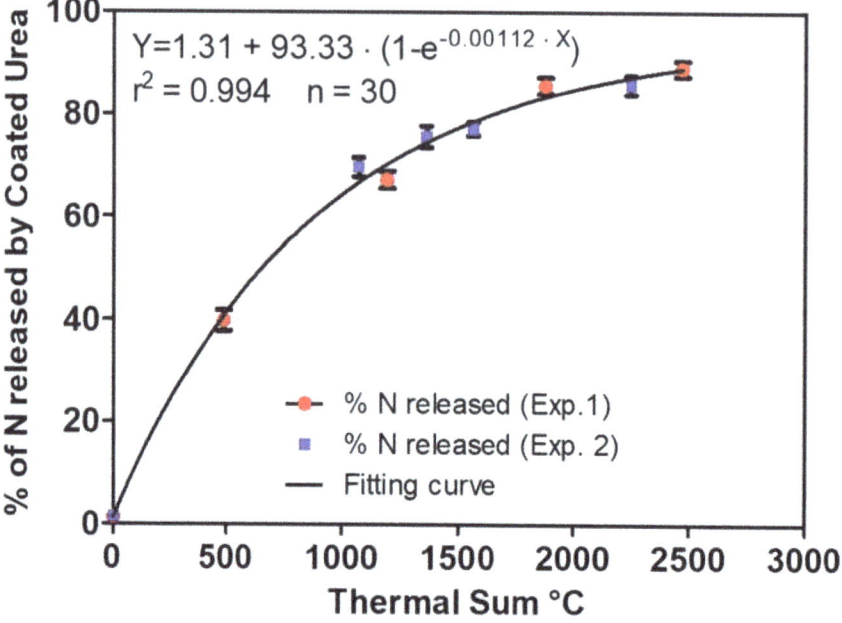

Figure 1. Percentage of N released by the granules of coated urea (CU) in Experiments 1 and 2, as a function of the cumulative daily average soil temperature (thermal sum).

In Experiment 3, the CUred treatment exhibited a similar water balance as the control (Table 4) and produced similar fruit biomass and yield, without affecting the quality parameters or the N content of the fruits (Tables 5 and 6). The amount of N leached was almost 3-fold lower with the coated fertilizer and a decrease was also observed in both plant N uptake and soil mineral N at the end of the experiment. The analysis of the CU granules recovered at the end of the trial revealed that 11% ureic N had not been released into the soil. As in Experiment 2, higher values of AE, PFP and PE indexes were obtained with the coated fertilizer (Table 8).

4. Discussion

All the treatments received the same amount of irrigation water, apart from low dissimilarities due to unavoidable inefficiencies in the irrigation system. The maximum differences in water supply were only 1.2% in Experiment 1, 3.0% in Experiment 2 and 1.5% in Experiment 3. Moreover, the leaching fraction was never lower than 13% (Table 4), which is indicative of a correct irrigation regime. With the only exception of the CUred treatment, all the treatments within the same experiment received the same total N amount.

4.1. Effect on the Crop (Yield and Quality)

Table 6 shows that in all the experiments the use of the DMPP fertilizer did not significantly affect the tomato yield compared with the control treatment. In contrast, both the CU40 and CU75-1 treatments in Experiment 1 improved the fruit amount and the CU75-2 treatment in Experiment 2 improved both the yield and the tomato quality. Although the differences were not always significant, at the highest urea doses we observed an increasing trend in all the parameters of fruit production in both Experiments 1 and 2. In each experiment, the different treatments did not affect the dry matter percentage of the fruits (Table 6) and the dry weight of the whole plants was also generally unaffected (Table 5). On the other hand, a different weight distribution among plant organs was observed with the different fertilizers; in Experiment 1, the leaf dry biomass was higher for the CON1 than for the high dose CU treatments, and the same behaviour was observed in Experiment 2, where also the N concentrations of leaf and stem tissues were higher for CON2 than for the CU75-2 treatment (Table 5). This outcome indicated a lower vegetative vigour for the CU-treated plants, which could be due to a reduced initial soil N availability and was consistent with a significantly lower evapotranspiration and a higher leaching fraction than those of the control and DMPP treatments (Table 4).

On the other hand, in Experiment 1 the application of coated urea at low concentration (CU20) produced a similar effect as DMPP20; although both treatments significantly lowered N leaching (Table 7), they determined an increase in leaf dry biomass and N concentration compared with CON1 (Table 5). Nitrogen is the main constituent responsible for vegetative growth and top dressing was initially applied as NH_4NO_3 with both treatments (Table 1). Hence, this outcome suggested that the plants vegetative behaviour was not effectively limited, due to a ready N availability in the root zone at the beginning of the growing period. In agreement with our findings, it was reported that in tomato high N levels increased plant vigour and delayed flower and fruit formation [38]. Similar results were reported also for different vegetable species, such as zucchini [39].

A limitation of plant vigour by the CU fertilizer was observed also in Experiments 2 and 3. Compared with CON2, the CU75-2 treatment increased both yield and fruit size and determined a similar N uptake; to a lesser extent, the same behaviour was observed also for the CU50 treatment, thereby suggesting that application of the coated fertilizer did not affect the plants ability to take up N from the soil. In Experiment 3, the reduction of the total N dose determined a strong decrease of N leaching compared with the control; thus, despite a slightly lower N uptake, the CUred treatment did not have any effect on the production (Tables 6 and 7).

4.2. N Use Efficiency and Agronomical Implications

In Experiment 1, all the values of the agronomical indexes were higher than the other trials, probably due to high light intensity conditions (approximately 5-fold higher than in Experiment 2) and high fruit yield during the spring season. In agreement with this outcome, [37,40] found that the REC index, which denotes the crop ability to absorb N from the soil, could be increased in processing tomato by good climatic conditions, since the crop could use more efficiently the N fertilizer available. Moreover, the lower ratio between crop N uptake and N supply that occurred in Experiments 2 and 3 could have contributed to reduce the NUE indexes as compared with Experiment 1. Several authors [37,41,42] reported that the NUE starts to decline when the N supply exceeds the crop N requirement. In all the experiments, the physiological index PE was not influenced by the type of fertilizer that was supplied to the plants (Table 8), indicating that the distinct treatments did not affect the physiological processes of N uptake and use. On the other hand, except for the CU20 treatment, in all the experiments the REC index was higher with CU than with the other fertilizers. A similar trend was observed in Experiments 2 and 3 for AE and PFP. The substantial increase of the agronomical indexes observed with the coated fertilizer can be explained by a higher fruit yield (Table 6), and in Experiment 3, by the reduction of the total N dose (Table 1). Several authors [7,43,44] reported NUE data for distinct vegetable cropping systems, either under greenhouse or in open-air conditions. With a fertilizer dose below 500 kg N/ha, the literature values of REC for greenhouse tomato ranged from 0.21 to 0.33 [7], which is in good agreement with those reported in Table 8 for Experiments 2 and 3. It was found that, along with yield and quality, the NUE was improved in potato fertilized with controlled release urea [45]. Similar results were obtained in wheat [46] and rice [47].

One possible drawback of CU application is the time gap between N release and N plant uptake [26,27]. Generally, the controlled release fertilizers are characterized by a release period, that is the time interval necessary for a fertilizer granule to release 80% of the inner nutrient at a fixed temperature (21 °C or 25 °C). Our study showed that the N release by the CU fertilizer was positively correlated with the cumulative daily average soil temperature (thermal sum) rather than with the time elapsed from transplanting both in spring and in autumn (Figure 1), despite the daily average temperature increased during the growing cycle in Experiment 1 and followed the opposite trend in Experiment 2. As expected, the crop development and the N uptake were also increased by higher temperatures in all the treatments. Therefore, the application of the CU fertilizer enabled us to effectively meet the plants nutritional needs, and our results demonstrated that the CU fertilizer could be used as the predominant N source, with simplification of the fertigation programs. However, to prevent a possible yield reduction due to calcium disorder (blossom-end rot), about 25–33% of the total N crop requirements should be beneficially satisfied by the application of calcium nitrate [48].

4.3. Effect on the Environment (N Leaching)

Compared with the conventional treatment, the use of DMPP fertilizer reduced N leaching only in Experiment 1 (Table 7), even though the nitrification inhibitor was expected to be less effective at higher temperature [49]. However, some authors [50] reported that the inhibiting efficiency of DMPP is modulated by several soil parameters acting simultaneously.

Both in Experiments 1 and 2, a lower evapotranspiration was observed for the high-dose CU treatments than for the other treatments. Because of similar irrigation, this was associated with higher values of water drainage and leaching fraction (Table 4). However, the CU treatments determined a lower N leaching (Table 7), in agreement with studies on several species, such as potato and corn [51], bell pepper [52] and rice [53]. This outcome suggested that CU application was effective in limiting N losses into drainage water. Following a similar trend with this result, a recent life cycle assessment (LCA) study on the impact of N fertilizers on the environment [8] reported the use of alternative coated N fertilizers as an effective strategy to reduce water pollution by eutrophication.

A reduced N loss by leaching with the CU fertilizer suggested the possibility to decrease the N dose commonly applied by growers. This hypothesis was tested in Experiment 3, where the CUred treatment employed -25% total N compared to the conventional fertilization. The data proved the effectiveness of the CU fertilizer, which enabled to decrease N leaching by about 65% (Table 7) without appreciable differences in tomato yield or quality (Table 6). Moreover, the results of Experiment 3 confirmed that with the CUred treatment, the combined effects of lower N supply and lower N loss allowed for the saving of considerable amounts of fertilizer, improving both economic costs and environmental impact. Specifically, in Experiment 3 the amount of fertilizer that could be saved with no influence on the production was up to 114.8 kg N/ha, that is about 30% of total N normally applied in tomato culture.

Concerning the N balance, our results showed that in Experiment 2, the plant growth was lower than expected, due to unexpectedly low light intensity in the autumn season (Table 2). In consequence, N input was higher than N output with both the stabilized and the coated fertilizer. On the other hand, both in Experiments 1 and 3, N input was always lower than N output, with a difference ranging from 24.0 to 43.4 kg N/ha. However, it is worth noting that the computation of N input reported in Table 7 did not include the N supply from soil organic matter mineralization during the growing period. This contribution could be estimated as 23 kg N/ha in Experiment 1 and 21 kg N/ha in Experiment 3, based on literature data for mineral N release in different types of soils [54]. By adding the estimated amounts to the N input, the overestimation of N output resulted well below 5% for all the treatments.

5. Conclusions

This study confirmed the effectiveness of the CU fertilizer in reducing N leaching from the soil both in spring and autumn growing cycles. At the same time, the results showed that with CU application both tomato yield and quality were maintained or even improved compared with conventional or stabilized fertilizers. Therefore, the CU treatments could satisfy the plants N requirement, preventing at the same time excess concentration of the element in the root zone. This outcome is consistent with the expected performance of controlled-release fertilizers, which should match the nutritional needs of plants better than the soluble or stabilized fertilizers, by providing a gradual N release in the soil. In contrast, with both the CON and DMPP treatments, the high availability of soluble N in the soil promoted vegetative behaviour, with a consequent increase in water use and a possible blooming delay.

The experiments indicated that N leaching could be effectively decreased by increasing the percentage of coated fertilizer and that the decrease of N leaching ranged from 9 to 28% of total N applied.

Further work (specifically, a proper validation trial) is needed to extend the results obtained in the greenhouse to the open field growing conditions. The main outcome of this study was that the limitation of N losses achieved using the coated fertilizer enabled a reduction of N application by 25% as compared with the growers' practice, without detrimental effects on the tomato production.

Author Contributions: Conceptualization, L.I., R.C. and A.P.; methodology, L.I. and R.C.; investigation, T.C. and L.B.; data curation, T.C., L.B., G.C. and F.F.; writing—original draft preparation, R.M., L.I. and C.T.; writing—review and editing L.I., R.M., A.P. and C.T.; visualization, R.M. and L.I.; supervision, L.I. and R.C. All authors have read and agreed to the published version of the manuscript.

Funding: This research received no external funding.

Acknowledgments: The authors wish to thank Chingoileima Maibam for the final English editing of the text.

Conflicts of Interest: The authors declare no conflict of interest.

References

1. Long, S.P.; Marshall-Colon, A.; Zhu, X.-G. Meeting the Global Food Demand of the Future by Engineering Crop Photosynthesis and Yield Potential. *Cell* **2015**, *161*, 56–66. [CrossRef] [PubMed]
2. Li, X.; Li, Q.; Xu, X.; Su, Y.; Yue, Q.; Gao, B. Characterization, swelling and slow-release properties of a new controlled release fertilizer based on wheat straw cellulose hydrogel. *J. Taiwan Inst. Chem. Eng.* **2016**, *60*, 564–572. [CrossRef]
3. Lu, C.; Tian, H. Global nitrogen and phosphorus fertilizer use for agriculture production in the past half century: Shifted hot spots and nutrient imbalance. *Earth Syst. Sci. Data* **2017**, *9*, 181–192. [CrossRef]
4. Martínez-Gaitán, C.; Granados, M.R.; Fernández, M.D.; Gallardo, M.; Thompson, R. Recovery of 15N Labeled Nitrogen Fertilizer by Fertigated and Drip Irrigated Greenhouse Vegetable Crops. *Agronomy* **2020**, *10*, 741. [CrossRef]
5. Thompson, R.; Incrocci, L.; Van Ruijven, J.; Massa, D. Reducing contamination of water bodies from European vegetable production systems. *Agric. Water Manag.* **2020**, *240*, 106258. [CrossRef]
6. Tei, F.; De Neve, S.; De Haan, J.; Kristensen, H.L. Nitrogen management of vegetable crops. *Agric. Water Manag.* **2020**, *240*, 106316. [CrossRef]
7. Ti, C.; Luo, Y.; Yan, X. Characteristics of nitrogen balance in open-air and greenhouse vegetable cropping systems of China. *Environ. Sci. Pollut. Res.* **2015**, *22*, 18508–18518. [CrossRef]
8. Da Costa, T.P.; Westphalen, G.; Nora, F.B.D.; Silva, B.D.Z.; Da Rosa, G.S.; De Zorzi, B. Technical and environmental assessment of coated urea production with a natural polymeric suspension in spouted bed to reduce nitrogen losses. *J. Clean. Prod.* **2019**, *222*, 324–334. [CrossRef]
9. Thomson, A.J.; Giannopoulos, G.; Pretty, J.; Baggs, E.M.; Richardson, D.J. Biological sources and sinks of nitrous oxide and strategies to mitigate emissions. *Philos. Trans. R. Soc. B Biol. Sci.* **2012**, *367*, 1157–1168. [CrossRef]
10. Thompson, R.; Martínez-Gaitan, C.; Gallardo, M.; Giménez, C.; Fernández, M. Identification of irrigation and N management practices that contribute to nitrate leaching loss from an intensive vegetable production system by use of a comprehensive survey. *Agric. Water Manag.* **2007**, *89*, 261–274. [CrossRef]
11. D'Alessandro, W.; Bellomo, S.; Parello, F.; Bonfanti, P.; Brusca, L.; Longo, M.; Maugeri, R. Nitrate, sulphate and chloride contents in public drinking water supplies in Sicily, Italy. *Environ. Monit. Assess.* **2012**, *184*, 2845–2855. [CrossRef] [PubMed]
12. Voogt, W.; Beerling, E.A.M.; Blok, C.; van der Maas, A.A.; van Os, E.A. The road to sustainable water and nutrient management in soil-less culture in Dutch greenhouse horticulture. In Proceedings of the NUTRIHORT: Nutrient Management, Nutrient Legislation and Innovative Techniques in Intensive Horticulture, Ghent, Belgium, 16–18 September 2013; Available online: https://edepot.wur.nl/290253 (accessed on 11 November 2020).
13. Brés, W. Estimation of Nutrient Losses from Open Fertigation Systems to Soil during Horticultural Plants Cultivation. *Pol. J. Environ. Stud.* **2009**, *183*, 341–345.

14. Chartzoulakis, K. Water resources management in the Island of Crete, Greece, with emphasis on the agricultural use. *Hydrol. Res.* **2001**, *3*, 193–205. [CrossRef]
15. The European Council. Council Directive 91/676/EEC 12/12/1991 concerning the protection of waters against pollution caused by nitrates from agricultural sources. *Off. J. Eur. Commun.* **1991**, *L375*, 1–8.
16. Massa, D.; Incrocci, L.; Maggini, R.; Carmassi, G.; Campiotti, C.A.; Pardossi, A. Strategies to decrease water drainage and nitrate emission from soilless cultures of greenhouse tomato. *Agric. Water Manag.* **2010**, *97*, 971–980. [CrossRef]
17. Van Grinsven, H.J.M.; Berge, H.F.M.T.; Dalgaard, T.; Fraters, B.; Durand, P.; Hart, A.; Hofman, G.; Jacobsen, B.H.; Lalor, S.T.J.; Lesschen, J.P.; et al. Management, regulation and environmental impacts of nitrogen fertilization in northwestern Europe under the Nitrates Directive; a benchmark study. *Biogeosciences* **2012**, *9*, 5143–5160. [CrossRef]
18. Wang, Z.; Li, S. Effects of Nitrogen and Phosphorus Fertilization on Plant Growth and Nitrate Accumulation in Vegetables. *J. Plant Nutr.* **2004**, *27*, 539–556. [CrossRef]
19. Ahluwalia, A.; Gladwin, M.; Coleman, G.D.; Hord, N.; Howard, G.; Kim-Shapiro, D.B.; Lajous, M.; Larsen, F.J.; Lefer, D.J.; McClure, L.A.; et al. Dietary Nitrate and the Epidemiology of Cardiovascular Disease: Report from a National Heart, Lung, and Blood Institute Workshop. *J. Am. Heart Assoc.* **2016**, *5*, e003402. [CrossRef]
20. Umar, S.; Iqbal, M. Nitrate accumulation in plants, factors affecting the process, and human health implications. A review. *Agron. Sustain. Dev.* **2007**, *27*, 45–57. [CrossRef]
21. Zhong, W.; Hu, C.; Wang, M. Nitrate and nitrite in vegetables from north China: Content and intake. *Food Addit. Contam.* **2002**, *19*, 1125–1129. [CrossRef]
22. The European Commission. Commission Regulation (EU) No. 1258/2011 amending Regulation (EC) No. 1881/2006 as regards maximum levels for nitrates in food stuffs. *Off. J. Eur. Union* **2011**, *L320*, 15–17.
23. Carson, L.C.; Ozores-Hampton, M. Methods for Determining Nitrogen Release from Controlled-release Fertilizers Used for Vegetable Production. *HortTechnology* **2012**, *22*, 20–24. [CrossRef]
24. Chalk, P.M.; Craswell, E.T.; Polidoro, J.C.; Chen, C. Fate and efficiency of 15Nlabelledslow- and controlled release fertilizers. *Nutr. Cycl. Agroecosyst.* **2015**, *102*, 167–178. [CrossRef]
25. Dubey, A.; Mailapalli, D.R. Zeolite coated urea fertilizer using different binders: Fabrication, material properties and nitrogen release studies. *Environ. Technol. Innov.* **2019**, *16*, 100452. [CrossRef]
26. Azeem, B.; KuShaari, K.; Man, Z.B.; Basit, A.; Thanh, T.H. Review on materials & methods to produce controlled release coated urea fertilizer. *J. Control. Release* **2014**, *181*, 11–21. [CrossRef]
27. Qiao, D.; Liu, H.; Yu, L.; Bao, X.; Simon, G.P.; Petinakis, E.; Chen, L. Preparation and characterization of slow-release fertilizer encapsulated by starch-based superabsorbent polymer. *Carbohydr. Polym.* **2016**, *147*, 146–154. [CrossRef]
28. Guertal, E. Slow-release Nitrogen Fertilizers in Vegetable Production: A Review. *HortTechnology* **2009**, *19*, 16–19. [CrossRef]
29. Naz, M.Y.; Sulaiman, S.A. Slow release coating remedy for nitrogen loss from conventional urea: A review. *J. Control. Release* **2016**, *225*, 109–120. [CrossRef]
30. Cataldo, D.A.; Maroon, M.; Schrader, L.E.; Youngs, V.L. Rapid colorimetric determination of nitrate in plant tissue by nitration of salicylic acid. *Commun. Soil Sci. Plant Anal.* **1975**, *6*, 71–80. [CrossRef]
31. Kempers, A.; Zweers, A. Ammonium determination in soil extracts by the salicylate method. *Commun. Soil Sci. Plant Anal.* **1986**, *17*, 715–723. [CrossRef]
32. Olsen, S.R.; Cole, C.V.; Watanabe, F.S.; Dean, L.A. *Estimation of Available Phosphorus in Soils by Extraction with NaHCO$_3$, USDA No. 939*; U.S. Department of Agriculture: Washington, DC, USA, 1954.
33. Thomas, G.W. Exchangeable Cations. In *Methods of Soil Analysis*, 2nd ed.; Page, A., Ed.; American Society of Agronomy, Inc.; Soil Science Society of America, Inc.: Madison, WI, USA, 1982; pp. 159–165. [CrossRef]
34. Ministero delle Politiche Agricole e Forestali. *Decreto Ministeriale del 13/09/1999, Approvazione dei "Metodi Ufficiali di Analisi Chimica del Suolo"*; Gazzetta Ufficiale della Repubblica Italiana Suppl. Ordin. n.248: Rome, Italy, 1999. (In Italian)
35. Omar, L.; Ahmed, O.H.; Majid, N.M.A. Improving Ammonium and Nitrate Release from Urea Using Clinoptilolite Zeolite and Compost Produced from Agricultural Wastes. *Sci. World J.* **2015**, *2015*, 574201. [CrossRef] [PubMed]

36. Pandey, R.K.; Ie, J.W.M.; Bako, Y. Nitrogen fertilizer response and use efficiency for three cereal crops in Niger Commun. *Soil Sci. Plan.* **2001**, *32*, 1465–1482. [CrossRef]
37. Elia, A.; Conversa, G. Agronomic and physiological responses of a tomato crop to nitrogen input. *Eur. J. Agron.* **2012**, *40*, 64–74. [CrossRef]
38. Haque, M.E.; Paul, A.K.; Sarker, J.R. Effect of Nitrogen and Boron on the Growth and Yield of Tomato (*Lycopersicum esculentum* L.). *Int. J. Bio-Resour. Stress Manag.* **2011**, *2*, 277–282.
39. Addae-Kagya, K.; Norman, J.C. The influence of nitrogen levels on local cultivars of eggplant (*Solanum integrifolium* L.). *Acta Hortic.* **1977**, *2*, 397–402. [CrossRef]
40. Tei, F.; Benincasa, P.; Guiducci, M. Critical nitrogen concentration in processing tomato. *Eur. J. Agron.* **2002**, *18*, 45–55. [CrossRef]
41. Hirel, B.; Lemaire, G. From Agronomy and Ecophysiology to Molecular Genetics for Improving Nitrogen Use Efficiency in Crops. *J. Crop. Improv.* **2006**, *15*, 213–257. [CrossRef]
42. Greenwood, D.J.; Hunt, J. Effect of nitrogen fertilizer on the nitrate contents of field vegetables grown in Britain. *J. Sci. Food Agric.* **1986**, *37*, 373–383. [CrossRef]
43. Jiang, H.M.; Zhang, J.; Yang, J.C.; Liu, Z.H.; Song, X.Z.; Jiang, L.H. Effects of models of N application on greenhouse tomato N uptake, utilization and soil NO_3–N accumulation. *J. Agro-Environ. Sci.* **2009**, *28*, 2623–2630. Available online: http://en.cnki.com.cn/Article_en/CJFDTOTAL-NHBH200912034.htm (accessed on 10 November 2020). (In Chinese).
44. Min, J.; Zhao, X.; Shi, W.M.; Xing, G.X.; Zhu, Z.L. Nitrogen balance and loss in a greenhouse vegetable system in South eastern China. *Pedosphere* **2011**, *21*, 464–472. [CrossRef]
45. Gao, X.; Li, C.; Zhang, M.; Wang, R.; Chen, B. Controlled release urea improved the nitrogen use efficiency, yield and quality of potato (*Solanum tuberosum* L.) on silt loamy soil. *Field Crop. Res.* **2015**, *181*, 60–68. [CrossRef]
46. Yang, Y.; Zhang, M.; Zheng, L.; Cheng, D.-D.; Liu, M.; Geng, Y.-Q. Controlled Release Urea Improved Nitrogen Use Efficiency, Yield, and Quality of Wheat. *Agron. J.* **2011**, *103*, 479–485. [CrossRef]
47. Shivay, Y.S.; Prasad, R.; Pal, M. Effect of Nitrogen Levels and Coated Urea on Growth, Yields and Nitrogen Use Efficiency in Aromatic Rice. *J. Plant Nutr.* **2015**, *39*, 875–882. [CrossRef]
48. Taylor, M.; Locascio, S.; Alligood, M. Blossom-end Rot Incidence of Tomato as Affected by Irrigation Quantity, Calcium Source, and Reduced Potassium. *HortScience* **2004**, *39*, 1110–1115. [CrossRef]
49. Yu, Q.; Ye, X.; Chen, Y.; Zhang, Z.; Tian, G. Influences of nitrification inhibitor 3,4-dimethyl pyrazole phosphate on nitrogen and soil salt-ion leaching. *J. Environ. Sci.* **2008**, *20*, 304–308. [CrossRef]
50. Zerulla, W.; Barth, T.; Dressel, J.; Erhardt, K.; Von Locquenghien, K.H.; Pasda, G.; Rädle, M.; Wissemeier, A. 3,4-Dimethylpyrazole phosphate (DMPP)—A new nitrification inhibitor for agriculture and horticulture. *Biol. Fertil. Soils* **2001**, *34*, 79–84. [CrossRef]
51. Shoji, S.; Delgado, J.; Mosier, A.; Miura, Y. Use of controlled release fertilizers and nitrification inhibitors to increase nitrogen use efficiency and to conserve air and water quality. *Comm. Soil Sci. Plant Anal.* **2001**, *32*, 1051–1070. [CrossRef]
52. Guertal, E.A. Preplant Slow-Release Nitrogen Fertilizers Produce Similar Bell Pepper Yields as Split Applications of Soluble Fertilizer. *Semigroup Forum* **2000**, *92*, 388. [CrossRef]
53. Kiran, J.K.; Khanif, Y.M.; Amminuddin, H.; Anuar, A.R. Effects of Controlled Release Urea on the Yield and Nitrogen Nutrition of Flooded Rice. *Commun. Soil Sci. Plant Anal.* **2010**, *41*, 811–819. [CrossRef]
54. Baroncelli, P.; Landi, S.; Marzialetti, P.; Scavo, N. Uso Razionale delle Risorse nel Florovivaismo: I Fertilizzanti. In *Quaderno ARSIA No. 2*; ARSIA—Agenzia Regionale per lo Sviluppo e l'Innovazione nel settore Agricolo-forestale: Firenze, Italy, 2004; p. 281. (In Italian)

Publisher's Note: MDPI stays neutral with regard to jurisdictional claims in published maps and institutional affiliations.

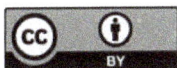

© 2020 by the authors. Licensee MDPI, Basel, Switzerland. This article is an open access article distributed under the terms and conditions of the Creative Commons Attribution (CC BY) license (http://creativecommons.org/licenses/by/4.0/).

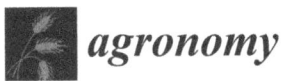

Article

Application of Single Superphosphate with Humic Acid Improves the Growth, Yield and Phosphorus Uptake of Wheat (*Triticum aestivum* L.) in Calcareous Soil

Muhammad Izhar Shafi [1,†], Muhammad Adnan [2], Shah Fahad [3,4,*,†], Fazli Wahid [2], Ahsan Khan [5], Zhen Yue [6], Subhan Danish [7,*], Muhammad Zafar-ul-Hye [7], Martin Brtnicky [8,9,10] and Rahul Datta [8,*]

1. Department of Soil and Environmental Sciences, The University of Agriculture, Peshawar 25000, Pakistan; mirzaizhar2008@aup.edu.pk
2. Department of Agriculture, The University of Swabi, Swabi 23561, Pakistan; madnanses@gmail.com (M.A.); fazliwahid@uoswabi.edu.pk (F.W.)
3. Hainan Key Laboratory for Sustainable Utilization of Tropical Bioresource, College of Tropical Crops, Hainan University, Haikou 570228, China
4. Department of Agronomy, The University of Haripur, Haripur 22620, Pakistan
5. Department of Zoology, The University of Swabi, Swabi 23561, Pakistan; ahsan@uoswabi.edu.pk
6. College of Life Science, Liniyi University, Liniyi 276000, China; yuezhen@lyu.edu.cn
7. Department of Soil Science, Faculty of Agricultural Sciences and Technology, Bahauddin Zakariya University, Multan 60800, Punjab, Pakistan; zafarulhye@bzu.edu.pk
8. Department of Agrochemistry, Soil Science, Microbiology and Plant Nutrition, Faculty of AgriSciences, Mendel University in Brno, Zemedelska 1, 61300 Brno, Czech Republic; martin.brtnicky@mendelu.cz
9. Department of Geology and Pedology, Faculty of Forestry and Wood Technology, Mendel University in Brno, Zemedelska 3, 61300 Brno, Czech Republic
10. Institute of Chemistry and Technology of Environmental Protection, Faculty of Chemistry, Brno University of Technology, Purkynova 118, 62100 Brno, Czech Republic
* Correspondence: shahfahad@uoswbai.edu.pk (S.F.); sd96850@gmail.com (S.D.); rahulmedcure@gmail.com (R.D.); Tel.: +420-773990283 (R.D.)
† Equally Contributing authors: Muhammad Izhar Shafi and Shah Fahad.

Received: 7 July 2020; Accepted: 11 August 2020; Published: 19 August 2020

Abstract: In calcareous soil, the significant portion of applied phosphorus (P) fertilizers is adsorbed on the calcite surface and becomes unavailable to plants. Addition of organic amendments with chemical fertilizers can be helpful in releasing the absorbed nutrients from these surfaces. To check out this problem, a field experiment was conducted for two years to determine the effect of P fertilizers and humic acid (HA) in enhancing P availability in soil and their ultimate effect on growth, yield and P uptake of wheat in calcareous soils. The experiment was comprised of five levels of P (0, 45, 67.5, 90 and 112.5 kg P_2O_5 ha^{-1}) as a single superphosphate (SSP) and 2 levels of locally produced humic acid (with and without HA) arranged in a two factorial randomized complete block design (RCBD) with three replications. Wheat plant height, spike length, number of grains per spike, 1000-grain weight, grain, straw and biological yield were significantly improved by the addition of HA with SSP. Very often, the performance of 67.5 kg P_2O_5 ha^{-1} with HA were either similar or better than 90 or even 112.5 kg P_2O_5 ha^{-1} applied without HA. Post-harvest soil organic matter, AB-DTPA extractable and water-soluble P, plant P concentration and its uptake were also significantly improved by the addition of HA with SSP compared to sole SSP application. It was evident that P efficiency could be increased with HA addition and it has the potential to improve crop yield and plants P uptake in calcareous soils.

Keywords: calcareous soil; humic acid; phosphorus uptake; single superphosphate; wheat

1. Introduction

Soil fertility and crop productivity are closely related to three main components of soil ecosystems: the bio-available soil nutrients, soil microbiota and organic matter content [1–5]. Phosphorus is 2nd most yield limiting nutrient after nitrogen in agricultural production across the world [6,7]. Phosphorus (P) plays many key functions in plant life especially in the storage and transfer of energy, photosynthesis, respiration, cell division, and enlargement. Plants take P in $H_2PO_4^-$ or HPO_4^{-2} forms from the soil solution. Application of phosphatic fertilizers in a balanced amount and at the correct time with good application techniques and management methods has good impacts on crop yield. However, responses to fertilization can be species and variety-dependent, which greatly influences nutrient accumulation and utilization in the plant [8,9]. Organic Fertilizer addition to soil increases risk of xenobiotic contamination [10–13].

Phosphorus deficiency is often a yield-limiting factor in agricultural soils, particularly in those having high carbonate contents, which reduces phosphorus solubility. In these conditions, achieving a target crop productivity generally demands the use of higher fertilizer rates as a way to account for that increased inefficiency. Besides being expensive [14], use of supra-optimum rates of chemical fertilizers in recent years has been frequently pointed as the reason behind in reduction in organic substances found within the soil [15]. Moreover, excessive usage of chemical fertilizers in agriculture has caused environmental issues like biological processes, physical destruction of the soil and nutritional imbalances [16]. In addition, research shows that increased corn and bean overall yields and quality can be obtained by using organic and chemical fertilizers simultaneously, which in turn aids to reducing the use of chemical fertilizers and improving soil health and overall sustainability [17].

Several studies reported that plant growth and development are greatly related with the movement of specific organic fractions present in both the soil solutions (known as dissolved organic matter) and soil matrix (soil organic matter). These fractions have been defined as humic substances and include humic acids, fulvic acids and humin [1,18]. The advantageous activities of these humic substances in relation to crop production has been attributed to two main effects [19,20]: the indirect effect on soil properties and fertility, related to the ability of these substances to form complexes or chelates with soil metals [14], which impacts soil structure, texture and nutrients availability [19]. While the direct regulating growth effect on plant hormones such as auxin, ethylene, nitric oxide, cytokinins, abscisic acid and reactive oxygen species [20].

Humic acid (HA) is an active ingredient of humus that can play an essential role in improved soil health and plant growth. Physically, it provides good soil structure and enhances the water holding capacity of the soil; biologically it enhances the growth of beneficial soil organisms, while chemically it acts as an adsorption and retention complex for inorganic plant nutrients [21]. Humic acid cannot be only found in soils, but also in peats, rivers, oceans and lignitic coals and can result from the biological decomposition and of organic matter. Humic substances can change the unavailable elements into available forms and can rupture Fe or Al bonded P in acidic soils and Ca in calcareous soils, rendering more soil P to be available for plant uptake. Humic acid can make complexes with Na, K, Mn, Zn, Ca, Fe, Cu and with a variety of other elements to overcome a particular element shortage in the soil. Thus, under certain conditions, the use of HA and its concomitant stimulating effect on various crops has received considerable attention [22]. Chemical composition of HA varies depending on the source and edaphoclimatic conditions where it was formed, but average HA composition contains 51–57% organic C, 4–6% N and 0.2 to 1% P that can be used both for plant nutrition and for improving soil physicochemical and biological parameters [21]. Additionally, HS was found to have a marked effect on the emergence of lateral roots, and the hyper induction of sites for lateral root emergence [23]. Research shows that the effect of Humic substances (HS) on plant growth depends on the source, concentration and molecular weight of humic fractions [24,25]. That is why the present study was conducted to evaluate the role of locally produced HA in enhancing P availability and wheat growth in calcareous soil amended with different P levels as SSP.

2. Materials and Methods

2.1. Experimental Procedure

A field study was conducted over two years, to investigate the effect of different levels of single superphosphate applied alone and in combination of HA on growth, yield and phosphorus uptake by wheat crop at the Research Farm of the University of Agriculture, Peshawar-Pakistan. The experimental farm is located at 34.01° N latitude, 71.35° E longitude at an altitude of 350 m above sea level in Peshawar valley. The soil in the experimental site was a silt loam, alkaline calcareous, low in organic matter and P contents (Table 1) and was also highly responsive to P application [26]. Treatments included the application of P at 0, 45, 67.5, 90 and 112.5 kg P_2O_5 ha^{-1} applied as Single Superphosphate (SSP) without and with the HA addition (i.e., 0 and 5 kg HA ha^{-1}). Humic acid was extracted from brown coal collected from Hyderabad, Pakistan in the laboratory of Soil and Environmental_Sciences, The University of Agriculture Peshawar, Pakistan by following the procedure of Hai and Mir [27]. The experiment was arranged as a two factorial [5 (P levels) and 2 (HA levels)] randomized complete block design (RCBD) with 3 replications. The required P fertilizer along with half recommended levels of N (120 kg ha^{-1}) and a full dose of K as 60 kg K_2O ha^{-1} were applied as urea and sulphate of potash respectively, before planting. The remaining half rate of N was applied with the first irrigation. Wheat (Triticum aestivum L.) variety "Atta Habib" having a seed rate of 100 kg ha^{-1} was sown through handrill with 30 cm row spacing in a plot size of 4 m × 5 m. All the agronomic practices and manual weed control were followed as per the standard advised procedure for all treatments uniformly. Plants were harvested at physiological maturity. The field was irrigated as per crop requirements.

Table 1. Characteristics of composite soil of the area and humic acid used in the experiment.

Properties	Concentration
Soil	
Sand (%)	25.00
Silt (%)	65.23
Clay (%)	7.00
Textural class	Silt loam
pH $_{(1:5)}$	7.9
EC $_{(1:5)}$ dS m^{-1}	0.20
Organic matter content (%)	0.72
AB DTPA extractable P (mg kg^{-1})	4.0
AB DTPA extractable K (mg kg^{-1})	110
Lime contents (%)	14.04
Humic acid	
Organic C (%)	50.4–60.3
Total N (%)	3.0–5.5
AB DTPA Extractable P (mg kg^{-1})	50.0–52.5
Zn (mg kg^{-1})	05.5–07.3
Mn (mg kg^{-1})	12.2–15.5
pH (1:5)	5.5–6.0

Data on plant height was determined by taking the height of five randomly selected plants from soil surface to the tip of each plant at physiological maturity in each treatment plot and then averaged. To determine the spike length, five spikes were randomly selected in each plot and their length was measured from base of rachis to the tip of uppermost spikelet. After that the spikes were threshed individually to determine grains per spike and their mean were taken as a grains spike^{-1}. Thousand grains weight was recorded by counting and weighing thousand grains randomly taken from each treatment plot. Grain yield was recorded after threshing of plants taken from central four rows in each treatment and then converted into kg ha^{-1} by using the following formula:

$$\text{Grain yield (kgha}^{-1}) = \frac{\text{Grain yield in kg obtained from harvested rows} \times 10000 \text{ m}^2}{(\text{Row lenght} \times \text{Row spacing in meter} \times \text{No. of rows})}$$

Biological yield (BY) was measured by weighing the entire harvested crop (un-threshed crop i.e., both grain and straw) in each treatment. The BY was then converted in to kg ha^{-1} with the following formula:

$$\text{Biological yield (kgha}^{-1}) \frac{\text{Biological yield in kg obtained from harvested rows} \times 10000 \text{ m}^2}{(\text{Row lenght} \times \text{Row spacing in meter} \times \text{No. of rows})} \quad (1)$$

Straw yield was calculated by subtracting grain yield from biological yield.

2.2. Samples Collection and Physicochemical Analysis

Soil samples were taken from (0–30 cm) of the soil used in the field experiment and were prepared for some physical and chemical analysis. Soil properties changes with land use [28–30]. The whole plant samples (shoots + grains) were randomly taken from each treatment plot after harvesting and were dried at 70 °C until constant mass weight. Then, dried samples were grounded to pass a 1-mm screen, as suggested by Weidhuner et al. [30–32] and samples were thoroughly mixed and stored for analysis. Soil EC and pH were quantified in 1:5 soil water suspensions by the procedure of Rhoades [33] and Thomas [34], respectively. Organic matter (O.M.) contents in soil were determined by dichromate oxidation as described by Nelson and Sommers [35], AB-DTPA extractable and water-soluble phosphorus concentration was measured by the standard procedures of Soltanpour and Schwab [36]. The soil was also analyzed for lime content by adopting the procedure of Loeppert and Suarez [37] while soil texture was measured by the procedure of Gee and Bauder [38]. Plant P concentration and its uptake by wheat were determined by the protocol of Jones et al. [39]. Characterization of soil and HA is provided in Table 1.

2.3. Statistical Analysis

Data were subjected to two way ANOVA analysis for the significance of treatment effects and means were separated using the least significant difference (LSD) test with significance set at $p \leq 0.05$ using Staistix 2000 statistical package [40].

3. Results

3.1. Plant Height (cm)

Application of different levels of P and HA produced significantly ($p \leq 0.05$) taller wheat plants than the plots where SSP without HA was applied. When averaged across the P levels, HA produced 84 cm taller plants as compared to 82 cm without HA. When average across the HA levels, the application of P levels at 90 kg P$_2$O$_5$ ha^{-1} produced maximum taller plants of height 88 cm and the decrease in plant height at a higher level of P indicates that 90 kg P$_2$O$_5$ ha^{-1} is the optimum dose in the given soil conditions. The interactive effect of HA and P levels was also significant. Maximum plant height 89 cm was observed where 90 kg P$_2$O$_5$ ha^{-1} with 5 kg HA ha^{-1} was applied, whereas a minimum of 77 cm was observed in control.

3.2. Spike Length (cm)

Spike length as influenced by the different levels of P and HA is given in Table 2. When averaged across HA, different levels of SSP significantly increased the spike length as compared to control. On average the maximum spike length (10.77 cm) was recorded in the treatments applied with

112.5 kg P_2O_5 ha^{-1} which was statistically higher than the spike length obtained at 67.5 and 45 kg P_2O_5 ha^{-1} but not significant from the plots treated with 90 kg P_2O_5 ha^{-1}. Application of HA also increased the spike length of wheat plants significantly, but the interactive effect of P and HA was non-significant with a range from 9.75 cm in control to 10.89 cm observed in treatments P at 90 kg P_2O_5 ha^{-1} with 5 kg HA ha^{-1}.

3.3. Grains Spike^{-1}

Data showed that both different doses of SSP and HA had a significant effect on the number of grains spike^{-1} (Table 2). The number of grains spike^{-1} significantly increased with each level of SSP over control. On average maximum, 58 grains spike^{-1} were observed in plots treated with 112.5 kg P_2O_5 ha^{-1} SSP that was statistically similar to those obtained at 90 kg P_2O_5 ha^{-1} SSP, whereas a minimum of 51 grain spike^{-1} was recorded in control. Application of HA also showed significant results with maximum grains spike^{-1} (56) in the plots receiving 5 kg HA ha^{-1} dose which was statistically higher than the plots treated without HA, while the interactive effect was non-significant with a maximum number of 60 grains spike^{-1} obtained from the plots treated with 90 kg P_2O_5 ha^{-1} with the application of HA.

3.4. 1000-Grain Weight

Table 2 shows the 1000-grain weight as influenced by the application of different levels of SSP with and without HA. The data revealed the increase in grain weight with increasing levels of P fertilizer and HA. The non-significant interaction revealed that HA increased the grain size irrespective of P levels. Similarly, when averaged across the HA, the application of 112.5 P_2O_5 ha^{-1} produced heavier grains amounting 46.05 g per 1000 seeds which was 25.64% heavier than control. When averaged across the P levels, application of HA produced heavier grains of 42.61 g which were statistically higher than the grain weight of the plots which receive no HA.

3.5. Grain Yield (kg ha^{-1})

The addition of HA and P levels significantly increased the grain yield over control. Application of HA showed an additional advantage over the sole application of SSP by increasing the grain yield from 3% in control to 16% at 90 kg P_2O_5 ha^{-1} suggesting an increase in P use efficiency with the application of HA with each increment in P level (Table 2). When averaged across HA, grain yield of 2947 kg ha^{-1} was recorded in the plots treated with 90 kg P_2O_5 ha^{-1} which was statistically higher than the grain yield obtained at 112.5, 67.5 and 45 kg P_2O_5 ha^{-1} indicating that the 90 kg P_2O_5 ha^{-1} could be the optimum level in the prevailing soil and climatic conditions for the wheat crop. The HA also showed significant results with grain yield of 2540 kg ha^{-1} over no HA application with grain yield of 2338 kg ha^{-1}.

Table 2. Effect of phosphorus and humic acid on the growth, yield and P nutrition of wheat under agro climatic conditions of Peshawar, Pakistan.

Phosphorus (kg P$_2$O$_5$ ha^{-1})	Humic Acid (kg ha^{-1})	Plant Height (cm)	Spike Length (cm)	Grains Spike^{-1}	1000-Grain Weight (g)	Grain Yield (kg ha^{-1})	Straw Yield (kg ha^{-1})	Biological Yield (kg ha^{-1})	Harvest Index (%)	Plant P Concentration (g kg^{-1})	P Uptake (kg ha^{-1})
0		78 ± 0.13 e	9.91 ± 0.10 c	51 ± 0.73 d	36.65 ± 0.23 e	1835 ± 33 e	2658 ± 28 d	4493 ± 214 e	41 ± 0.60 ab	2.5 ± 0.04 d	11.54 ± 0.33 e
45		81 ± 0.03 d	10.20 ± 0.18 b	53 ± 0.50 c	39.95 ± 0.32 d	2237 ± 64 d	3480 ± 109 c	5717 ± 242 d	39 ± 1.21 b	2.9 ± 0.10 c	17.02 ± 0.67 d
67.5		83 ± 0.06 c	10.34 ± 0.01 b	56 ± 0.17 b	42.00 ± 0.45 c	2500 ± 36 c	3864 ± 23 b	6364 ± 229 c	39 ± 0.23 b	3.1 ± 0.06 bc	19.91 ± 0.44 c
90		88 ± 0.26 a	10.67 ± 0.09 a	58 ± 0.44 a	44.87 ± 0.67 b	2947 ± 18 a	3927 ± 97 b	6874 ± 369 b	43 ± 0.71 a	3.1 ± 0.07 b	21.41 ± 0.71 b
112.5		87 ± 0.03 b	10.77 ± 0.07 a	58 ± 0.33 a	46.05 ± 0.20 a	2678 ± 13 b	4549 ± 53 a	7227 ± 267 a	36 ± 0.32 c	3.3 ± 0.09 a	24.30 ± 0.84 a
LSD ($p \leq 0.05$)		0.63	0.28	1.33	0.81	95.597	180.96	154.39	2.033	0.1421	1.157
	0	82 ± 0.07 b	10.27 ± 0.08 b	54 ± 0.41 b	41.20 ± 0.40 b	2338 ± 37 b	3609 ± 46	5947 ± 1053 b	39 ± 0.68	2.9 ± 0.04 b	17.71 ± 0.34 b
	5	84 ± 0.05 a	10.48 ± 0.12 a	56 ± 0.18 a	42.61 ± 0.29 a	2540 ± 25 a	3782 ± 81	6322 ± 1106 a	40 ± 0.63	3.1 ± 0.07 a	19.97 ± 0.62 a
LSD ($p \leq 0.05$)		0.40	0.18	0.84	0.51	60.461	ns	97.644	ns	0.0898	0.733
0	0	77 ± 0.23 h	9.75 ± 0.05	51 ± 0.88	35.73 ± 0.26	1807 ± 43 f	2534 ± 90	4341 ± 65 h	42 ± 1.37	2.5 ± 0.03	11.11 ± 0.24
	5	78 ± 0.23 g	10.06 ± 0.17	52 ± 0.58	37.57 ± 0.23	1862 ± 23 f	2782 ± 54	4644 ± 77 g	40 ± 0.18	2.5 ± 0.05	11.98 ± 0.45
45	0	80 ± 0.23 f	10.04 ± 0.27	52 ± 1.00	39.40 ± 0.40	2168 ± 57 e	3377 ± 114	5545 ± 80 f	39 ± 1.35	2.9 ± 0.03	16.19 ± 0.15
	5	81 ± 0.24 e	10.36 ± 0.23	54 ± 1.02	40.50 ± 0.40	2306 ± 70 d	3582 ± 122	5888 ± 141 e	39 ± 1.11	3.0 ± 0.17	17.86 ± 1.20
67.5	0	81 ± 0.23 e	10.31 ± 0.10	55 ± 0.33	41.40 ± 0.67	2439 ± 74 cd	3763 ± 84	6202 ± 20 d	39 ± 1.25	2.9 ± 0.04	18.66 ± 0.20
	5	85 ± 0.35 d	10.37 ± 0.10	58 ± 0.33	42.60 ± 0.36	2561 ± 26 c	3965 ± 125	6526 ± 121 c	39 ± 0.84	3.2 ± 0.09	21.16 ± 0.72
90	0	86 ± 0.44 c	10.44 ± 0.11	56 ± 0.58	43.83 ± 0.49	2731 ± 35 b	3882 ± 35	6613 ± 61 c	41 ± 0.29	2.9 ± 0.05	19.49 ± 0.53
	5	89 ± 0.15 a	10.89 ± 0.10	60 ± 0.33	45.90 ± 0.86	3163 ± 69 a	3972 ± 174	7135 ± 109 b	44 ± 1.63	3.3 ± 0.09	23.33 ± 0.89
112.5	0	85 ± 0.31 d	10.83 ± 0.06	58 ± 0.02	45.63 ± 0.33	2547 ± 30 c	4490 ± 22	7037 ± 38 b	36 ± 0.28	3.2 ± 0.13	23.10 ± 1.03
	5	88 ± 0.37 b	10.71 ± 0.14	58 ± 0.67	46.47 ± 0.45	2808 ± 29 b	4607 ± 90	7415 ± 62 a	38 ± 0.71	3.4 ± 0.06	25.50 ± 0.72
LSD ($p \leq 0.05$)		0.89	ns	ns	ns	135	ns	218	ns	ns	ns

Means with same letters are not significantly different from each other. The ±values represent stander error of the mean ($n = 3$) while, ns stands for non-significant difference at $p \leq 0.05$.

3.6. Straw Yield (kg ha^{-1})

Wheat straw yield as influenced by different levels of SSP with and without HA is presented in Table 2. With an increase in P level, the straw yield significantly increased over control except for 67.5 and 90 kg P$_2$O$_5$ ha^{-1} which were statistically similar. The maximum straw yield of 4549 kg ha^{-1} was recorded from the treatments applied with 112.5 kg P$_2$O$_5$ ha^{-1} which was 71% higher than control. This increase signifies the function of P in crop growth and productivity in the tested soil and climatic conditions, however, the role of HA was found non-significant. The interactive effect of P levels and HA was also non-significant with maximum straw yield of 4607 kg ha^{-1} was observed in the plots treated with 112.5 kg P$_2$O$_5$ ha^{-1} and HA, while minimum (2534 kg ha^{-1}) was in case of control.

3.7. Biological Yield (kg ha^{-1})

Both the P levels, HA and their interaction significantly ($p \leq 0.05$) increased the biological yield of wheat (Table 2). The interaction of P levels with HA exhibited that biological yield increases with increasing application of P but HA application further intensify such improvement. On average, each increment of P produced higher biological yield than the preceding lower dose indicating the role of P in increasing the crop growth in the given soil and climatic conditions. The maximum biological yield (7227 kg ha^{-1}) was recorded in the plots treated with 112.5 kg P$_2$O$_5$ ha^{-1} that was statistically higher than the plots applied with 90, 67.5 and 45 kg P$_2$O$_5$ ha^{-1} (Table 3 and Figure 1A). The data regarding biological yield also revealed that the increase over control with 90 kg P$_2$O$_5$ kg ha^{-1} and HA was 64% which was close to 62% increase observed with 112.5 kg P$_2$O$_5$ ha^{-1} applied without HA suggesting that P application dose could be reduced with HA (Figure 1B). Similarly, when averaged across the P levels, the HA application produced 6322 kg biological yield ha^{-1} on dry weight basis which was significantly higher than the plots which does not receive HA advocating the increasing role of P with HA. A remarkable percent increase of 6.2%, 5.2%, 7.9% and 5.4% in biological yield was observed with the addition of HA and P levels over the sole application of P levels.

Table 3. Effect of different levels of phosphorus and humic acid on post-harvest soil properties of wheat under field conditions of Peshawar, Pakistan.

P Levels (kg P$_2$O$_5$ ha^{-1})	Humic Acid Levels (kg ha^{-1})	OM (%)	Extractable P (mg kg^{-1})	WSP (mg kg^{-1})	Extractable K (mg kg^{-1})
0		0.83 ± 0.02 c	5.05 ± 0.06 e	0.139 ± 0.01 e	86 ± 0.58 e
45		1.00 ± 0.01 b	5.93 ± 0.07 d	0.155 ± 0.02 d	97 ± 0.88 d
67.5		1.04 ± 0.05 b	6.88 ± 0.15 c	0.185 ± 0.01 c	107 ± 1.01 c
90		1.13 ± 0.02 a	7.78 ± 0.12 b	0.206 ± 0.01 b	121 ± 0.51 b
112.5		1.16 ± 0.04 a	8.68 ± 0.10 a	0.232 ± 0.01 a	134 ± 0.84 a
LSD ($p \leq 0.05$)		0.063	0.121	0.016	2.461
	0	0.95 ± 0.02 b	6.12 ± 0.12 b	0.165 ± 0.01 b	102 ± 0.19 b
	5	1.11 ± 0.03 a	7.61 ± 0.08 a	0.201 ± 0.02 a	116 ± 1.01 a
LSD ($p \leq 0.05$)		0.040	0.076	0.015	1.556
0	0	0.83 ± 0.03 f	4.20 ± 0.06 j	0.135 ± 0.01 f	81 ± 1.45 h
	5	0.82 ± 0.02 f	5.90 ± 0.06 h	0.144 ± 0.01 ef	91 ± 1.47 g
45	0	0.89 ± 0.04 ef	5.07 ± 0.09 i	0.144 ± 0.01 ef	90 ± 0.88 g
	5	1.11 ± 0.03 cd	6.80 ± 0.07 f	0.165 ± 0.02 de	103 ± 0.91 e
67.5	0	0.93 ± 0.06 e	6.05 ± 0.21 g	0.171 ± 0.01 d	98 ± 1.01 f
	5	1.15 ± 0.04 bc	7.67 ± 0.09 d	0.198 ± 0.01 c	116 ± 1.73 c
90	0	1.04 ± 0.01 d	7.10 ± 0.15 e	0.180 ± 0.02 cd	112 ± 1.45 d
	5	1.22 ± 0.04 ab	8.47 ± 0.12 b	0.233 ± 0.01 b	130 ± 0.89 b
112.5	0	1.08 ± 0.03 cd	8.13 ± 0.12 c	0.198 ± 0.01 c	127 ± 1.20 b
	5	1.24 ± 0.04 a	9.23 ± 0.09 a	0.266 ± 0.03 a	141 ± 0.58 a
LSD ($p \leq 0.05$)		0.0886	0.171	0.222	3.480

The mean while tanders Means with same letters are not significantly different from each other. OM and WSP stand for organic matter and water soluble P respectively. The ± values represent stander error of the mean ($n = 3$).

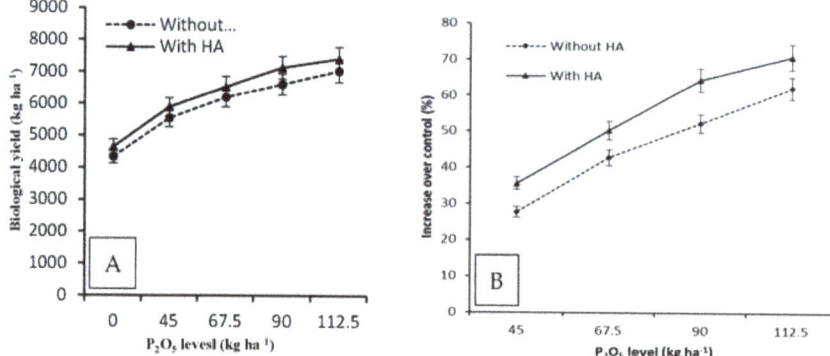

Figure 1. Comparative increase in biological yield of wheat after the application of SSP with and without HA; observed values (**A**) and increase over control (**B**).

3.8. Harvest Index (%)

Application of different P levels significantly affect the harvest index of wheat crop, where the HA addition and interaction of P levels and HA non-significantly affect the harvest index of wheat plants (Table 2). When averaged across the HA levels, maximum harvest index of 43% was observed in the plots that received 90 kg P_2O_5 ha^{-1}, whereas lowest harvest index of 36% was noted in plots that receive 112.5 kg P_2O_5 ha^{-1} in the form of SSP.

3.9. Plant Phosphorus Concentration (g kg^{-1})

Both P levels and HA showed significant effects and increased plant phosphorous concentration (Table 2). The application of 112.5 kg P_2O_5 ha^{-1} enhanced the plant shoots [P] in leaves with a value of 3.3 g kg^{-1} which was statistically higher than other treatments. On average maximum plant [P] of 3.1 g kg^{-1} was observed in the plots applied with 5 kg HA ha^{-1} which was statistically higher than 2.9 g kg^{-1} observed in plots that receive no HA. The interactive effect of P levels with HA was non-significant with maximum P concentration of 3.4 g kg^{-1} in plots where 112.5 kg P_2O_5 ha^{-1} was used with HA, while the minimum of 2.5 g kg^{-1} was noted in control plots.

3.10. Phosphorous Uptake by the Plant (kg ha^{-1})

Regarding the P-uptake of wheat plants, the addition of different levels of SSP with HA showed superior results over sole SSP application (Table 2). When averaged across the HA, maximum P uptake of 24.30 kg ha^{-1} was noted in plots that were treated with 112.5 kg P_2O_5 ha^{-1}, followed by 21.41 kg ha^{-1} in plots received 90 kg P_2O_5 ha^{-1}, whereas, the minimum was noted in control plots. When averaged across P levels, the maximum P uptake of 19.97 kg ha^{-1} which was 13% higher than uptake in plots treated without HA (Figure 2A). Regarding different P levels, addition of HA increases the P uptake from 10.3 to 21.2% as compared to plots where P levels were applied without HA. The interaction of P levels and HA was non-significant with the maximum uptake of 25.50 kg ha^{-1} observed with 112.5 kg P_2O_5 ha^{-1} applied with HA. The total uptake of P at 90 kg P_2O_5 ha^{-1} applied with HA (23.33 kg ha^{-1}) was similar to uptake of 23.10 kg ha^{-1} at 112.5 kg P_2O_5 ha^{-1} without HA suggesting the increase in P use efficiency and reduction in P requirements for optimum crop growth and yield. Similarly, the percent increase over control with HA-SSP at 67.5 kg ha^{-1} was 90.5% that was more than the percent increase over control at 90 kg SSP alone (75.4%) confirming the fact that P use efficiency increased with HA application (Figure 2B).

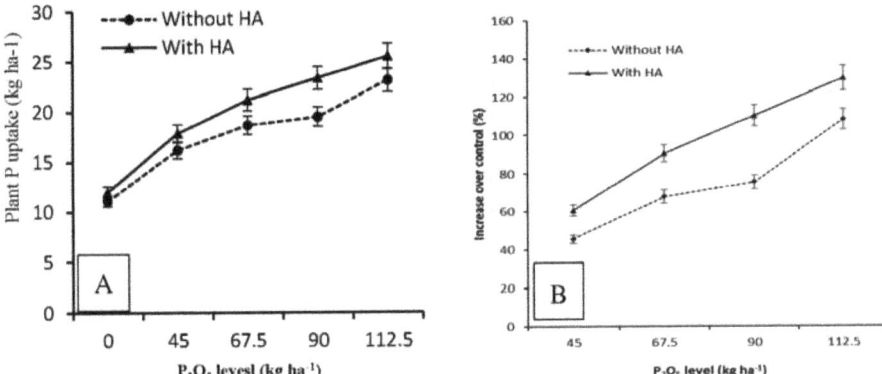

Figure 2. Comparative increases in plant P uptake after the application of SSP with and without HA; observed values (**A**) and Increase over control (**B**).

3.11. Soil Organic Matter

Soil organic matter (SOM) content was significantly affected by P levels, HA and their interaction. Treatments receiving SSP and HA had significantly ($p \leq 0.05$) higher organic matter than sole SSP levels at each increment of P levels from 45 to 112.50 kg P_2O_5 ha^{-1} (Table 3). When averaged across P levels, the HA had 1.11% organic matter which was significantly higher than 0.95% calculated for plots received no HA. Similarly, when averaged across the HA, the maximum soil organic matter contents of 1.16% was observed in plots treated with higher doses of SSP of 112.5 kg P_2O_5 ha^{-1} that was statistically identical to 1.13% observed in the plots treated with 90 kg P_2O_5 ha^{-1} but higher than other treatments and control. The interactive effect of HA and SSP was significant with the highest organic matter contents of 1.24% in plots treated with 112.5 kg P_2O_5 ha^{-1} and HA, and the lowest of 0.82% was noted in control. It was evident from the interaction (HA*P) that SOM increased with the application of HA regardless of P rate except in control and plots treated with 45 kg P_2O_5 ha^{-1} where SOM content was similar for with and without HA treated plots. The organic matter content observed for 112.50 kg P_2O_5 ha^{-1} without HA was at par to 67.5 kg P_2O_5 ha^{-1} with HA which were significantly lower than plots amended with 90 kg P_2O_5 ha^{-1} with HA. Similarly, OM observed at 45 kg P_2O_5 ha^{-1} with HA was statistically similar to that observed for 67.5 kg P_2O_5 ha^{-1} without HA. These finding suggested that, HA application can preserved soil organic matter content when applied with SSP.

3.12. AB-DTPA Extractable Phosphorus

Results showed that treatments receiving HA + SSP had significantly ($p \leq 0.05$) more soil AB-DTPA extractable P than SSP alone at each increment of P levels from 45 to 112.50 kg P_2O_5 ha^{-1} (Table 3). When averaged across the P levels, HA-SSP produced 7.61 mg P kg^{-1} which was significantly higher than 6.12 mg P kg^{-1} observed in no HA plots. Addition the SSP with HA increased the post-harvest soil AB-DTPA P over alone SSP levels with a mean value of 24.3%. Similarly, when averaged across the fertilizer HA, the AB-DTPA extractable P increased with each increment of P. The mean maximum AB-DTPA ext. P of 8.68 mg kg^{-1} was recorded in treatments applied with 112.5 kg P_2O_5 ha^{-1} that was statistically higher than the phosphorous content of other treatments. The minimum AB-DTPA ext. P with a value of 5.05 mg kg^{-1} was observed in control. The interactive effect of SSP and HA was also significant showing increases with an increase in P levels. The maximum AB-DTPA ext. P of 9.23 mg kg^{-1} was recorded in plots receiving 120 kg P_2O_5 ha^{-1} as HA + SSP while the minimum of (4.20 mg kg^{-1}) was recorded in control.

3.13. Water-Soluble phosphorus

Analysis of variance (ANOVA) revealed that P levels, humic acid and their interaction significantly affected soil water soluble P. Water-soluble phosphorus significantly ($p \leq 0.05$) increased with HA and P levels (Table 3). HA treated plots, when averaged across P levels, maintained higher water-soluble P of (0.201 mg kg^{-1}) than plots receiving no HA which had 0.165 mg kg^{-1} water-soluble P, on an average basis. The percent increase in water-soluble phosphorous with HA+SSP levels over respective sole P levels ranged from 6.7% in control to 34.3% in treatments receiving 112.5 kg P$_2$O$_5$ ha^{-1} suggesting higher release from HA+SSP than commercially available SSP. The interactive effect of HA and SSP was significant with maximum water-soluble P of (0.266 mg kg^{-1}) observed in 112.5 kg P$_2$O$_5$ ha^{-1} as HA-SSP while a minimum of (0.135 mg kg^{-1}) was recorded in control. The significant interaction of HA*P demonstrated that, WSP increased with increasing P level, however, this increase was more in plot treated with 5 ton HA ha^{-1} compared to control HA at respective P levels. Furthermore, with respect to WSP the response of 45 kg P$_2$O$_5$ ha^{-1} with HA was significantly better than 67.5 kg P$_2$O$_5$ ha^{-1} without HA and the performance of 67.5 kg P$_2$O$_5$ ha^{-1} with HA was at par to 90 kg P$_2$O$_5$ ha^{-1} without HA. It was also evident that 90 and 112.5 kg P$_2$O$_5$ ha^{-1} with HA performed similar which was significantly superior than 112.5 kg P$_2$O$_5$ ha^{-1} without HA. Thus, it can be deduced that, HA enhances P availability in soil amended with P as chemical fertilizers.

4. Discussion

Application of P levels with humic acid (HA) produced significantly taller wheat plants than sole P application at each increment of P levels from 45 to 112.50 kg P$_2$O$_5$ ha^{-1}, whereas the interactive effect of P and HA was also significant. The increase over control with 67.5 kg P$_2$O$_5$ kg ha^{-1} and HA was 10.4% which was close to 11.7% increases observed with the application of 90 kg P$_2$O$_5$ ha^{-1} alone indicating that P application dose could be reduced with HA. Such differential increases revealed that P use efficiency was increased with HA over sole application of P as commercial SSP fertilizer and as such could reduce the farmer input cost without compromise on yield and crop productivity. These results revealed that the linear increase in plant height could be achieved with P increased levels and HA applications. Ahmad et al. [26] also suggested that plant height can be increased with a higher P rate application. Khattak and Dost [41] also reported the increase in plant height with HA which has suggested that the application of HA with different fertilizers may cause beneficial effects on plant growth and nutrients uptake. This could be associated with the capability of HA to improve the biochemical environment of soil by promoting soil enzymatic activities, microbial activities and population, cation exchange capacity and water retention of soil that ultimately enhance the plant growth and nutrients uptake. These results were also in accordance with Tahir et al. [42] who reported that the application of HA significantly improved the plant height. The application HA with SSP improved the quality of wheat produced as indicated by grain size and weight. Combine application of SSP and HA produced higher 1000-grain weight than SSP alone at each P level, while their interaction remained non-significant at $p \leq 0.05$. These results advocated the role of P in increasing the size and quality of seed in the present study. These results were similar to the study of Kaleem et al. [9] who reported that maximum phosphorus dose enhanced the number of grains spike^{-1}, tillers number, thousand-grain weights and grain yield due to the highest accumulation of photosynthates in the plants and increased grain ripening which resulted in heavier grains. The results were also in close consistency with the findings of Ibrahim et al. [43] who stated that wheat 1000 grains weight could be increased significantly with the combined application of chemical and organic fertilizers. Wheat spike length and grains per spike showed almost similar trend and an increase was observed with increasing P and HA levels. Addition of HA with all P levels showed increased spike length except 112.5 kg P$_2$O$_5$ ha^{-1} which showed a decrease of 1.11%. This negative increase may be associated with the imbalance in plant nutrients caused by increased concentration of phosphorus. It is an established fact that higher doses of one nutrient can have detrimental effect on the absorption of others and as such reduce the crop performances. The results also depicted that balance ratio of P fertilizers is essential to obtain higher yield of wheat against the common farmer's practice in the area who do not bother to keep in mind the balance of different fertilizers at the time of sowing [9]. These improvements revealed that application of P with HA improved the storage of photosynthates in the plants. This accumulation of photosynthates in plants enhances the enzymatic, microbial and catalytic activities in plants and thus produces higher grains spike^{-1}, grain yield, straw yield and biomass as well [9]. Results regarding the grain yield showed that the percent increases of 41.7% with HA and 67.5 kg P_2O_5 ha^{-1} is closely resembled to 40.9 and 51% obtained with SSP alone at 90 and 112.5 kg P_2O_5 ha^{-1}, respectively, revealing a reduction in P requirements and increase in P fertilizer use efficiency with the addition of HA. A similar effect was noted by Khattak and Dost [41] who stated that the combined use of fertilizers and HA could increase the yield of different crops and reduce the crop fertilizer requirements without compromise on yields and quality. The substantial increase in wheat yield over control with SSP and HA suggested its potential use as an effective P fertilizer. The increase in grain yields with P levels is a well-established fact in P deficient soils. The HA would have increased the P availability by making its soluble complexes and stimulating plant growth [24] as well as by providing a good physicochemical and biological environment of the soils to the plants [21]. Proliferation of rhizobacteria also played an imperative role in better uptake of phosphorus when applied in the presence of organic carbon [44–47]. Improvement in straw and biological yield revealed that a significant increase in straw and biological yield could be obtained by the application of phosphorus and HA [27]. The increase in growth parameter and yield may be related with the stimulating effect of P and HA on plant growth by the assimilation of major and minor elements, enzyme activation and/or inhibition, changes in membrane permeability, protein synthesis that ultimately enhances the biomass or biological production [48,49]. The results were also in consistence with Sarir et al. [50] and Sharif et al. [51] who reviewed that HA application can improve biological yield up to a prominent level. Data regarding the P concentration in plant shoots suggested that the application of SSP with HA increased the plant P concentration as 3.5, 10.4, 6.9 and 6.3% with 45, 67.5, 90 and 112.5 kg P_2O_5, respectively, over the same levels of SSP alone indicating that HA increased the P use efficiency and uptake of plants. The results of the study were similar to the study of Khattak and Dost [41] who reported that HA increased the plant growth and nutrients uptake capability through the improvement of soil enzymatic system and microbial activities and population ultimately making the soil conditions favourable for plant uptake. The results of the study can also be supported by the results of Majumdar et al. [52] who stated that the application of rock phosphate mixed with different organic manures could increase P concentration in plants significantly. The higher P concentration in plant leaves with the application of HA along with SSP was in line with the study of Cooper et al. [53] and Atiyeh et al. [54]. They stated that the addition of HA in the soils enhanced the root growth as well as the proliferation, branching, and initiation of root hairs and thus able the roots towards more nutrient capturing and increase nutrient concentrations in the plants. A lot of studies showed an increase in root length, root number and root branching with the application of HA. However, the increase in root growth is generally more noticeable than shoot growth [55]. Pettit [56] also reported a prominent increase of root initiation and increased root growth with the application humic and fulvic acids to the soil ultimately increasing the nutrient concentrations in plant tissues. The uptake of P indicated that the observed increases in wheat growth and yield with SSP levels and HA in the present study. The increase in P uptake with increasing P levels is an accepted fact [57] and the additional advantage with HA is in consistence with the findings of Erdal et al. [55] who stated a prominent accumulation of nutrients in the plant with the application of organic materials along with mixing of inorganic fertilizers. These results can also be supported by Sharif et al. [51] who reported that P and N uptake could be increased with the addition of P fertilizers (SSP) along with organic materials. The results regarded the soil organic matter contents indicated that both SSP and HA could improve the soil organic matter content. The improvement in the organic matter could be attributed to higher biomass and bumper root growth and as such more leftover fraction as also indicated by close resemblance between plant biomass and soil organic matter. These results are in line with the findings of Sharif et al. [51] who reported that the use of inorganic fertilizers along with organic fertilizers (humic acid and FYM) increased soil organic matter content. Similar findings were reported by Tamayo et al. [58] and Han et al. [59], who stated an increase in soil organic carbon with the use of chemical fertilizer along with the organic. The data regarding the AB-DTPA extractable P revealed that the increase over control with 67.5 kg P_2O_5 kg ha^{-1} and HA was 83% which was more than 70% increases observed with 90 kg P_2O_5 ha^{-1} applied alone suggesting that P application dose could be reduced with the HA. The results of the study are similar to the findings of [60] who reported that the application of HA to acidic and alkaline soil decreases the P complex formation and dissolves the insoluble and unavailable P thus enhance the availability of phosphorus to the plants. Similar results were reported by Sharif et al. [51] and Majumdar et al. [52] who stated that phosphorus concentration could be increased with the application of rock phosphate (RP) along with the mixing of different organic materials. An increase in water-soluble P is related to the accessibility of phosphorus added to the soil as well as with HA which decreases the P fixation and provides more water-soluble P for plants. These results were in uniformity with the findings of several researchers [26,61–65]. They reported that the supplementation of P from various P sources including rock phosphate and HA application increased the soil solution P whereas the high pH and lime contents in calcareous soils reduced it by making its insoluble complexes. Like other organic materials, the HA make soluble complexes with P and increase its concentration in the soil solution. However, plant and microbial exudates neutralized the rhizosphere by producing (H^+) as a result of cation uptake can increase the availability of P in the soil.

5. Conclusions

Application of P as SSP fertilizer and humic acid (HA) significantly improved wheat growth, yields, P uptake and post-harvest soil AB-DTPA extractable and water-soluble P contents. The interactive effect of P and HA were found significant for plant height, grain and biological yield and soil AB-DTPA extractable P and K. The significant superiority of SSP and HA over sole SSP at almost every application rate suggested improvement in P fertilizer use efficiency with HA. The grain yield obtained at 67.5 kg P_2O_5 ha^{-1} with HA was statistically comparable to 112.5 kg P_2O_5 ha^{-1} applied as commercial SSP suggested that the input expenditures of fertilizer may be reduced up to 50% by combine application of chemical fertilizers with HA. Similarly, HA with SSP maintained higher AB-DTPA extractable, water-soluble P, soil organic matter contents, plant P concentrations and P uptake over commercial SSP in the soil, which further signifies the importance of HA in enhancing P availability.

Author Contributions: Formal analysis, A.K.; Investigation, S.F.; Methodology, F.W.; Project administration, Z.Y.; Software, S.D. and R.D.; Supervision, Z.Y.; Validation, S.D.; M.Z.-u.-H.; and M.B.; Writing—original draft, M.A.; Writing—review & editing, M.I.S., S.F., M.B. and R.D. All authors have read and agreed to the published version of the manuscript.

Funding: "This work was supported by the 1. Program for "Shandong Provincial Natural Science Foundation of China (ZR2018BC012)". 2. Project of Technology Agency of the Czech Republic "TH02030169".

Acknowledgments: The authors would like to acknowledge the financial support of the Shandong Provincial Natural Science Foundation of China for this study.

Conflicts of Interest: The authors declare no conflict of interest.

References

1. MacCarthy, P.; Clapp, C.; Malcolm, R.; Bloom, P. Humic substances in soil and crop sciences: Selected readings. In Proceedings of the Symposium Cosponsored by the International Humic Substances Society, Chicago, IL, USA, 2 December 1985.
2. Magdoff, F.; Weil, R.R. *Soil Organic Matter in Sustainable Agriculture*; CRC Press: Boca Raton, FL, USA, 2004.
3. Kumar, S.; Lai, L.; Kumar, P.; Valentín Feliciano, Y.M.; Battaglia, M.L.; Hong, C.O.; Owens, V.N.; Fike, J.; Farris, R.; Galbraith, J. Impacts of Nitrogen Rate and Landscape Position on Soils and Switchgrass Root Growth Parameters. *Agron. J.* **2019**, *111*, 1046–1059. [CrossRef]

4. Kumar, P.; Lai, L.; Battaglia, M.L.; Kumar, S.; Owens, V.; Fike, J.; Galbraith, J.; Hong, C.O.; Farris, R.; Crawford, R.; et al. Impacts of nitrogen fertilization rate and landscape position on select soil properties in switchgrass field at four sites in the USA. *CATENA* **2019**, *180*, 183–193. [CrossRef]
5. Adnan, M.; Fahad, S.; Zamin, M.; Shah, S.; Mian, I.A.; Danish, S.; Zafar-Ul-hye, M.; Battaglia, M.L.; Naz, R.M.M.; Saeed, B.; et al. Coupling phosphate-solubilizing bacteria with phosphorus supplements improve maize phosphorus acquisition and growth under lime induced salinity stress. *Plants* **2020**, *9*, 900. [CrossRef] [PubMed]
6. Afif, E.; Matar, A.; Torrent, J. Availability of Phosphate Applied to Calcareous Soils of West Asia and North Africa. *Soil Sci. Soc. Am. J.* **1993**, *57*, 756–760. [CrossRef]
7. Ketterings, Q.; Czymmek, K. Removal of Phosphorus by Field Crops. *Agron. Fact Sheet* **2007**, *28*.
8. Alam, S. Wheat yield and P fertilizer efficiency as influenced by rate andintegrated use of chemical and organic fertilizers. *Pakistan J. Soil Sci.* **2003**, *22*, 72–76.
9. Kaleem, S.; Ansar, M.; Ali, M.A.; Sher, A.; Ahmad, G.; Rashid, M. Effect of Phosphorus on the Yield and Yield Components of Wheat Variety " Inqlab-91 " Under Rainfed Conditions. *Sarhad J. Agric.* **2009**, *25*, 1989–1992.
10. Molaei, A.; Lakzian, A.; Haghnia, G.; Astaraei, A.; Rasouli-Sadaghiani, M.; Teresa Ceccherini, M.; Datta, R. Assessment of some cultural experimental methods to study the effects of antibiotics on microbial activities in a soil: An incubation study. *PLoS ONE* **2017**, *12*, e0180663. [CrossRef]
11. Molaei, A.; Lakzian, A.; Datta, R.; Haghnia, G.; Astaraei, A.; Rasouli-Sadaghiani, M.; Ceccherini, M.T. Impact of chlortetracycline and sulfapyridine antibiotics on soil enzyme activities. *Int. Agrophysics* **2017**, *31*, 499. [CrossRef]
12. Meena, R.S.; Kumar, S.; Datta, R.; Lal, R.; Vijayakumar, V.; Brtnicky, M.; Sharma, M.P.; Yadav, G.S.; Jhariya, M.K.; Jangir, C.K. Impact of agrochemicals on soil microbiota and management: A review. *Land* **2020**, *9*, 34. [CrossRef]
13. Brtnicky, M.; Dokulilova, T.; Holatko, J.; Pecina, V.; Kintl, A.; Latal, O.; Vyhnanek, T.; Prichystalova, J. Datta, R. Long-Term Effects of Biochar-Based Organic Amendments on Soil Microbial Parameters. *Agronomy* **2019**, *9*, 747. [CrossRef]
14. Battaglia, M.; Groover, G.; Thomason, W. *Harvesting and Nutrient Replacement Costs Associated with Corn Stover Removal in Virginia*; Virginia Tech: Blacksburg, VA, USA, 2018.
15. Ibrikci, H.; Ryan, J.; Ulger, A.C.; Buyuk, G.; Cakir, B.; Korkmaz, K.; Karnez, E.; Ozgenturk, G.; Konuskan, O. Maintenance of phosphorus fertilizer and residual phosphorus effect on corn production. *Nutr. Cycl. Agroecosystems* **2005**, *72*, 279–286. [CrossRef]
16. Albayrak, S.; Camas, N. Effects of Different Levels and Application Times of Humic Acid on Root and Leaf Yield and Yield Components of Forage Turnip (Brassica rapa L.). *J. Agron.* **2005**, *4*, 130–133. [CrossRef]
17. Majidian, M.; Ghalavand, A.; Karimian, N.; Haghighi, A. Effects of water stress, nitrogen fertilizer and organic fertilizer in various farming systems in different growth stages on physiological characteristics, physical characteristics, quality and chlorophyll content of maize single cross hybrid 704. *Iran. Crop Sci. J.* **2006**, *10*, 303–330.
18. Stevenson, F.J. *Humus Chemistry: Genesis, Composition, Reactions*; John Wiley & Sons: Hoboken, NJ, USA, 1994; ISBN 0-471-59474-1.
19. Chen, Y.; Aviad, T. Effects of Humic Substances on Plant Growth. In *Humic Substances in Soil and Crop Sciences: Selected Readings*; Soil Science Society of America: Madison, WI, USA, 1990; pp. 161–186.
20. Jorquera, M.; Inostroza, N.; Lagos, L.; Barra, P.; Marileo, L.; Rilling, J.; Campos, D.; Crowley, D.; Richardson, A.; Mora, M.L. Bacterial community structure and detection of putative plant growth-promoting rhizobacteria associated with plants grown in Chilean agro-ecosystems and undisturbed ecosystems. *Biol. Fertil. Soils* **2014**, *50*, 1141–1153. [CrossRef]
21. Brannon, C.A.; Sommers, L.E. Preparation and characterization of model humic polymers containing organic phosphorus. *Soil Biol. Biochem.* **1985**, *17*, 213–219. [CrossRef]
22. Malik, K.A.; Bhatti, N.A.; Kauser, F. Effect of Soil Salinity on Decomposition and Humification of Organic Matter by Some Cellulolytic Fungi. *Mycologia* **1979**, *71*, 811. [CrossRef]
23. Canellas, L.P.; Olivares, F.L. Physiological responses to humic substances as plant growth promoter. *Chem. Biol. Technol. Agric.* **2014**, *1*, 3. [CrossRef]

24. Nardi, S.; Pizzeghello, D.; Gessa, C.; Ferrarese, L.; Trainotti, L.; Casadoro, G. A low molecular weight humic fraction on nitrate uptake and protein synthesis in maize seedlings. *Soil Biol. Biochem.* **2000**, *32*, 415–419. [CrossRef]
25. Francioso, O.; Sanchez-Cortes, S.; Tugnoli, V.; Ciavatta, C.; Sitti, L.; Gessa, C. Infrared, raman, and nuclear magnetic resonance (1H, 13C, and 31P) spectroscopy in the study of fractions of peat humic acids. *Appl. Spectrosc.* **1996**, *50*, 1165–1174. [CrossRef]
26. Ahmad, M.; Khan, M.J.; Muhammad, D. Response of maize to different phosphorus levels under calcareous soil conditions. *Sarhad J. Agric.* **2013**, *29*, 43–48.
27. Hai, S.; Mir, S. The lignitic coal derived humic acid and the prospective utilization in Pakistan's agriculture and industry. *Sci. Technol. Dev.* **1998**, *17*, 32–40.
28. Marfo, T.D.; Datta, R.; Pathan, S.I.; Vranová, V. Ecotone Dynamics and Stability from Soil Scientific Point of View. *Diversity* **2019**, *11*, 53. [CrossRef]
29. Danso Marfo, T.; Datta, R.; Vranová, V.; Ekielski, A. Ecotone Dynamics and Stability from Soil Perspective: Forest-Agriculture Land Transition. *Agriculture* **2019**, *9*, 228. [CrossRef]
30. Yadav, G.S.; Datta, R.; Imran Pathan, S.; Lal, R.; Meena, R.S.; Babu, S.; Das, A.; Bhowmik, S.N.; Datta, M.; Saha, P. Effects of conservation tillage and nutrient management practices on soil fertility and productivity of rice (*Oryza sativa* L.)–rice system in north eastern region of India. *Sustainability* **2017**, *9*, 1816. [CrossRef]
31. Weidhuner, A.; Afshar, R.K.; Luo, Y.; Battaglia, M.; Sadeghpour, A. Particle size affects nitrogen and carbon estimate of a wheat cover crop. *Agron. J.* **2019**, *111*, 3398–3402. [CrossRef]
32. Datta, R.; Vranová, V.; Pavelka, M.; Rejsek, K.; Formánek, P. Effect of soil sieving on respiration induced by low-molecular-weight substrates. *Int. Agrophysics* **2014**, *28*, 119–124. [CrossRef]
33. Rhoades, J.D. Salinity: Electrical Conductivity and Total Dissolved Solids. In *Methods of Soil Analysis, Part 3, Chemical Methods*; Sparks, D.L., Page, A.L., Helmke, P.A., Loeppert, R.H., Soltanpour, P.N., Tabatabai, M.A., Johnston, C.T., Sumner, M.E., Eds.; Soil Science Society of America: Madison, WI, USA, 1996; Volume 5, pp. 417–435.
34. Thomas, G.W. Soil pH and soil acidity. In *Methods of Soil Analysis, Part 3: Chemical Methods*; John Wiley & Sons: Madison, WI, USA, 1996; Volume 5, pp. 475–490.
35. Nelson, D.W.; Sommers, L.E. Total Carbon, Organic Carbon, and Organic Matter. In *Methods of Soil Analysis: Part 2 Chemical and Microbiological Properties*; Page, A.L., Ed.; American Society of Agronomy; Crop Science Society of America, and Soil Science Society of America: Madison, WI, USA, 1982; pp. 539–579.
36. Soltanpour, P.N.; Schwab, A.P. A new soil test for simultaneous extraction of macroand micro-nutrients in alkaline soils. *Commun. Soil Sci. Plant Anal.* **1977**, *8*, 195–207. [CrossRef]
37. Loeppert, R.H.; Suarez, D.L. Carbonate and Gypsum. In *Methods of Soil Analysis, Part 3, Chemical Methods*; Soil Science Society of America: Madison, WI, USA, 2018; Volume 9, pp. 181–197.
38. Gee, G.W.; Bauder, J.W. Particle-Size analysis. In *Methods of Soil Analysis: Part 1—Physical and Mineralogical Methods*; Klute, A., Ed.; Soil Science Society of America: Madison, WI, USA, 1986; pp. 383–411.
39. Jones, J.B.; WolfH, B.; Mills, H.A. *Plant Analysis Handbook: A Practical Sampling, Preparation, Analysis, and Interpretation Guide*; Micro-Macro Publishing Inc.: Athens, GA, USA, 1991.
40. Steel, R.G.; Torrie, J.H.; Dickey, D.A. *Principles and Procedures of Statistics: A Biometrical Approach*, 3rd ed.; McGraw Hill Book International Co.: Jurong West, Singapore, 1997.
41. Khattak, R.A.; Dost, M. Seed cotton yield and nutrient concentrations as influenced by lignitic coal derived humic acid in salt-affected soils. *Sarhad J. Agric.* **2010**, *26*, 43–49.
42. Tahir, M.; Khurshid, M.; Khan, M.; Abbasi, M.; Kazmi, M. Lignite-derived humic acid effect on growth of wheat plants in different soils. *Pedosphere* **2011**, *21*, 124–131. [CrossRef]
43. Ibrahim, M.; Hassan, A.U.; Iqbal, M.; Valeem, E.E. Response of wheat growth and yield to various levels of compost and organic manure. *Pakistan J. Bot.* **2008**, *40*, 2135–2141.
44. Danish, S.; Younis, U.; Akhtar, N.; Ameer, A.; Ijaz, M.; Nasreen, S.; Huma, F.; Sharif, S.; Ehsanullah, M. Phosphorus solubilizing bacteria and rice straw biochar consequence on maize pigments synthesis. *Int. J. Biosci.* **2015**, *5*, 31–39. [CrossRef]
45. Zafar-ul-Hye, M.; Danish, S.; Abbas, M.; Ahmad, M.; Munir, T.M. ACC deaminase producing PGPR *Bacillus amyloliquefaciens* and *Agrobacterium fabrum* along with biochar improve wheat productivity under drought stress. *Agronomy* **2019**, *9*, 343. [CrossRef]

46. Danish, S.; Zafar-ul-Hye, M.; Mohsin, F.; Hussain, M. ACC-deaminase producing plant growth promoting rhizobacteria and biochar mitigate adverse effects of drought stress on maize growth. *PLoS ONE* **2020**, *15*, e0230615. [CrossRef]
47. Danish, S.; Zafar-ul-Hye, M. Co-application of ACC-deaminase producing PGPR and timber-waste biochar improves pigments formation, growth and yield of wheat under drought stress. *Sci. Rep.* **2019**, *9*, 5999. [CrossRef]
48. Datta, R.; Anand, S.; Moulick, A.; Baraniya, D.; Pathan, S.I.; Rejsek, K.; Vranova, V.; Sharma, M.; Sharma, D.; Kelkar, A. How enzymes are adsorbed on soil solid phase and factors limiting its activity: A Review. *Int. Agrophysics* **2017**, *31*, 287. [CrossRef]
49. Datta, R.; Kelkar, A.; Baraniya, D.; Molaei, A.; Moulick, A.; Meena, R.S.; Formanek, P. Enzymatic degradation of lignin in soil: A review. *Sustainability* **2017**, *9*, 1163. [CrossRef]
50. Sarir, M.; Akhlaq, M.; Zeb, A.; Sharif, M. Comparison of various organic manures with or without chemicalfertilizers on the yield and components of maize. *Sarhad J. Agric.* **2005**, *21*, 237–245.
51. Sharif, M.; Burni, T.; Wahid, F.; Khan, F.; Khan, S.; Khan, A.; Shah, A. Effect of rock phosphate composted with organic materials on yield and phosphorus uptake of wheat and mung bean crops. *Pak. J. Bot.* **2013**, *45*, 1349–1356.
52. Majumdar, B.; Venkatesh, M.; Kumar, K. Effect of rock phosphate, superphosphate and their mixtures with FYM on soybean and soil-P pools in a typic hapludalf of Meghalaya. *J. Indian Soc. Soil Sci.* **2007**, *55*, 167–174.
53. Cooper, R.J.; Liu, C.; Fisher, D.S. Influence of humic substances on rooting and nutrient content of creeping bentgrass. *Crop Sci.* **1998**, *38*, 1639–1644. [CrossRef]
54. Atiyeh, R.M.; Lee, S.; Edwards, C.A.; Arancon, N.Q.; Metzger, J.D. The influence of humic acids derived from earthworm-processed organic wastes on plant growth. *Bioresour. Technol.* **2002**, *84*, 7–14. [CrossRef]
55. Erdal, İ.; Bozkurt, M.A.; Çimrin, K.M.; Karaca, S.; Sağlam, M. Effects of Humic Acid and Phosphorus Applications on Growth and Phosphorus Uptake of Corn Plant (*Zea mays* L.) Grown in a Calcareous Soil. *Turkish J. Agric. For.* **2000**, *24*, 663–668.
56. Pettit, R.E. Organic matter, humus, humate, humic acid, fulvic acid and humin: Their importance in soil fertility and plant health. *CTI Res.* **2004**, 1–17.
57. Jiang, Z.Q.; C.N., F.; Huang, L.L.; Guo, W.S.; Zhu, X.K.; Peng, Y.X. Effects of phosphorus application on dry matter production and phosphorus uptake in wheat (*Triticum aestivum* L.). *Plant Nutr. Fertil. Sci.* **2006**, *12*, 32–38.
58. Tamayo, V.; Munoz, A.; Diaz, A. Organic fertilizer application to maize on alluvial soils in a moderate climate. *Actual. Corpoica* **1997**, *108*, 19–249.
59. Han, X.; Wang, S.; Veneman, P.L.M.; Xing, B. Change of organic carbon content and its fractions in black soil under long-term application of chemical fertilizers and recycled organic manure. *Commun. Soil Sci. Plant Anal.* **2006**, *37*, 1127–1137. [CrossRef]
60. Ulukan, H. Effect of soil applied humic acid at different sowing times on some yield components in wheat (Triticum spp.) hybrids. *Int. J. Bot.* **2008**, *4*, 164–175. [CrossRef]
61. Kaya, C.; Akram, N.A.; Ashraf, M.; Sonmez, O. Exogenous application of humic acid mitigates salinity stress in maize (*Zea mays* L.) plants by improving some key physico-biochemical attributes. *Cereal Res. Commun.* **2018**, *46*, 67–78. [CrossRef]
62. Sonmez, O.; Pierzynski, G.M.; Frees, L.; Davis, B.; Leikam, D.F.; Sweeney, D.W.; Janssen, K.A. A field-based assessment tool for phosphorus losses in runoff in Kansas. *J. Soil Water Conserv.* **2009**, *64*, 212–222. [CrossRef]
63. Naseer, M.; Muhammad, D. Direct and residual effect of Hazara rock phosphate (HRP) on wheat and succeeding maize in alkaline calcareous soils. *Pak. J. Bot.* **2014**, *46*, 1755–1761.
64. Liu, C.; Cooper, R.J.; Bowman, D.C. Humic acid application affects photosynthesis, root development, and nutrient content of creeping bentgrass. *HortScience* **1998**, *33*, 1023–1025. [CrossRef]
65. Malik, K.A.; Azam, F. Effect of humic acid on wheat (Triticum aestivum L.) seedling growth. *Env. Exp Bot.* **1985**, *25*, 245–252. [CrossRef]

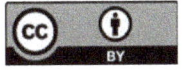

© 2020 by the authors. Licensee MDPI, Basel, Switzerland. This article is an open access article distributed under the terms and conditions of the Creative Commons Attribution (CC BY) license (http://creativecommons.org/licenses/by/4.0/).

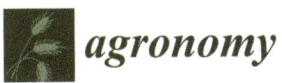

Article

Solubility and Efficiency of Rock Phosphate Fertilizers Partially Acidulated with Zeolite and Pillared Clay as Additives

Ana Paula Bettoni Teles, Marcos Rodrigues and Paulo Sergio Pavinato *

College of Agriculture Luiz de Queiroz—ESALQ-USP, Av. Pádua Dias, 11, Piracicaba-SP 13418-900, Brazil; ana.bettoni@usp.br (A.P.B.T.); rodrigues.m@alumni.usp.br (M.R.)
* Correspondence: pavinato@usp.br; Tel.: +55-19-3417-2136

Received: 24 April 2020; Accepted: 24 June 2020; Published: 27 June 2020

Abstract: Soluble phosphates are the most common sources currently used in crop production in tropical soils; however, they present low efficiency and are more expensive than natural rock phosphates. The objective was to develop new phosphate fertilizers with slow solubility through the partial acidification of rock phosphates (RPs), incorporating materials with adsorption characteristics to favor slow dissolution and prevent phosphorus (P) fixation in the soil. Three rock phosphates, Araxá (ARP), Bayovar (BRP) and Morocco (MRP), were evaluated at two acidulation levels (25 and 50% Ac.) and two additives; pillared clays (PILC) and zeolites (Zeo), plus triple superphosphate (TSP) and a control (nil-P). The soil diffusion was evaluated in concentric rings in Petri dishes. Solubility was evaluated in leaching columns and sampled in layers from surface for P forms in the soil profile. The relative agronomic efficiency (RAE) was evaluated in maize. Greater diffusion was provided by TSP, followed by BRP and MRP both with 50% Ac. + Zeo, and MRP with 50% Ac. + PILC. Percolated P was more pronounced under TSP, followed by RPs (BRP and MRP) with 50% Ac. + Zeo. BRP and MRP + 50% Ac. were the most promising sources with RAE above 74% compared to TSP.

Keywords: phosphorus sources; P solubilization; P acidulation; relative agronomic efficiency

1. Introduction

Phosphorus (P) plays an important role in plant metabolism, since it is involved in processes such as cell energy transfer, respiration and photosynthesis [1], making it an essential and irreplaceable element. Plants absorb P from the soil solution as phosphate ions, mainly $H_2PO_4^-$ [2]. However, soils usually have low levels of plant-available P, especially in tropical regions. This is a result of adsorption and precipitation reactions, and its high affinity with soil constituents [3]. Given this limited P availability, agricultural production is highly dependent on the use of fertilizers.

Phosphate fertilizers are produced from rock phosphate (RP), a natural non-renewable resource. About 80% of the RP mined annually is used for fertilizer production and, considering the current level of consumption, it is expected that reserves will vanish in three centuries time [2,4]. The possibility of exhaustion of this resource may compromise global food production [5]. The most used phosphate sources in agriculture are those that are highly water soluble, with fast dissolution in the soil which favors precipitation and adsorption. Approximately three days after the application of these sources in the soil, a large part of their P (more than half in some cases) is transformed into non-labile forms [6,7], substantially reducing their efficiency when applied to crops. Therefore, the future availability of P depends on the development of new technologies or soil management practices to improve its efficiency.

Considering this reference to the motivation to improve P efficiency, partial acidulation of RP is a technological development already in existence [8] that can be of help. In the processing of partially acidulated phosphates, a small amount of sulfuric or phosphoric acid reacts with RP in order to breakdown part of the hydroxyapatite (insoluble P) into monocalcium phosphate (soluble P), and thereby obtain a fast dissolution product [9]. Moreover, the incorporation of minerals with high phosphate adsorption capacity and/or high cation exchange capacity (CEC), such as pillared clays (PILC) and zeolites, into partially acidulated phosphates shows promise to improve agronomic efficiency [10,11]. The premise is that the initial P release will saturate the acidic sites of the PILC before adsorption, which act as a vehicle for slow and gradual dissolution into soil solution. Furthermore, when calcium (Ca) from RP is released after dissolution, it can be held by negative charges of the PILC or zeolites, favoring the solubilization of acid-unreacted RP, which also prevents Ca-P retrogradation [10,11].

Thus, we hypothesized herein that new phosphate fertilizers with slower and more synchronized solubility according to plant demand are more efficient than completely acidulated commercial sources. This study aimed to develop new crop efficient sources of phosphate fertilizers with gradual solubility using partial acidulation (25 and 50% of total solubilization) in the following distinct rock phosphates—Araxá (ARP), Bayovar (BRP) and Morocco (MRP)—and also adding high reactivity minerals such as pillared clay (PILC) and zeolites (Zeo), thus enabling the evaluation of the potential pH change in the soil, soil P diffusion; P solubilization and P agronomic efficiency.

2. Materials and Methods

2.1. Phosphate Rocks and Additives

Two high-reactivity sources of RP (Bayovar from Peru and BG4 from Morocco) and one low-reactivity source (Araxá from Brazil) were used as raw material for the production of partially acidulated phosphate fertilizers. Their chemical parameters and composition and total P_2O_5, 2% citric acid soluble P (P_{CA} 2%) and water soluble concentrations of each RP are presented in Table 1. Additionally, zeolites and pillared clay (PILC) were used as additives in the phosphate fertilizers for improving the dissolution, also characterized in Table 1.

Table 1. Chemical characteristics of the rock phosphates (RPs) used and total chemical composition by X-ray fluorescence, cation exchange capacity (CEC) and maximum P adsorption capacity (MPAC) of pillared clays and zeolites.

Rock Phosphate				Phosphorus (P_2O_5)					
		Total		P_{CA} 2% (1:100; w/v)				H_2O	
				%					
Araxá (ARP)		29.9		5.7				0.03	
Bayovar (BRP)		28.9		14.8				0.02	
Morocco (MRP)		30.0		9.0				0.08	
Additives	SiO_2	Al_2O_3	K_2O	Fe_2O_3	MgO	TiO_2	Na_2O	CEC	MPAC [3]
				%				$mmol_c\ kg^{-1}$	$mg\ kg^{-1}$
Pillared clay	35.7	23.7	0.2	6.6	4.0	0.5	0.04	676 [1]	5527
Zeolite	51.3	14.6	1.5	1.9	3.3	0.2	0.9	1450 [2]	31

[1] Determined according to the USDA-NRCS [12]; [2] determined according to Farkaš et al. [13]; [3] determined according to Alvarez et al. [14].

Natural zeolite, a mineral composed of intertwined tetrahedra, was obtained from Slovakia, provided by the Celta Brazil company. The zeolites were ground and passed through a 60 mesh sieve to increase the specific surface area. The clays used for pillarization came from a natural rock rich in montmorillonite (bentonite), supplied by Bentonit União Nordeste S.A., commercially known as Brasgel. For the pillarization process, the bentonite was finely milled, fractionated and purified in order to eliminate its coarser fractions and decrease its impurities. Purification of the material was carried out by removing iron oxides following the dithionite-citrate-bicarbonate method [15]. Next, the material was dispersed with Na_2CO_3 0.1 g L^{-1} solution with continuous stirring for approximately 12 h and fractionated by sedimentation to obtain the clay fraction (<2 µm).

The purified clay was pillared based on the methodology described by Narayanan and Deshpande [16]. The pillaring solution was obtained by using constant dripping of 0.4 mol L^{-1} NaOH in a solution of 0.2 mol L^{-1} $AlCl_3 \cdot 6H_2O$ under constant stirring at room temperature. At the end of the drip, the solution remained under stirring for a period of 15 h, with the first two hours at a temperature of 60 °C and the remaining time at room temperature (25 °C). For clay intercalation, the pillaring solution was then dripped at a maximum rate of 5 mL min^{-1} in a clay suspension of 1% (w/w), under vigorous stirring. After this, the material was continuously stirred for a period of 20 h. The resulting product was washed with deionized water to remove all free chlorine, oven dried at 60 °C and calcinated at 350 °C. In order to confirm pillarization, the final product was submitted to X-ray diffractometry (XRD), in a Miniflex II Desktop X-Ray Diffractometer Rigaku apparatus, with CuKα radiation, using the powder blade method. When saturated with sodium, the natural clay had a basal spacing of 1.4 nm. After the intercalation of aluminum polyhidroxication (pillarization) and calcination at 350 °C, it was observed that the clay reached a basal space of 1.8 nm, evidencing that the pillarization had been effective (Figure 1).

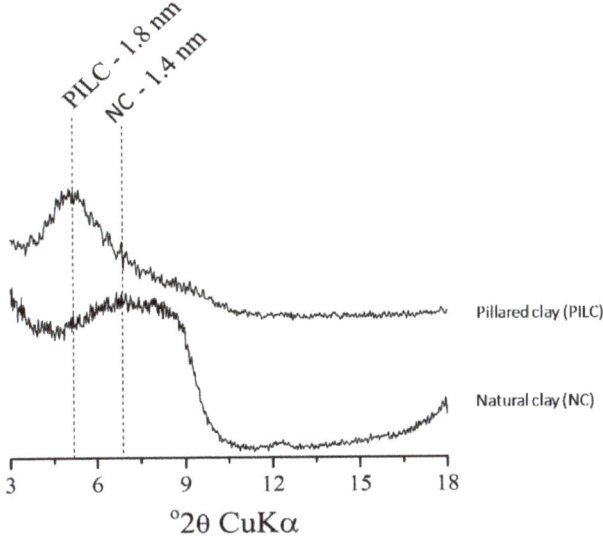

Figure 1. X-ray diffractograms of natural clay and pillared clay after calcination at 350 °C.

2.2. Fertilizer Production

Both minerals, PILC and zeolites, were mixed with each RP in a proportion of 9% of the final volume, followed by partial acidification with sulfuric acid corresponding to 25 and 50% of the proportional commercial acidulation of soluble phosphates, such as simple superphosphate. The resulting mixture was cured for seven days, then oven dried, ground and passed through a 60 mesh sieve and granulated in a wet dish granulator, which consisted of the application of a dextrin-based binder solution (10% w/v) to the dry blend to obtain the granules. The final products were oven dried at 45 °C until reaching a constant weight and then standardized into granules of 2–3 mm diameter.

2.3. Chemical Analysis

Twelve new products were obtained with the combinations mentioned above, which were characterized in terms of total P_2O_5 extracted with concentrated nitric acid + hydrochloric acid, and P_2O_5 soluble in water (H_2O), soluble in neutral ammonium citrate + water (NAC + H_2O) and soluble in 2% citric acid (P_{CA}), according to the methodologies of the Brazilian Ministry of Agriculture, Livestock and Supply [17] (Table 2).

Table 2. Characterization for the total P_2O_5, water soluble, neutral ammonium citrate + water (NAC + H_2O) and 2% citric acid (P_{CA} 2%) soluble P of phosphate fertilizers partially acidulated plus the additives pillared clay (PILC) and zeolite (Zeo).

Fertilizers	Treatment	Phosphorus Level (P_2O_5)			
		Total	H_2O	NAC + H_2O	P_{CA} 2%
		%			
ARP + PILC + 50% acidulation	1	20.1	2.6	7.6	5.5
ARP + PILC + 25% acidulation	2	23.3	1.4	5.0	4.7
ARP + Zeo + 50% acidulation	3	20.3	2.1	9.2	5.6
ARP + Zeo + 25% acidulation	4	23.5	1.4	5.0	4.8
BRP + PILC + 50% acidulation	5	21.7	3.3	6.9	8.1
BRP + PILC + 25% acidulation	6	23.6	1.3	4.6	8.4
BRP + Zeo + 50% acidulation	7	21.2	6.3	8.0	11.0
BRP + Zeo + 25% acidulation	8	23.7	1.7	3.9	6.2
MRP + PILC + 50% acidulation	9	21.6	3.6	6.4	8.9
MRP + PILC + 25% acidulation	10	23.7	1.1	3.6	7.8
MRP + Zeo + 50% acidulation	11	22.0	6.1	6.1	9.6
MRP + Zeo + 25% acidulation	12	24.0	2.2	3.2	7.4

ARP = Araxá rock phosphate; BRP = Bayovar rock phosphate; MRP = Morocco rock phosphate.

2.4. X-Ray Diffraction Analysis

All the final products (phosphate fertilizers) were characterized in terms of the mineralogical composition and structural changes that occurred in the RPs after acidification by means of X-ray diffraction (XRD). For this purpose, the powder blade method was used and the diffractograms were generated using the Miniflex II Desktop X-Ray Diffractometer Rigaku, with CuKα radiation, with an analysis interval of 5° to 60° 2θ.

2.5. Phosphorus Diffusion in Petri Dishes

Phosphorus diffusion from fertilizer granules was evaluated in plastic Petri dishes (8.6 cm in diameter and 1.1 cm tall) containing 78 g of dry soil with four replications, following a methodology described by Degryse and McLaughlin (2014) [18]. The soil was a loamy sand Hapludox [19] or Latossolo Vermelho Amarelo distrófico according to the Brazilian classification system [20]. In order to increase the soil base saturation to 70%, $CaCO_3$ and $MgCO_3$ were applied at a ratio of 3:1, respectively. The soil properties after liming are listed in Table 3.

Soil in Petri dishes was moistened with deionized water up to 60% of the soil water holding capacity. Plates were then sealed with plastic film, covered with aluminum foil and left to equilibrate the soil solution for 24 h at 26 °C. The next day, they were opened and a granule of each fertilizer, corresponding to each treatment (Table 2) containing about 5.0 mg P, was placed exactly in the center of the plate, and lightly pressed into the soil. Next, they were again sealed with plastic film and covered with aluminum foil to prevent water loss and light incidence. They were then incubated at a temperature of 26 °C, for five weeks. One no-P fertilizer treatment and one treatment containing triple superphosphate (TSP) were also incubated as controls. Each treatment was replicated four times.

After incubation, Petri dishes were dismantled and the soil was sampled in concentric circles around the granule. The radii of the soil layers sampled were 0–7.75; 7.75–13.5; 13.5–25.5 and 25.5–43 mm, starting from the center (granule). Samples were dried at 40 °C and sieved (<2 mm) to determine the total and available P and the pH in water (ratio 1:10). Total P was determined by acid digestion with $H_2SO_4 + H_2O_2$, following the methodology proposed by Olsen and Sommers [21]. Available P was determined by anion exchange resin (membranes), following the first step of the procedure proposed by Hedley et al. [22]. Concentration of P in the extracts was colorimetrically determined by the blue-molybdate method [23].

Table 3. Chemical, physical and mineralogical characteristics of the soil used in diffusion study.

Granulometry			CBD		Oxalate		MPAC
Clay	Silt	Sand	Fe_d	Al_d	Fe_{ox}	Al_{ox}	
		g kg^{-1}					mg kg^{-1}
75	37	888	5.13	0.99	0.31	1.39	157
pH	P resin	S	H + Al	Ca^{2+}	Mg^{2+}	K^+	BS	CEC	V
$CaCl_2$	mg dm^{-3}			mmol$_c$ dm^{-3}					%
5.2	4	142	12	21	6	1.7	28.7	40.7	71

MPAC = maximum phosphorus adsorption capacity; CBD = citrate-bicarbonate-dithionite; Fe_d and Al_d = iron and aluminum, respectively, extracted by the dithionite-citrate-bicarbonate method; Fe_{ox} and Al_{ox} = iron and aluminum, respectively, extracted by the acid ammonium oxalate method; BS = base sum; CEC = cation exchange capacity; V = base saturation.

2.6. Soil Columns P Solubilization

Fertilizer solubility was evaluated in leaching thermoplastic acrylic columns with an internal diameter of 2.1 cm and a height of 25 cm. Nylon caps were fitted to the bottom of the column with a hole in the center where plastic hoses were attached to collect leaked water. Above each column, 300 mL bottles were attached, adapted to drip water constantly, controlling the flow. Fifty grams of dry soil were added to each column equivalent to reaching up to nearly 10 cm in height in the column. Original soil properties are presented in Table 4. Next, it was saturated with distilled water. Subsequently, fertilizers corresponding to each treatment were added at 100 mg P per column to the top soil surface. The treatments evaluated herein were: T1–12 (Table 2) as well as pure phosphates ARP(T13); BRP(T14); MRP(T15); TSP(T16) and a control (T17). Deionized water was percolated through the columns at a rate of 20 mL day^{-1} in the first 25 days. After that, the same amount was used every three days until 60 days had elapsed. The content of P was determined in leachates by the blue-molybdate method, following Murphy and Riley [23].

Table 4. Chemical, physical and mineralogical characteristics of the soil used in the column solubilization study.

Granulometry			CBD		Oxalate		MPAC
Clay	Silt	Sand	Fe_d	Al_d	Fe_{ox}	Al_{ox}	
		g kg^{-1}					mg kg^{-1}
180	90	730	9.11	1.99	0.27	1.41	295
pH	OM	P resin	Al^{3+}	H + Al	Ca^{2+}	Mg^{2+}	K^+	BS	CEC	m	V
$CaCl_2$	g dm^{-3}	mg dm^{-3}			mmol$_c$ dm^{-3}						%
5.1	3	<3	<2	11	9	3	<0.9	12.1	23.1	14	52

MPAC = maximum P adsorption capacity; CBD = citrate-bicarbonate-dithionite; Fe_d and Al_d = iron and aluminum, respectively, extracted by the dithionite-citrate-bicarbonate method; Fe_{ox} and Al_{ox} = iron and aluminum, respectively, extracted by the acid ammonium oxalate method; OM = organic matter; BS = base sum; CEC = cation exchange capacity; m = aluminum saturation; V = base saturation.

At the end of the incubation period, the columns were disassembled and the soil sampled in the following layers of 0–1; 1–2; 2–3; 3–6 and 6–10 cm, starting from the top. Samples were oven dried at 40 °C and sieved (<2 mm) and chemical P fractionation was performed according to the methodology proposed by Hedley et al. [22], with modifications by Condron et al. [24]. The last extractor (0.5 mol L^{-1} NaOH), because of lack of interest for our purpose, was skipped. The P concentration in extracts was determined by the blue-molybdate method [23]. The compartments estimated with the respective fractions were as follows: labile, which includes the inorganic P extracted by anion exchange resin (Pi_{AER}) plus inorganic and organic P extracted by 0.5 mol L^{-1} NaHCO$_3$ (Pi_{BIC} and Po_{BIC}); moderately labile, which includes the inorganic and organic P extracted by 0.1 mol L^{-1} NaOH ($Pi_{Hid0.1}$ and $Po_{Hid0.1}$) more inorganic P extracted by HCl (Pi_{HCl}); and non-labile, composed of the residual acid digestion ($P_{residual}$).

2.7. Plant Growth-Pot Experiment

The agronomic efficiency of the phosphate fertilizers generated in our lab was evaluated in a greenhouse pot study using a maize (*Zea mays* L.) hybrid 2B587 from Dow Seeds as a test crop. Soil and treatments used here were the same from the previously mentioned column P solubilization test. The experimental design was completely randomized with four replicates, in plastic pots with 3 L capacity, coated with plastic bags containing 3 kg of soil.

Phosphate treatments were added at the rate of 60 mg kg^{-1} soil, based on the total P content of each fertilizer. The basic sowing fertilization for all pots consisted of 20 mg kg^{-1} of N as ammonium nitrate (32% N) and 60 mg kg^{-1} of K$_2$O as polyhalite (14% of K$_2$O) in a uniform hand mixture in the total soil volume. Thirty milliliters per pot of micronutrients solution were added containing: 0.81 mg kg^{-1} B (H$_3$BO$_3$ p.a.), 1.56 mg kg^{-1} Fe (Fe (NO$_3$)$_2$.9H$_2$O p.a.), 3.66 mg kg^{-1} Mn (MnSO$_4$.H$_2$O p.a.), 4.0 mg kg^{-1} Zn (ZnSO$_4$.7H$_2$O p.a.), 1.33 mg kg^{-1} Cu (CuSO$_4$.5H$_2$O p.a.) and 0.15 mg kg^{-1} Mo ((NH$_4$)$_6$Mo$_7$O$_{24}$.4H$_2$O p.a.). Twenty days after sowing, this was complemented with 40 mg kg^{-1} of N as ammonium nitrate solution and another 30 mL per pot of the same micronutrient solution.

Each pot was sown with five maize seeds, later leaving the two best plants growing for 45 days. At the end, maize shoots and roots were harvested. Roots were washed in distilled water. Both plant parts were oven dried at 65 °C until constant dry mass (DM). After determining the DM of the shoot and root, the tissue was ground to determine the foliar P content through nitric-perchloric digestion [25] and to estimate accumulated total P.

The agronomic efficiency of the phosphate fertilizers was estimated in relation to the high water solubility commercial source (TSP), and therefore named, relative agronomic efficiency (RAE), obtained from the following equation:

$$RAE_i = (Y_i - Y_0/Y_{TSP} - Y_0) * 100 \quad (1)$$

where Y_i is the DM produced by source *i*, Y_{TSP} the DM produced by the commercial source (TSP) and Y_0 is the DM produced by the control treatment (no P addition).

2.8. Statistical Analysis

All data were submitted to normality analysis (Shapiro–Wilk test) and homoscedasticity (Barlett's test) at 5% of error probability and then to variance analysis (ANOVA). The Scott–Knott test at 5% was used for comparisons between treatments. Statistical analysis was performed using the ExpDes statistical package [26] in the R computational statistical environment [27].

3. Results and Discussion

3.1. Mineralogical and Structural Changes in Fertilizers

X-ray diffraction was performed to visualize changes in the mineral structure and its arrangement in RPs after partial acidification and incorporation of PILC and zeolites. Notably, in pure phosphates (ARP, BRP and MRP), there was a dominance of apatite, with some quartz present only in MRP. After acidulation, the intensity of the apatite peaks and the appearance of calcium sulfates, such as gypsum and bassanite, were observed. In RPs treated by 25% acidulation, the decrease in apatite peaks was less intense than those treated by 50% acidulation. Furthermore, calcium sulfate peaks became more intense under the highest acidification level, as a consequence of the sulfuric acid reaction (Figure 2). When the reaction was 100%, it was described as follows:

$$Ca_{10}(PO_4)_6F_2 + 7H_2SO_4 + 6.5H_2O \rightarrow 3Ca(H_2PO_4) \cdot H_2O + 7CaSO_4 \cdot 1/2H_2O + 2HF \tag{2}$$

When the amount of acid used was not sufficient to react 100% of the apatite, we obtained the so-called partially acidulated phosphates [9], as obtained in this study, and the apatite peaks did not disappear completely. Aside from this, the presence of zeolites or PILC as additives did not interfere in the phosphate peaks presented in diffractograms (Figure 2).

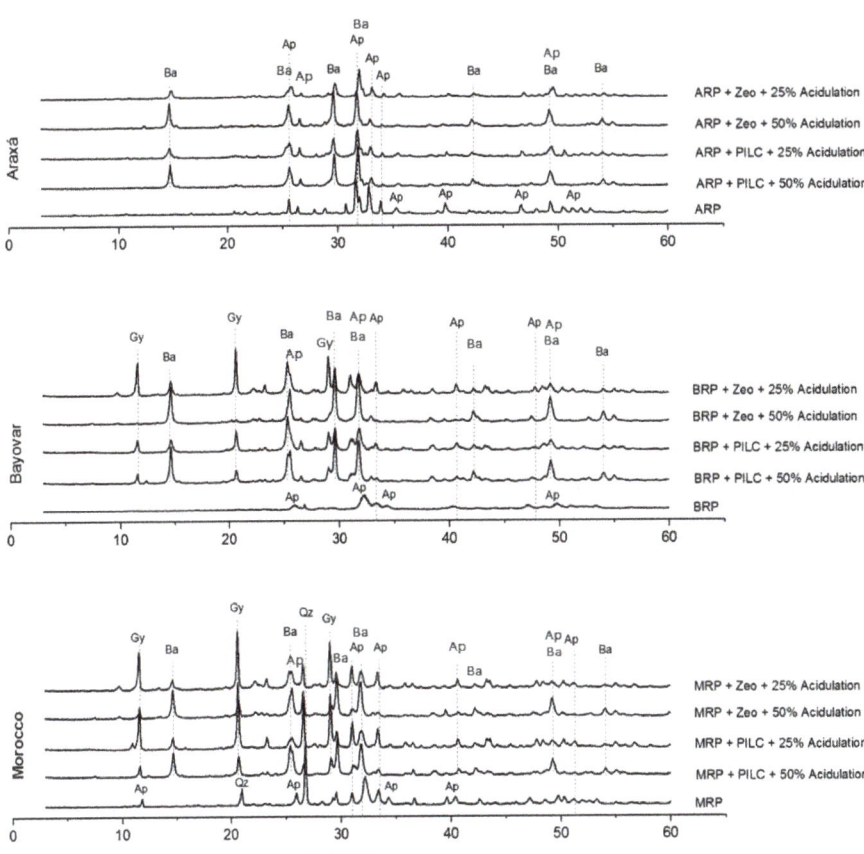

Figure 2. X-ray diffractograms of pure and acidulated RP (25 and 50% ac.) with the incorporation of pillared clay (PILC) or zeolite (Zeo), powder blades. ARP = Araxá Rock Phosphate; BRP = Bayovar Rock Phosphate; MRP = Morocco Rock Phosphate; PILC = pillared clay; Zeo = zeolite. Identified minerals: Ap = apatite; Qz = quartz; Gy = gypsum; Ba = bassanite.

The BRP diffractogram showed apatite peaks of lower crystallinity when compared to other pure phosphates (ARP and MRP). This is evidenced by wider peaks and lower intensity due to the occurrence of isomorphic substitutions of phosphate by carbonate in the mineral structure [28]. As a consequence, BRP was more susceptible to solubilization, with apatite peaks almost disappearing after its partial acidification, even at the lowest rate (25% ac.) (Figure 2). These results are in accordance with Mattiello et al. [28] and Santos et al. [29], who both studied the generation of phosphate fertilizers from the acidic residues of the metallurgical industry and different RPs, including BRP and ARP, and observed the greater vulnerability of BRP to acidulation when compared to other non-reactive RPs such as ARP.

According to Dorozhkin [30], several factors may influence the solubility of apatite and among them the most relevant are the composition of the rock, the particle size and the strength and composition of the acid used to solubilize. In this study, the smaller amount of sulfuric acid used (25%) was enough to alter the crystalline structure of all RPs, generating calcium sulfates (gypsum and bassanite) and transforming part of the apatite into more soluble forms (e.g., monocalcium phosphate). The presence of more soluble forms of P in these partially acidulated products was detected by the greater solubility in water (Table 2) when compared to the pure RPs, whose solubility in water was nearly zero (Table 1). Thus, even under less acidulation, increments in agronomic efficiency according to the structural changes promoted in relation to the pure phosphates were expected and will be discussed below.

3.2. Phosphorus Diffusion

3.2.1. Changes in Soil pH by Phosphate Fertilizers

All treatments, including TSP, increased the pH around the granule in relation to control (Figure 3). In the first layer, where the effect was more pronounced, the greatest increases were observed under TSP and almost all reactive RPs (T5, T6, T7, T9, T11 and T12), with the exception of treatments 8 and 10. Therefore, the capacity of these fertilizers to change the soil pH does not seem to be related to the presence of PILC and zeolites in their formulation, but to the higher solubility of phosphates. In corroboration, Cesar [31], when evaluating the diffusion of P from several phosphate sources in two contrasting textured tropical soils, observed that all phosphate sources, including pure TSP and those associated with BRP, were able to increase the pH close to the fertilizer granule.

According to Hettiarachchi et al. [32], after soluble or partially soluble phosphate fertilizer deposition in the soil, the granules' first action is to absorb water. This water moves towards the pores of the granules predominantly by capillarity flow and vapor transfer, and from there a series of reactions begins and one of the first items to change is the pH. Commonly, it is expected that partially acidulated phosphates and TSP decrease soil pH near the granule because of the acidic nature of their saturated solution [33], and the displacement of H^+ from the surface of the colloids to the soil solution caused by the increase in Ca concentration [34]. This acidifying effect of the dissolution of fertilizers containing monocalcium phosphate has already been reported in other studies. Lombi et al. [35], studying the lability, mobility and solubility of different phosphate fertilizers in calcareous and non-limestone soils, observed a significant decrease in soil pH up to a distance of 13.5 mm from the granule. Similar results were reported by them in another study carried out only on calcareous soils [36]. Silva [37] evaluated the diffusion of P from traditional fertilizers with reduced solubility in Entisol and observed that all fertilizers containing monocalcium phosphate were able to decrease the soil pH near the application point. Nascimento et al. [38] when studying the diffusion of P from calcium, magnesium and ammonium phosphates in soils of Brazil (Ultisol) and the United States (Mollisol), observed that calcium phosphate (TSP) was able to decrease the pH in all situations; however, this decrease was more significant in the soil with an initial pH of 8.0 (alkaline). In addition to the acidic characteristics of this source and the displacement of H^+ from the CEC to the soil solution induced by the increase in Ca concentration, the authors explain, based on the work of Cerozi and Fitzsimmons [39], that phosphate ions present three protonation constants (pH 2.1, 7.2 and 12.6). Thus, when the phosphate ion is added to soils with a pH higher than 7.2, there is a tendency for this ion to deprotonate, i.e., to donate H^+ to the solution, leading to a decrease in soil pH.

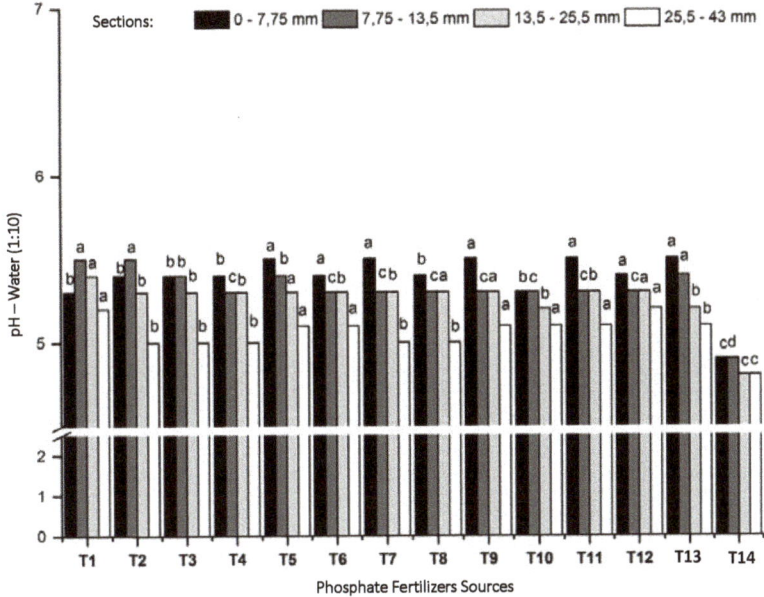

Figure 3. Soil pH as function of fertilizer source and soil layer after five weeks of incubation. Mean values followed by the same letter in the same layer do not differ by *t*-test (Scott-Knott, $P < 0.05$). T1 = ARP + PILC + 50% Ac.; T2 = ARP + PILC + 25% Ac; T3 = ARP + Zeo + 50% Ac; T4 = ARP + Zeo + 25% Ac.; T5 = BRP + PILC + 50% Ac.; T6 = BRP + PILC + 25% Ac.; T7 = BRP + Zeo + 50% Ac; T8 = BRP + Zeo + 25% Ac; T9 = MRP + PILC + 50% Ac.; T10 = MRP + PILC + 25% Ac.; T11 = MRP + Zeo + 50% Ac.; T12 = MRP + Zeo + 25% Ac.; T13 = TSP (triple superphosphate); T14 = control. ARP = Araxá rock phosphate; BRP = Bayovar rock phosphate; MRP = Morocco rock phosphate; PILC = pillared clay; Zeo = zeolite.

Giving due credit to substantial evidence that the soil pH around the granule would decrease with the dissolution of phosphate fertilizers, the contradictory results observed here can be explained by the specific adsorption reactions of P on the surface of Fe and Al oxides, which potentially released OH^- into the soil solution [40]. It is important to highlight that the majority of the soils in which there was a decrease in pH around the granules were calcareous or alkaline soils, with distinct characteristics from our study. Thus, the contrasting results can be attributed to these differences, since in soils with high pH, the precipitation of P with Ca becomes one of the main mechanisms of P immobilization [32], which does not release OH^- into the soil solution, as is the case with adsorption to Fe and Al oxyhydroxides [40].

3.2.2. Available and Total P after Fertilizer Diffusion

TSP was the source with the highest soil available P content up to 25.5 mm from the granule (Figure 4a). Partial acidulated fertilizers (50% ac.) produced from BRP and MRP containing PILC and zeolites in the formulation (T5, T7, T9 and T11) also presented superior values of available P in the first layer (<7.75 mm) compared to other sources. According to Williams [41], soil P movement depends, among other factors, on the composition of the fertilizer granule. Thus, in the second layer (7.75–13.5 mm), fertilizers from BRP and MRP containing zeolite resulted in higher P resin contents when compared to the same phosphates containing PILC, within the same level of acidulation (T5 < T7; T6 < T8; T9 < T11; T10 < T12). In the third layer (13.5–25.5 mm), this behavior was observed only in phosphates produced from BRP at 50% acidulation (T5 < T7) (Figure 4a). The highest P diffusion under products containing zeolite is attributed to its lower MPAC (31 mg kg^{-1}) when compared to PILC (5527 mg kg^{-1}). In the case of products containing PILC, the P released by acidulation may possibly have bound to its clay acidic sites, inhibiting P movement in the soil.

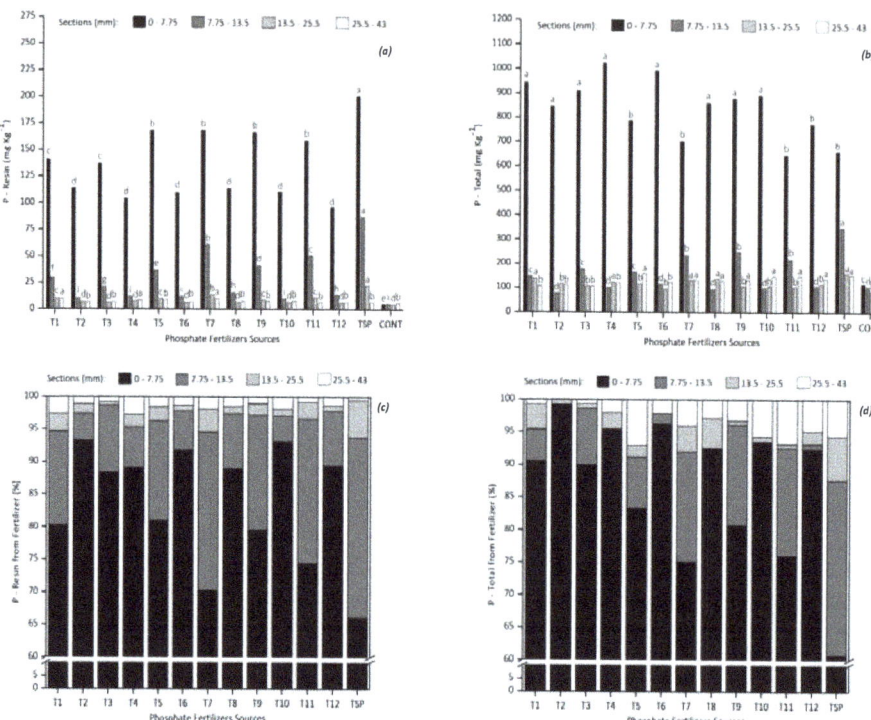

Figure 4. Soil available P (resin) (**a**) and total P content (**b**) in samples at distinct distances from the fertilizer granule application (radii of 0–7.75, 7.75–13.5, 13.5–25.5, and 25.5–43 mm) after five weeks of incubation. Mean values followed by the same letter for each soil layer do not differ by t-test (Scott–Knott, $P < 0.05$). Percent distribution of available P (**c**) and total P (**d**) from fertilizer in each layer (% P$_f$S$_{1-4}$) calculated according to the equation proposed by Lombi et al. [35]: %P$_f$S$_i$ = [(P$_f$)S$_i$ * W$_i$/Σi = 1 − 4((P$_f$)S$_i$ * W$_i$], where i is the layer of the petri dish (1 to 4); (P$_f$)Si is the content of available or total P as a function of the fertilizer addition; and Wi the mass of soil in a particular layer. (P$_f$)Si was calculated by subtracting the mean of the control treatment of the other treatments with fertilizers. T1 = ARP + PILC + 50% Ac.; T2 = ARP + PILC + 25% Ac; T3 = ARP + Zeo + 50% Ac; T4 = ARP + Zeo + 25% Ac.; T5 = BRP + PILC + 50% Ac.; T6 = BRP + PILC + 25% Ac.; T7 = BRP + Zeo + 50% Ac; T8 = BRP + Zeo + 25% Ac; T9 = MRP + PILC + 50% Ac.; T10 = MRP + PILC + 25% Ac.; T11 = MRP + Zeo + 50% Ac.; T12 = MRP + Zeo + 25% Ac. TSP = triple superphosphate; CONT = control; ARP = Araxá rock phosphate; BRP = Bayovar rock phosphate; MRP = Morocco rock phosphate; PILC = pillared clay; Zeo = zeolite.

No difference in available P was observed between control (T14) and the sources produced (T1–T12) in the last layer (25.5–43 mm), except for treatments T1, T4 and T7 whose differences are most likely due to small analytical variations (Figure 4a). Hardly any P from fertilizers would reach this distance and still remain available due to their strong interactions with the soil clay minerals [18]. In general, the phosphates produced from ARP with 50% ac. containing PILC or zeolites (T1 and T3) provided the lowest levels of available P up to a distance of 13.5 mm when compared to BRP and MRP, at the same level of acidulation (T5, T7, T9 and T11). However, within the less acidulated group (25%

ac.), there were no major differences between them (T2, T4, T6, T8, T10 and T12), especially in the first layer (0–7.75 mm) (Figure 4a).

All the RPs with 50% ac. presented higher available P up to 13.5 mm from the granule when compared with 25% ac. Apatite is the main mineral present in RPs (Figure 2), and its dissolution is facilitated in acidic medium [42]; thus, the more H^+ enters the system, the greater its dissolution. More than 65% of the available P from our fertilizers was restricted to the first layer (<7.75 mm), similar to TSP although a completely soluble source (Figure 4c). In general, the available P in soil decreased gradually with the distance from the granule. Overridingly, in the literature, there are reports of small movements of P from phosphate fertilizers in soil [18,35,36,43,44], confirming that only a small portion of the soil (few millimeters) is actually influenced by P fertilizers.

The results of total P content in each distance from the granule represent the diffusion of P from fertilizers in five weeks of incubation (Figure 4b). In general, the phosphate sources that resulted in the lowest total P in the first layer (<7.75 mm), regardless of the control, were also the ones that resulted in the highest P content in the adjacent layer (7.75–13.5 mm) (T7, T11 and TSP). More than 90% of total P from phosphate sources derived from ARP at both acidulation levels (T1–T4) and from reactive RP (BRP and MRP) with 25% ac. (T6, T8, T10 and T12) was restricted to the first 7.75 mm from the granule. The source with the greatest diffusion was TSP, even though more than 60% remained close to the granule (<7.75 mm) (Figure 4d).

In general, partially acidulated phosphates containing zeolite promoted more total P diffusion when compared to the same phosphates containing PILC, at the same level of acidulation (T1 < T3; T2 < T4; T5 < T7; T6 < T8; T9 < T11; T10 < T12) (Figure 4d). As already mentioned, this greater diffusion with zeolites is attributed to its smaller MPAC. Possibly, P released from the dissolution of RPs + PILC was potentially bound to the acidic sites of its own clay, limiting P movement in the soil. Silva [37] evaluated the diffusion of P from reduced solubility phosphate fertilizers in Cerrado soil using the SEM-EDXA (Scanning Electron Microscope with Energy Dispersive X-ray Analyzer) technique to determine the elemental composition of the granules before and after a period of soil contact. The results show that approximately 50% of P remained within the fertilizer granule even after five weeks of incubation in most of the evaluated products. He also verified the presence of ions such as Ca, Fe and Al in the constitution of these granules after the incubation, which may explain their small dissolution.

A certain level of soil moisture is fundamental to adequate fertilizer dissolution. However, once the fertilizer granules are in contact with the soil, two forces will regulate P availability; firstly, the water flows towards the granule by negative osmotic potential, carrying with it numerous chemical species such as Ca^{2+}, Al^{3+}, Fe^{2+}, Mg^{2+}, etc. This explains the presence of several elements inside the granules after incubation which were not part of their original composition, as observed by Silva [37]. Secondly, dissolved elements from the granule move to outside the surrounding areas of lower concentration. At this time, due to the high affinity of P with various metals, insoluble compounds such as P-Al and P-Fe precipitates, for example, may form [32,37], which justifies the weak diffusion and great permanence of P close to the fertilizer granule (<7.75 mm). Another fact is the movement of the companion ion [45], in this case especially Ca. For more intense P diffusion into the soil solution, more Ca dissolution and movement is required, preferably outside the granule region, which was not intensified in our study because of the static incubation, without solution flow, in agreement with the results already reported by Silva [37].

Moreover, the movement of P depends on fertilizer characteristics, such as the size of their particles/granules and their composition, and a series of soil properties, such as compaction, moisture level and mineralogical composition [41]. Thus, Benbi and Gilkes [46] studied the movement of P from TSP in two soils with high and low MPAC. After four weeks of fertilizer application, the added P was retained up to 80 mm away from the fertilizer granule in both soils. Within this 80 mm boundary, they also observed that P retention occurs in three different zones; one refers to the local of fertilizer granule, another one to the region next to the granule where precipitation and adsorption reactions predominate near the maximum limits, and the last is the most external where P is adsorbed to the soil at lower levels than its MPAC. These different zones of P accumulation are in agreement with the restricted available P diffusion observed here in our study.

3.3. Solubilization of Fertilizers in Soil Columns

3.3.1. Leaching Potential

The presence of P in leached solution was not detected in the control treatment. Moreover, no P was detected in the leached solutions containing pure RPs (ARP, BRP and MRP), which testifies to the zero water solubility of these sources (Table 1). Therefore, it is assumed that all the P contained in the leached water derives from the lab treatments applied to these RPs (Figure 5).

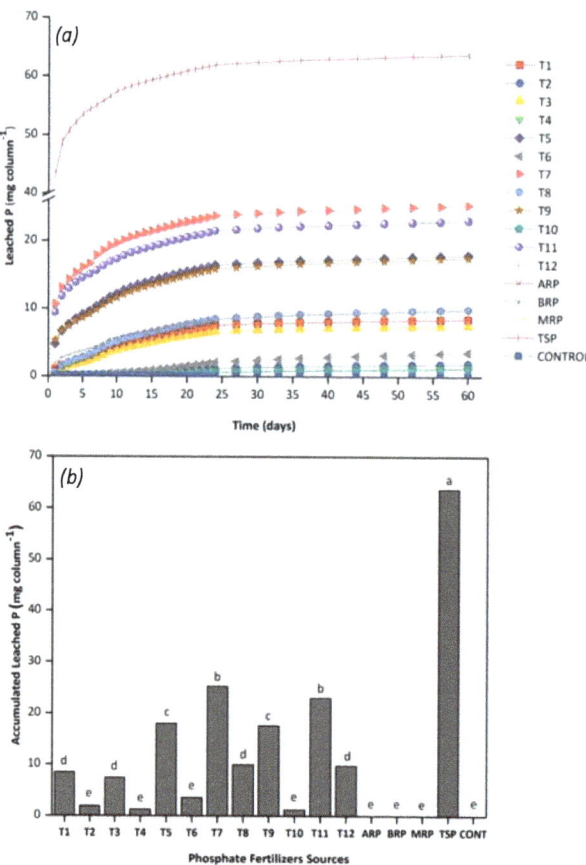

Figure 5. Phosphorus leaching from phosphate fertilizers over time (**a**) and accumulated leached P after 60 days of incubation (**b**). Mean values followed by the same letter do not differ by *t*-test (Scott–Knott, $P < 0.05$). T1 = ARP + PILC + 50% Ac.; T2 = ARP + PILC + 25% Ac; T3 = ARP + Zeo + 50% Ac; T4 = ARP + Zeo + 25% Ac.; T5 = BRP + PILC + 50% Ac.; T6 = BRP + PILC + 25% Ac.; T7 = BRP + Zeo + 50% Ac; T8 = BRP + Zeo + 25% Ac.; T9 = MRP + PILC + 50% Ac.; T10 = MRP + PILC + 25% Ac.; T11 = MRP + Zeo + 50% Ac.; T12 = MRP + Zeo + 25% Ac.; ARP = Araxá rock phosphate; BRP = Bayovar rock phosphate; MRP = Morocco rock phosphate; TSP = triple superphosphate; CONT = control. PILC = pillared clay; Zeo = zeolite.

According to the acidulation level and additives incorporated in each source evaluated herein, distinct amounts of P were detected in the leachate through the soil columns over the 60 days' incubation period (T1–T12) (Figure 5a). In total, five groups were identified; the first group, involving treatments T2, T4, T6 and T10, was classified as insoluble phosphates, meaning that these treatments were not able to promote leaching of P sufficient to differentiate from pure RPs and control, varying from 1.2 to 3.5 mg P per column over the 60 days' incubation period. The second group, consisting of treatments T1, T3, T8 and T12, represented fertilizers with reduced solubility, sufficient to be different from the insoluble ones, with the P leached ranging from 7.4 to 10.0 mg P per column. The third group consisted of treatments T5 and T9, whose leaching was 18.0 and 17.5 mg of P per column, respectively, and the fourth group, composed of treatments T7 and T11, registered 25.2 and 23.0 mg of P per column, respectively. These last two groups, involving treatments with high reactive RPs, are potentially viable alternatives for overcoming the totally soluble sources due to the slower dissolution of P into solution. TSP, the one with the highest P loss in leached solution (64 mg of P per column), constituted the fifth and last group (Figure 5b).

According to the P solubilization and leaching patterns observed for all the fertilizers evaluated here (except for the insoluble ones—group 1), it is possible to identify two distinct phases (Figure 5a). The first phase consisted of the first 10 days, when more than 50% of P had already leached. From the 10th day onwards, there was a significant decrease in the P content in the leaching solution, comprising a second leaching phase. These two phases are explained by the high P affinity to the soil constituents. When released from fertilizer, the P will potentially bind to the surface of Fe and Al oxides. Initially, the soft energy of these bonds still allows for P percolation through the profile (first phase). Subsequently, the concentration of P in leachate decreases due to the increase in energy ("aging") of P linkage (bidentate and binucleate bonds), inhibiting P leaching in the solution [44].

Clearly, the acidulation levels were the major factors responsible for the dissolution of RPs and, consequently, for the differences in P levels detected in leachate (Figure 5b). However, the presence of PILC restricted the leaching of P, mainly in the treatments from reactive RPs (T5, T6, T9 and T10), due to its high MPAC (5527 mg kg^{-1}) when compared to treatments with Zeolite in the same RPs (T7, T8, T11 and T12).

3.3.2. Phosphorus Lability

For better comprehension of the P dynamics and its accumulation in soils, sequential extraction with distinct strength solutions has become a fundamental tool [47–50]. The "P fractionation" procedure allows for evaluating the forms and distribution of this nutrient in the soil according to the fractions extracted, as well as the fate of P applied via fertilizers, in order to identify changes in soil nutrient dynamics. All the fertilizers studied, including pure RPs, were able to increase the labile P fractions in the soil profile after 60 days of incubation. In the first layer (0–1 cm) ARP + PILC + 50% ac. (T1) provided the highest levels of labile P when compared to other sources, in the following decreasing sequence: T1 > TSP = T3 = T5 = T9 > T2 = T4 = T7 = T9 > T6 = T10 > T8 > T12 > T14 = T15 > T13 > T17 (Figure 6a and Appendix A). In deeper layers, in general, sources with 50% ac. recorded the highest increases in soil labile P pool, but were much less expressive than in the 0–1 cm layer (Figure 6b–e).

There was great accumulation of moderate labile P throughout the profile under our fertilizer sources (T1–T12), detaching the first layer (0–1 cm), where it represented more than 88% of the total P (Figure 6a and Appendix A). In general, it was observed that 50% ac. resulted in higher contents of P extracted by 0.1 mol L^{-1} NaOH and lower contents of P extracted by 1 mol L^{-1} HCl when compared to 25% ac. (Appendix C). Based on these observations, it is clear that P solubilized from fertilizers was rapidly bound to mineral compounds in our test soil. Thus, its availability over time will be compromised by the strength of the reaction (monodentate, bidentate and/or binucleate bonds). Nevertheless, the sources produced from the same RPs containing incorporated PILC had a higher content of P extracted with 0.1 mol L^{-1} NaOH than those containing zeolites at the same level of acidulation (25 or 50% ac.) (Appendix C). This is mainly due to the presence of AlOH and

AlOH$_2$ groups in PILC that are able to adsorb a large amount of P (PILC MPAC = 5527 mg kg^{-1}) [51]. Some plant species are capable of acquiring P from this moderately labile inorganic P fraction via different mechanisms such as mycorrhizal association or P-solubilizing rhizosphere exudates [52,53].

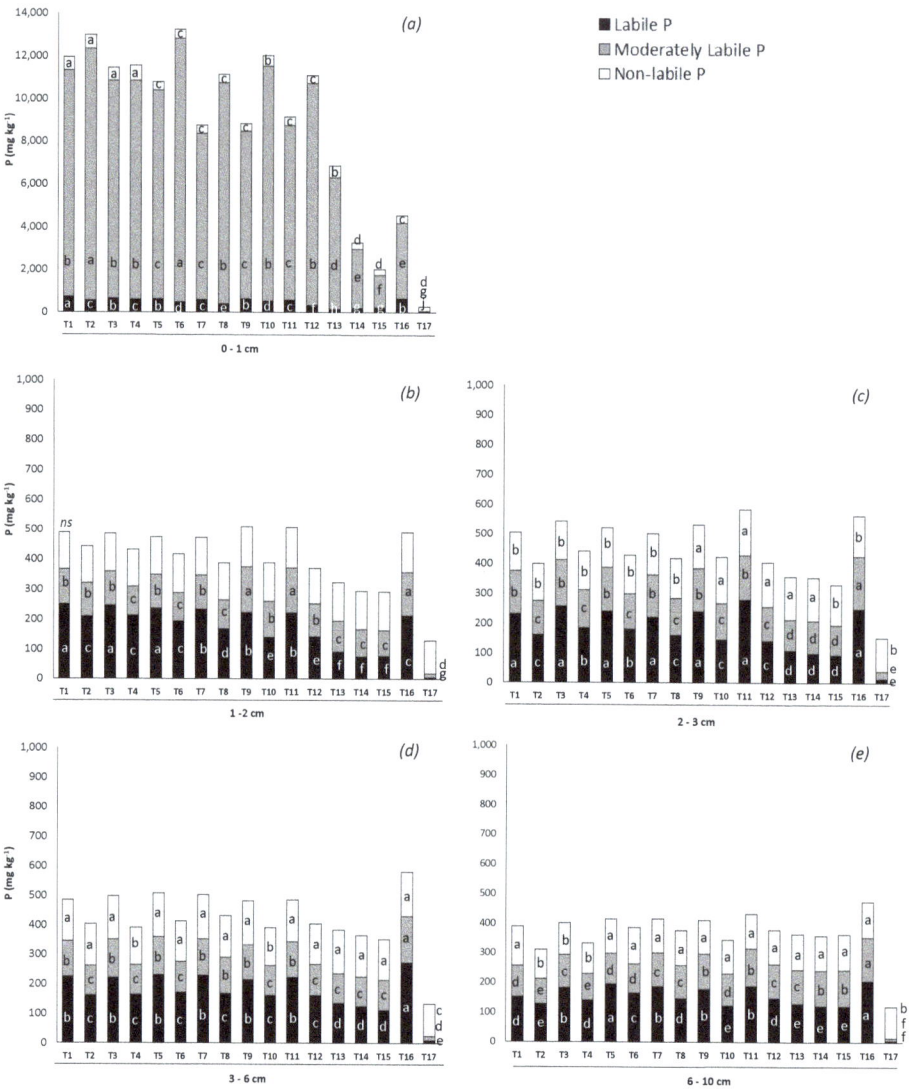

Figure 6. Labile, moderately labile and non-labile P pools in different soil layers of the column, 0–1 (**a**), 1–2 (**b**), 2–3 (**c**), 3–6 (**d**) and 6–10 cm (**e**), in response to phosphate fertilizers application after 60 days. Mean values followed by the same letter do not differ by *t*-test (Scott–Knott, P < 0.05). ns, not significant. T1 = ARP + PILC + 50% Ac.; T2 = ARP + PILC + 25% Ac; T3 = ARP + Zeo + 50% Ac; T4 = ARP + Zeo + 25% Ac.; T5 = BRP + PILC + 50% Ac.; T6 = BRP + PILC + 25% Ac.; T7 = BRP + Zeo + 50% Ac; T8 = BRP + Zeo + 25% Ac.; T9 = MRP + PILC + 50% Ac.; T10 = MRP + PILC + 25% Ac.; T11 = MRP + Zeo + 50% Ac.; T12 = MRP + Zeo + 25% Ac.; T13 = ARP (Araxá rock phosphate); T14 = BRP (Bayovar rock phosphate); T15 = MRP (Morocco rock phosphate); T16 = TSP (triple superphosphate); T17 = control. PILC = pillared clay; Zeo = zeolite.

In the first soil layer (0–1 cm), the total P content ranged from 2.007 (T15) to 13.242 (T6) mg kg^{-1} (Figure 6a). The residual fertilizer granules were homogenized to the soil at this layer when sampling, justifying this large amount of total P. According to Silva [37], after a short time in contact with the soil, approximately 50% of the P remains inside the fertilizer granule. The permanence of P within or surrounding the granule, as observed in this study, was due to the incomplete dissolution of the partially acidulated phosphates, proved by the significant participation of P extracted by HCl, which refers to Ca-phosphates (Appendix C). The formation of insoluble compounds such as P-Al and P-Fe or the adsorption of P onto the surface of Fe and Al sesquioxides also contributed to this accumulation, evidenced by the Pi fraction extracted by 0.1 mol L^{-1} NaOH (Appendix C). Under TSP, although a soluble source, P accumulation was also observed in this top layer due to its high affinity to the surface of Fe and Al sesquioxides. The retrogradation process (P-Ca) also restricted the movement of P from TSP, but to a lesser extent than the other sources (Figure 6a, Appendix C).

The non-labile P pool was the least influenced by our treatments (Figure 6). When analyzing the participation of each compartment in the total P in our soil, it was observed that under no fertilizer (control), the non-labile P represented the greatest part of the total P throughout the profile (74–89%). Several studies in tropical soils similarly reported this expressive proportion of non-labile P due to the high energy binding between phosphate and functional groups of Fe and Al sesquioxides [47–49,54–56]. Although there was an accumulation of non-labile P in the 0–1 cm layer under fertilizer application, its proportion to the total P was very small (3.2–13.4%) compared to other layers evaluated, and the sources that provided the highest accumulations were those produced from ARP (T1–T4), given its much lower reactivity compared to other sources (BRP and MRP) (Figure 6a). For other layers, non-labile P participation varied from 25 to 44.3% of the total P, but was not clearly influenced by any specific source/treatment (Figure 6b–e).

3.4. Agronomic Efficiency

At maize harvest (45 days after sowing), plants had typical symptoms of P deficiency under control (T17) and under pure RP treatments ARP (T13) and MRP (T15). Reduced growth and purplish, dark brown or dried leaves were the main symptoms observed (Appendix E). The difference in development between treatments was expressive, plants that received TSP looked healthy and better than other treatments, but all the partially acidulated phosphate sources with the incorporation of PILC and zeolites were able to promote greater maize growth than control and pure RPs.

Pure sources of ARP (T13) and MRP (T15) did not provide sufficient P for maize plants to express their initial growth potential, showing performances similar to the control for all the parameters evaluated (shoot and root DM, and accumulated P in shoot and root), resulting in very low RAE (0.8 and 10.6%, respectively) (Table 5). Therefore, the use of these RPs for direct application as fertilizer is not feasible. Partial acidulation (25 or 50% ac.) and incorporation of PILC or zeolites into their formulations resulted in significant increases in all plant parameters, with RAE ranging from 26.8 (T2) to 85.4% (T11).

The pure source BRP (T14) was able to differentiate from the control in plant growth parameters, with an RAE of 36.6% (Table 5). When BRP was acidulated by 25% (T6 and T8), it was not enough to significantly increase plant response. Similar results were also detected for ARP and MRP under 25% ac. (T2, T4, T10 and T12). However, it is worth mentioning that there was a physical difference between these fertilizers when BRP was applied in the powder/bran form, the same way that it is commercialized, and the phosphates that received 25% acidulation were applied as granules. The higher the phosphate contact with the soil, i.e., the greater its specific surface area, the greater its dissolution due to the higher contact of phosphate with the H^{+} protons present in the soil [57–60].

Among the lab fertilizers produced in our study, treatments T5 and T11 were the ones that provided RAE nearly similar to TSP (89 and 85%, respectively). Both received 50% acidulation, but T5 was produced from BRP with PILC and T11 was produced from MRP with zeolites. Treatments T7 (BRP + Zeo + 50% Ac.) and T9 (MRP + PILC + 50% Ac.) also resulted in good RAE indexes (74 and

76%, respectively). In view of these results, 50% acidulation may be a profitable alternative to improve fertilizer efficiency when using sedimentary RPs for crop production. Otherwise, additives PILC and zeolite do not seem to be effective in increasing P agronomic efficiency (Table 5).

Table 5. Dry matter yield and accumulated P content in shoot and root of maize under phosphate sources partially acidulated with incorporation of pillared clays or zeolites.

Treatments	Dry Matter (g)		Accumulated P (mg pot^{-1})		RAE (%)
	Shoot	Root	Shoot	Root	
T1	7.8 d	4.5 b	3.7 c	2.6 c	56.9
T2	4.1 e	3.0 c	2.1 c	1.5 c	26.8
T3	5.8 e	5.6 b	3.2 c	4.5 b	40.7
T4	4.4 e	3.7 c	2.4 c	2.1 c	29.3
T5	11.8 b	6.8 a	6.4 b	3.6 b	89.4
T6	5.7 e	4.7 b	2.8 c	2.3 c	39.8
T7	10.0 c	7.0 a	4.8 b	6.5 a	74.8
T8	5.9 e	4.8 b	3.2 c	2.2 c	41.5
T9	10.2 c	7.8 a	5.9 b	4.8 b	76.4
T10	4.9 e	3.7 c	2.7 c	1.9 c	33.3
T11	11.3 b	7.2 a	4.9 b	4.2 b	85.4
T12	5.0 e	4.1 c	2.6 c	1.6 c	34.1
T13	0.9 f	0.9 d	0.5 d	0.4 d	0.8
T14	5.3 e	3.9 c	3.0 c	1.8 c	36.6
T15	2.1 f	2.1 d	1.2 d	0.9 d	10.6
T16	13.1 a	5.8 b	14.3 a	3.9 b	100.0
T17	0.8 f	0.6 d	0.3 d	0.1 d	–

Means followed by the same letter in the column do not differ from each other by the Scott–Knott test at 5% probability. RAE = relative agronomic efficiency. T1 = ARP + PILC + 50% Ac.; T2 = ARP + PILC + 25% Ac; T3 = ARP + Zeo + 50% Ac; T4 = ARP + Zeo + 25% Ac.; T5 = BRP + PILC + 50% Ac.; T6 = BRP + PILC + 25% Ac.; T7 = BRP + Zeo + 50% Ac; T8 = BRP + Zeo + 25% Ac; T9 = MRP + PILC + 50% Ac.; T10 = MRP + PILC + 25% Ac.; T11 = MRP + Zeo + 50% Ac.; T12 = MRP + Zeo + 25% Ac.; T13 = ARP (Araxá rock phosphate); T14 = BRP (Bayovar rock phosphate); T15 = MRP (Morocco rock phosphate); T16 = TSP (triple superphosphate); T17 = control. PILC = pillared clay; Zeo = zeolite.

Numerous published research studies on the effectiveness of partially acidulated phosphate fertilizers found conflicting results [57,61–66]. This is attributed to differences in the physical form of application (powder versus granular), the products used for acidulation, the type of soil used to test the fertilizers and the doses tested [57,67]. From our study, it is possible to confirm that the type of RP used as raw material for the production of a partially acidulated phosphate also influences its effectiveness.

In fact, our previous incubation experiments (diffusion and solubilization) showed better results from sources containing zeolites (greater P diffusion and solubilization). This high P availability of fertilizers containing zeolite reflected in higher RAE only for MRP under 50% ac. (T11). In sources under 25% ac., the difference between zeolite and PILC products in similar RP sources was negligible. However, as solution soluble P can be easily adsorbed in a short period of time, the slower solubilization under the presence of PILC or even zeolite may play an important effect for better plant P utilization over time.

We confirmed here the very low diffusion of P in the soil. Therefore, we can say that the phosphate fertilizer placement can strongly influence its agronomic efficiency, and application techniques should be considered when thinking about improving the phosphate fertilizer use efficiency. A study conducted by Nkebiwe et al. [68], summarizing current techniques for N and P fertilizer placement in soil, showed that overall, fertilizer placement led to 3.7% higher yield, 3.7% higher nutrient concentration and 11.9% higher nutrient content in above-ground parts than fertilizer broadcast in soil surface. In fact, understanding the dynamics of P when fertilizers are applied in soil by different placement strategies and the use of new technologies may help to utilize P more efficiently.

4. Conclusions

The highest values of relative agronomic efficiency (>74%) were obtained with 50% acidulation of reactive RPs from Peru (BRP) and from Morocco (MRP) (T5, T7, T9; T11). Thus, these sources can be considered as being better suited alternatives for overcoming high solubility sources when searching for a product with more gradual P release into the soil. In the same trend, fertilizers produced from BRP and MRP with 50% acidulation containing zeolite in the formulation (T7 and T11) provided the highest diffusion and percolation of P in the soil profile, although still much lower than TSP. Otherwise, even zeolite and PILC seem not effective in increasing P agronomic efficiency.

All the fertilizers were able to increase the labile and moderately labile P fractions in the soil profile after 60 days of incubation. However, in the top layer, close to the fertilizer (0–1 cm), the sources containing PILC with 50% acidulation provided higher labile P contents when compared to zeolite, at the same level of acidulation and even RP source (T1 > T3, T5 > T7, T9 > T11). TSP was the most effective in percolating P in the soil profile, even in labile or moderate labile pools.

Author Contributions: Conceptualization, A.P.B.T. and P.S.P.; methodology, A.P.B.T., M.R. and P.S.P.; data curation, A.P.B.T.; statistical analysis, M.R.; writing—original draft preparation, A.P.B.T.; writing—review and editing, P.S.P. and M.R.; validation, A.P.B.T., M.R. and P.S.P. All authors have read and agreed to the published version of the manuscript.

Funding: This research did not receive any specific grant from funding agencies in the public, commercial, or not-for-profit sectors. The authors are grateful to Coordination for the Improvement of Higher Education Personnel (CAPES), which supported the scholarship to the first author.

Conflicts of Interest: The authors declare no conflicts of interest.

Appendix A

Table A1. Labile, moderately labile and non-labile P pools in the surface soil layer of the column in response to phosphate fertilizer application after 60 days.

Treatments	Labile P	Moderately Labile P	Non-Labile P
		mg Kg^{-1}	
		0–1 cm	
T1	709.6 a	10618.3 b	620.6 a
T2	555.2 c	11779.9 a	654.2 a
T3	647.9 b	10206.3 b	600.1 a
T4	588.6 c	10268.8 b	705.1 a
T5	609.3 b	9797.2 c	387.8 c
T6	479.8 d	12343.4 a	419.2 c
T7	583.3 c	7776.2 c	395.4 c
T8	390.4 e	10360.9 b	392.1 c
T9	624.7 b	7840.0 c	357.4 c
T10	520.6 d	11000.6 b	499.3 b
T11	567.0 c	8171.4 c	396.4 c
T12	329.3 f	10381.0 b	380.2 c
T13	140.5 h	6152.8 d	573.0 b
T14	191.0 g	2773.1 e	300.0 d
T15	213.6 g	1523.4 f	269.7 d
T16	638.8 b	3548.3 e	361.8 c
T17	21.9 i	41.4 g	197.9 d

Mean values followed by the same letter do not differ by t-test (Scott-Knott, P < 0.05). ns, not significant. T1 = ARP + PILC + 50% Ac.; T2 = ARP + PILC + 25% Ac.; T3 = ARP + Zeo + 50% Ac.; T4 = ARP + Zeo + 25% Ac.; T5 = BRP + PILC + 50% Ac.; T6 = BRP + PILC + 25% Ac.; T7 = BRP + Zeo + 50% Ac; T8 = BRP + Zeo + 25% Ac; T9 = MRP + PILC + 50% Ac.; T10 = MRP + PILC + 25% Ac.; T11 = MRP + Zeo + 50% Ac.; T12 = MRP + Zeo + 25% Ac.; T13 = ARP (Araxá rock phosphate); T14 = BRP (Bayovar rock phosphate); T15 = MRP (Morocco rock phosphate); T16 = TSP (triple superphosphate); T17 = control. PILC = pillared clay; Zeo = zeolite.

Appendix B

Table A2. Labile fractions of inorganic and organic P in the soil extracted by anion exchange resin (P_{AER}) and 0.5 mol L^{-1} $NaHCO_3$ (Pi_{BIC} and Po_{BIC}) in different layers of the columns according to the sources of phosphate fertilizers.

Sources	PRTA					PiBIC				PoBIC			
	0–1 cm	1–2 cm	2–3 cm	3–6 cm	6–10 cm	0–1 cm	1–2 cm	2–3 cm	3–6 cm	6–10 cm	0–1 cm	1–2 cm	2–3 cm	3–6 cm	6–10 cm
T1	220.7 a	132.6 a	139.5 b	129.7 b	89.6 d	400.9 a	74.2 b	75.3 c	80.2 a	51.1 d	88.6 a	42.9 a	16.8 a	14.5 b	10.6 a
T2	183.9 b	108.0 b	95.7 c	93.3 c	72.7 e	322.3 c	70.7 b	61.6 d	49.6 b	39.3 e	48.8 b	30.0 b	3.7 b	17.6 a	14.9 a
T3	190.6 b	132.5 a	151.4 b	132.1 b	107.1 b	396.2 a	81.0 a	86.0 b	76.6 a	59.8 b	61.0 a	32.2 b	20.1 a	11.9 b	14.5 a
T4	184.6 b	111.6 b	106.1 c	98.6 c	83.5 d	336.5 b	68.8 b	66.5 d	51.4 b	42.1 e	67.3 a	31.3 b	12.4 b	13.4 b	14.4 a
T5	208.1 a	133.1 a	154.8 b	140.0 b	123.8 a	369.7 b	79.5 a	80.9 c	77.5 a	59.1 b	61.1 a	32.4 b	19.7 a	24.6 a	19.6 a
T6	157.4 b	106.4 b	104.5 c	98.6 c	097.6 c	269.8 d	59.5 c	62.6 d	54.4 b	50.7 d	52.5 b	25.9 b	12.9 b	18.4 a	15.4 a
T7	207.0 a	132.0 a	137.0 b	132.8 b	113.1 b	280.8 d	72.2 b	76.3 c	76.1 a	58.6 b	95.4 a	27.9 b	7.7 b	19.1 a	13.8 a
T8	139.9 c	88.6 c	96.6 c	98.3 c	86.2 d	156.4 e	60.4 c	61.0 d	55.4 b	48.1 d	94.0 a	18.5 c	2.8 b	14.2 b	10.8 a
T9	245.7 a	137.8 a	143.1 b	130.7 b	112.5 b	312.8 c	74.4 b	70.2 d	67.8 a	53.4 c	66.0 a	10.2 d	26.4 a	15.9 b	11.0 a
T10	171.2 b	83.0 c	86.0 c	89.7 c	71.3 e	296.6 c	50.9 d	50.0 e	50.3 b	35.7 f	52.6 b	5.0 d	10.2 b	21.0 a	15.2 a
T11	217.0 a	140.3 a	186.6 a	137.4 b	119.8 a	269.0 d	72.1 b	76.7 c	74.1 a	54.3 c	80.9 a	7.8 d	16.4 a	10.5 b	14.2 a
T12	136.6 a	88.3 c	77.7 c	92.3 c	92.7 c	120.8 f	46.0 e	38.0 f	49.8 b	41.1 e	71.7 a	7.0 d	26.5 a	18.7 a	13.5 a
T13	72.4 d	50.2 d	55.4 d	67.3 d	76.0 e	34.7 g	35.4 f	33.6 f	39.8 c	39.8 e	33.3 b	5.1 d	20.1 a	28.4 a	12.2 a
T14	100.4 d	39.0 d	49.1 d	63.9 d	70.2 e	51.3 g	31.0 f	36.1 f	42.9 c	39.5 e	39.1 b	5.3 d	13.8 b	17.4 a	10.7 a
T15	134.2 c	39.3 d	49.1 d	57.5 d	67.0 e	37.1 g	31.0 f	33.3 f	39.5 c	39.5 e	42.1 b	6.4 d	11.5 b	14.6 b	12.9 a
T16	229.7 a	130.5 a	139.4 b	157.4 a	128.8 a	361.2 b	72.3 b	94.0 a	87.9 a	63.5 a	47.8 b	9.6 d	15.4 a	26.4 a	12.9 a
T17	0.7 e	0.5 e	0.2 e	0.3 e	0.4 f	4.0 h	3.7 g	5.4 g	6.0 d	2.3 g	17.0 b	1.1 d	8.1 b	3.5 b	2.7 b

Means followed by the same letter in the column do not differ from each other by the Scott-Knott test at 5% probability. T1 = ARP + PILC + 50% Ac.; T2 = ARP + PILC + 25% Ac; T3 = ARP + Zeo + 50% Ac; T4 = ARP + Zeo + 25% Ac.; T5 = BRP + PILC + 50% Ac; T6 = BRP + PILC + 25% Ac.; T7 = BRP + Zeo + 50% Ac; T8 = BRP + Zeo + 25% Ac; T9 = MRP + PILC + 50% Ac.; T10 = MRP + PILC + 25% Ac; T11 = MRP + Zeo + 50% Ac.; T12 = MRP + Zeo + 25% Ac.; T13 = ARP (Araxá rock phosphate); T14 = BRP (Bayovar rock phosphate); T15 = MRP (Morocco rock phosphate); T16 = TSP (triple superphosphate); T17 = control. PILC = pillared clay; Zeo = zeolite.

Appendix C

Table A3. Moderately labile fractions of inorganic and organic P in the soil extracted by 0.1 mol L^{-1} NaOH (Pi$_{Hid0.1}$ and Po$_{Hid0.1}$) and 1 mol L^{-1} HCl (P$_{HCl}$) in different layers of the columns in function sources of phosphate fertilizers.

Sources	Moderately Labile P (mg kg^{-1})															
	Pi$_{Hid0.1}$					Po$_{Hid0.1}$					P$_{HCl}$					
	0–1 cm	1–2 cm	2–3 cm	3–6 cm	6–10 cm	0–1 cm	1–2 cm	2–3 cm	3–6 cm	6–10 cm	0–1 cm	1–2 cm	2–3 cm	3–6 cm	6–10 cm
T1	2227.6 b	91.9 b	92.8 a	82.5 c	66.8 e	771.3 a	22.0 c	49.3 b	36.9 b	31.9 b	7619.2 b	3.0 a	1.7 c	1.5 b	5.5 a
T2	1348.3 c	89.6 b	77.3 c	69.5 e	57.6 f	302.1 c	18.6 c	36.0 c	29.2 b	23.2 c	10129.4 a	3.1 a	1.3 d	1.4 b	3.5 a
T3	2690.5 a	99.5 a	100.8 a	90.2 b	78.5 c	831.9 a	10.2 d	51.9 b	38.9 b	28.3 b	6683.8 b	3.6 a	1.7 c	1.7 b	4.6 a
T4	914.8 d	89.7 b	87.1 b	72.0 d	63.5 e	414.5 c	4.8 d	38.8 c	27.5 b	20.1 c	8939.4 a	2.9 a	1.2 d	1.5 b	4.9 a
T5	1340.6 c	99.8 a	102.1 a	91.7 b	76.3 c	518.5 b	16.8 c	49.4 b	39.1 b	22.0 c	6879.2 b	3.5 a	1.8 c	2.0 b	5.2 a
T6	907.1 d	90.7 b	82.1 b	73.3 d	72.6 d	264.8 c	1.2 d	35.2 c	28.2 b	21.6 c	11171.3 a	2.6 a	1.5 c	2.2 a	4.5 a
T7	677.2 d	99.9 a	97.0 a	87.2 b	88.7 b	308.5 c	11.2 d	42.7 c	35.4 b	22.6 c	6790.4 b	3.2 a	1.8 c	1.9 b	1.6 b
T8	359.4 e	87.0 b	84.1 b	77.2 d	87.8 b	292.3 c	8.2 d	37.3 c	42.2 b	22.8 c	9709.0 a	2.0 b	1.7 c	1.5 b	1.0 b
T9	1049.0 d	96.3 a	104.6 a	84.0 c	88.6 b	261.0 c	53.2 a	37.5 c	31.0 b	29.8 b	6529.9 b	1.8 b	2.0 b	2.9 a	1.0 b
T10	850.0 d	82.0 c	78.3 c	72.4 d	74.1 d	222.4 c	37.8 b	41.9 c	26.7 b	32.9 b	9928.1 a	0.7 c	1.4 d	1.7 b	0.7 b
T11	307.0 e	90.7 b	97.0 a	88.4 b	90.7 b	357.6 c	58.7 a	50.0 b	31.3 b	34.6 b	7506.7 b	1.2 c	2.0 b	2.0 b	1.2 b
T12	186.6 e	73.6 d	75.2 c	73.7 d	79.0 c	343.1 c	35.7 b	37.7 c	30.2 b	34.1 b	9851.1 a	0.7 c	1.3 d	1.4 b	0.9 b
T13	66.2 f	62.6 e	64.2 d	64.3 e	77.8 c	296.5 c	38.9 b	37.3 c	31.9 b	34.9 b	5789.9 b	1.7 b	2.6 a	2.8 a	2.0 b
T14	57.6 f	54.7 f	61.7 d	67.2 e	77.1 c	276.3 c	33.8 b	44.7 c	29.4 b	39.7 b	2439.1 c	2.1 b	2.7 a	2.9 a	2.2 b
T15	45.5 f	54.1 f	59.8 d	64.1 e	72.9 d	282.0 c	29.5 b	38.5 c	35.0 b	47.6 a	1195.8 d	1.9 b	2.5 a	2.7 a	2.3 b
T16	2136.6 b	97.3 a	101.2 a	99.4 a	96.5 a	511.7 b	45.3 a	72.3 a	57.0 a	49.7 a	899.8 d	1.8 b	2.4 a	2.6 a	1.9 b
T17	12.4 f	12.3 g	10.3 e	11.3 f	10.6 g	28.5 d	0.3 d	14.9 d	2.6 c	0.0 d	0.5 e	0.1 c	0.1 e	0.3 c	0.3 b

Means followed by the same letter in the column do not differ from each other by the Scott-Knott test at 5% probability. T1 = ARP + PILC + 50% Ac; T2 = ARP + PILC + 25% Ac; T3 = ARP + Zeo + 50% Ac; T4 = ARP + Zeo + 25% Ac; T5 = BRP + PILC + 50% Ac; T6 = BRP + PILC + 25% Ac; T7 = BRP + Zeo + 50% Ac; T8 = BRP + Zeo + 25% Ac; T9 = MRP + PILC + 50% Ac; T10 = MRP + PILC + 25% Ac; T11 = MRP + Zeo + 50% Ac; T12 = MRP + Zeo + 25% Ac; T13 = ARP (Araxá rock phosphate); T14 = BRP (Bayovar rock phosphate); T15 = MRP (Morocco rock phosphate); T16 = TSP (triple superphosphate); T17 = control. PILC = pillared clay; Zeo = zeolite.

Appendix D

Table A4. Residual fraction ($P_{residual}$) of P in the soil, considered non-labile, in different layers of the columns according to the sources of phosphate fertilizers.

Sources	Non-Labile P (mg kg^{-1}) $P_{residual}$				
	0–1 cm	1–2 cm	2–3 cm	3–6 cm	6–10 cm
T1	620.6 a	122.5 ^{ns}	128.6 b	138.8 a	133.0 a
T2	654.2 a	122.3	123.7 b	142.7 a	99.0 b
T3	600.0 a	126.5	130.6 b	146.4 a	107.4 b
T4	705.1 a	122.8	129.0 b	127.2 b	104.1 b
T5	387.7 c	125.8	131.3 b	148.5 a	112.6 a
T6	419.1 c	129.5	129.7 b	137.6 a	123.4 a
T7	395.3 c	125.3	138.3 b	149.9 a	116.3 a
T8	392.1 c	123.0	133.9 b	142.5 a	118.9 a
T9	357.4 c	135.0	148.0 a	149.4 a	114.4 a
T10	499.3 b	128.1	155.0 a	129.7 b	115.1 a
T11	396.4 c	136.0	155.4 a	141.3 a	117.5 a
T12	380.1 c	118.6	147.8 a	138.1 a	117.0 a
T13	572.9 b	128.1	144.5 a	149.4 a	121.0 a
T14	300.0 d	127.2	146.2 a	141.1 a	119.1 a
T15	269.7 d	129.3	136.0 b	138.3 a	120.5 a
T16	361.7 c	133.0	138.1 b	149.4 a	119.8 a
T17	94.8 d	111.4	113.5 b	109.8 c	106.7 b

Means followed by the same letter in the column do not differ from each other by the Scott-Knott test at 5% probability. ns = not significant. T1 = ARP + PILC + 50% ac.; T2 = ARP + PILC + 25% ac.; T3 = ARP + Zeo + 50% ac.; T4 = ARP + Zeo + 25% ac.; T5 = BRP + PILC + 50% ac.; T6 = BRP + PILC + 25% ac.; T7 = BRP + Zeo + 50% ac.; T8 = BRP + Zeo + 25% ac.; T9 = MRP + PILC + 50% ac.; T10 = MRP + PILC + 25% ac.; T11 = MRP + Zeo + 50% ac.; T12 = MRP + Zeo + 25% ac.; T13 = ARP (Araxá rock phosphate); T14 = BRP (Bayovar rock phosphate); T15 = MRP (Morocco rock phosphate); T16 = TSP (triple superphosphate); T17 = control. PILC = pillared clay; Zeo = zeolite.

Appendix E

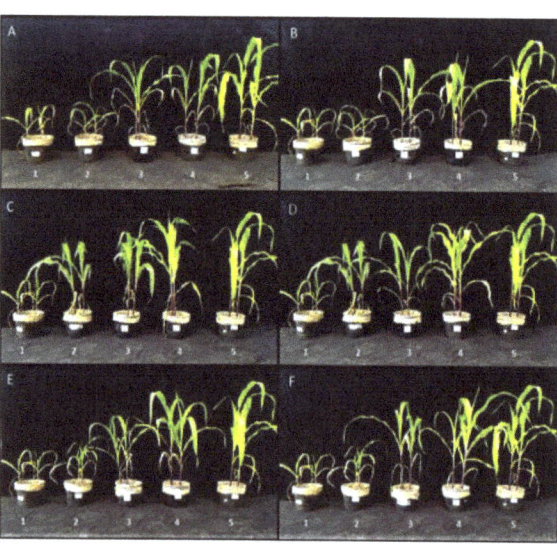

Figure A1. Maize plants at harvest (45 days growth) showing the differences between treatments. (**A**) 1 = Control (T17); 2 = ARP (T13); 3 = ARP + PILC + 25% ac. (T2); 4 = ARP + PILC + 50% ac. (T1);

5 = TSP (T16). (**B**) 1 = Control (T17); 2 = ARP (T13); 3 = ARP + Zeo + 25% ac. (T4); 4 = ARP + Zeo + 50% ac. (T3); 5 = TSP (T16). (**C**) 1 = Control (T17); 2 = BRP (T14); 3 = BRP + PILC + 25% ac. (T6); 4 = BRP + PILC + 50% ac. (T5); 5 = TSP (T16). (**D**) 1 = Control (T17); 2 = BRP (T14); 3 = BRP + Zeo + 25% ac. (T8); 4 = BRP + Zeo + 50% ac. (T7); 5 = TSP (T16). (**E**) 1 = Control (T17); 2 = MRP (T15); 3 = MRP + PILC + 25% ac. (T10); 4 = MRP + PILC + 50% ac. (T9); 5 = TSP (T16). (**F**) 1 = Control (T17); 2 = MRP (T15); 3 = MRP + Zeo + 25% ac. (T12); 4 = MRP + Zeo + 50% ac. (T11); 5 = TSP (T16). ARP = Araxá rock phosphate; BRP = Bayovar rock phosphate; MRP = Morroco rock phosphate; TSP = triplo superphosphate; PILC = pillared clay; Zeo = zeolite.

References

1. Lambers, H.; Plaxton, W.C. Phosphorus: Back to the roots. In *Phosphorus Metabolism in Plants*; Plaxton, W.C., Lambers, H., Eds.; Wiley-Blackwell: Hoboken, NJ, USA, 2015; pp. 3–22.
2. Roberts, T.L.; Johnston, A.E. Phosphorus use efficiency and management in agriculture. *Resour. Conserv. Recy.* **2015**, *105*, 275–281. [CrossRef]
3. Shen, J.; Yuan, L.; Zhang, J.; Li, H.; Bai, Z.; Chen, X.; Zhang, W.; Zhang, F. Phosphorus dynamics: From soil to plant. *Plant Physiol.* **2011**, *156*, 997–1005. [CrossRef]
4. [USGS] United States Geological Survey. 2015 Minerals Yearbook: Phosphate Rock [Advance Release]. 2015. Available online: https://minerals.usgs.gov/minerals/pubs/commodity/phosphate_rock/myb1-2015-phosp.pdf (accessed on 13 March 2019).
5. Jarvie, H.P.; Sharpley, A.N.; Flaten, D.; Kleinman, P.J.A.; Jenkins, A.; Simmons, T. The pivotal role of phosphorus in a resilient water–energy–food security nexus. *J. Environ. Qual.* **2015**, *44*, 1049–1062. [CrossRef]
6. Pagliari, P.H.; Strock, J.S.; Rosen, C.J. Changes in soil pH and extractable phosphorus following application of Turkey manure incinerator ash and triple superphosphate. *Commun. Soil Sci. Plant Anal.* **2010**, *41*, 1502–1512. [CrossRef]
7. Rajput, A.; Panhwar, Q.A.; Naher, U.A.; Rajput, S.; Hossain, E.; Shamshuddin, J. Influence of incubation period, temperature and different phosphate levels on phosphate adsorption in soil. *Am. J. Agric. Biol. Sci.* **2014**, *9*, 251–260. [CrossRef]
8. Biswas, D.R.; Narayanasamy, G. Characterization of Partially Acidulated Phosphate Rocks. *J. Indian Soc. Soil Sci.* **1995**, *43*, 618–623.
9. Cekinski, E. Fertilizantes Fosfatados [Phosphate fertilizers]. In *Tecnologia de Produção de Fertilizantes [Fertilizer Production Technology]*; Cekinski, E., Calmonovici, C.E., Bichara, J.M., Fabiani, M., Giulietti, M., Castro, M.L.M.M., Silveira, P.B.M., Pressionotti, Q.S.H.C., Guardani, R., Eds.; Instituto de Pesquisas Tecnológicas: São Paulo, Brazil, 1990; pp. 95–129. (In Portuguese)
10. Pickering, H.W.; Menzies, N.W.; Hunter, M.N. Zeolite/rock phosphate—A novel slow release phosphorus fertiliser for potted plant production. *Sci. Hortic.* **2002**, *94*, 333–343. [CrossRef]
11. Wu, P.-X.; Liao, Z.-W. Study on structural characteristics of pillared clay modified phosphate fertilizers and its increase efficiency mechanism. *J. Zhejiang Univ. Sci. B* **2005**, *6*, 195–201. [CrossRef]
12. [USDA-NRCS] United States Department of Agriculture—Natural Resources Conservation Service. *Soil Survey Laboratory Methods Manual (SSIR 42)*, 4th ed.; USDA-NRCS: Washington, DC, USA, 2004.
13. Farkas, A.; Rozic, M.; Barbaric-Mikocevic, Z. Ammonium exchange in leakage waters of waste dumps using natural zeolite from the Krapina region, Croatia. *J. Hazard. Mater.* **2005**, *117*, 25–33. [CrossRef]
14. Alvarez, V.V.H.; Novais, R.F.; Dias, L.E.; Oliveira, J.A. Determinação e uso do fósforo remanescente [Determination and use of phosphorus remnants]. *Soc. Bras. Ciênc. Solo Inf. Rep.* **2000**, *25*, 27–33. (In Portuguese)
15. Mehra, O.P.; Jackson, M.L. Iron oxide removal from soils and clays by a dithionite-citrate system buffered with sodium bicarbonate. *Clay Clay Miner.* **1960**, *7*, 317–327. [CrossRef]
16. Narayanan, S.; Deshpande, K. Alumina pillared montmorillonite: Characterization and catalysis of toluene benzylation and aniline ethylation. *Appl. Catal. A-Gen.* **2000**, *193*, 17–27. [CrossRef]
17. [MAPA] Ministério da Agricultura Pecuária e Abastecimento—Brasil [Ministry of Agriculture, Livestock, and Supply—Brazil]. *Manual de Métodos Analíticos Oficiais para Fertilizantes, Corretivos, Inoculantes, Substratos*

e Contaminantes [Official Analytical Methods Manual for Correctives, Inoculants, Substrates and Contaminants]; MAPA: Brasília, Brazil, 2007. (In Portuguese)
18. Degryse, F.; Mclaughlin, M.J. Phosphorus Diffusion from Fertilizer: Visualization, Chemical Measurements, and Modeling. *Soil Sci. Soc. Am. J.* **2014**, *78*, 832–842. [CrossRef]
19. [USDA-NRCS] United States Department of Agriculture—Natural Resources Conservation Service. *Soil Taxonomy: A Basic System of Soil Classification for Making and Interpreting Soil Surveys*, 2nd ed.; Agriculture Handbook, 436; USDA-NRCS: Washington, DC, USA, 1999.
20. [EMBRAPA] Empresa Brasileira de Pesquisa Agropecuária [Brazilian Agricultural Research Corporation]. *Sistema Brasileiro de Classificação de Solos [Soil Classification System in Brazil]*, 3rd ed.; Embrapa Soils: Rio de Janeiro, Brazil, 2013. (In Portuguese)
21. Olsen, S.R.; Sommers, L.E. Phosphorus. In *Methods of Soil Analysis: Chemical and Microbiological Properties*; Page, A.L., Ed.; American Society of Agronomy: Madison, WI, USA, 1982; pp. 403–430.
22. Hedley, M.J.; Stewart, J.W.B.; Chauhan, B.S. Changes in inorganic and organic soil phosphorus fractions induced by cultivation practices and by laboratory incubations. *Soil Sci. Soc. Am. J.* **1982**, *46*, 970–976. [CrossRef]
23. Murphy, J.; Riley, J.P. A modified single solution method for the determination of phosphate in natural waters. *Anal. Chim. Acta* **1962**, *27*, 31–36. [CrossRef]
24. Condron, L.M.; Goh, K.M.; Newman, R.H. Nature and distribution of soil phosphorus as revealed by a sequential extraction method followed by 31P nuclear magnetic resonance analysis. *Eur. J. Soil Sci.* **1985**, *36*, 199–207. [CrossRef]
25. Malavolta, E.; Vitti, G.C.; Oliveira, S.A. *Avaliação do Estado Nutricional das Plantas: Princípios E Aplicações [Assessment of the Nutritional Status of Plants: Principles and Applications]*, 2nd ed.; Potafos: Piracicaba, Brazil, 1997. (In Portuguese)
26. Ferreira, E.B.; Cavalcanti, P.P.; Nogueira, D.A. ExpDes: Experimental Designs Package. R Package Version 1.1.2. 2013. Available online: https://cran.r-project.org/web/packages/ExpDes.pt/index.html (accessed on 6 October 2018).
27. R Core Team. *R: A language and Environment for Statistical Computing*; R Foundation for Statistical Computing: Vienna, Austria, 2017; Available online: https://www.R-project.org (accessed on 6 October 2018).
28. Mattiello, E.M.; Resende Filho, I.D.P.; Barreto, M.S.; Soares, A.R.; Silva, I.R.; Vergütz, L.; Melo, L.C.A.; Soares, E.M.B. Soluble phosphate fertilizer production using acid effluent from metallurgical industry. *J. Environ. Manag.* **2016**, *166*, 140–146. [CrossRef]
29. Santos, W.O.; Hesterberg, D.; Mattiello, E.M.; Vergütz, L.; Barreto, M.S.C.; Silva, I.R.; Souza Filho, L.F.S. Increasing Soluble Phosphate Species by Treatment of Phosphate Rocks with Acidic Waste. *J. Environ. Qual.* **2016**, *45*, 1988–1997. [CrossRef]
30. Dorozhkin, S.V. Dissolution mechanism of calcium apatites in acids: A review of literature. *World J. Methodol.* **2012**, *2*, 1–17. [CrossRef]
31. Cesar, F.R.C.F. Eficiência Agronômica de Misturas no Mesmo Grânulo de Fosfatos Acidulados, Fosfatos Naturais e Enxofre Elementar [Efficiencies in Agronomics of Same Granule Mixtures in Acidulated Phosphates, Natural Phosphates, and Elementary Sulphurs]. Ph.D. Thesis, Luiz de Queiroz College of Agriculture—University of São Paulo, Piracicaba, Brazil, 2016. (In Portuguese).
32. Hettiarachchi, G.M.; Lombi, E.; McLaughlin, M.J.; Chittleborough, D.; Self, P. Density changes around phosphorus granules and fluid bands in a Calcareous Soil. *Soil Sci. Soc. Am. J.* **2006**, *70*, 960–966. [CrossRef]
33. Lindsay, W.L.; Frazier, A.W.; Stephenson, H.F. Identification of reaction products from phosphate fertilizers in soils. *Soil Sci. Soc. Am. J.* **1962**, *26*, 446–452. [CrossRef]
34. Montalvo, D.; Degryse, F.; Mclaughlin, M.J. Fluid Fertilizers Improve Phosphorus Diffusion but not Lability in Andisols and Oxisols. *Soil Sci. Soc. Am. J.* **2014**, *78*, 214. [CrossRef]
35. Lombi, E.; Mclaughlin, M.J.; Johnston, C.; Armstrong, R.D.; Holloway, R.E. Mobility, solubility and lability of fluid and granular forms of P fertiliser in calcareous and non-calcareous soils under laboratory conditions. *Plant Soil* **2004**, *269*, 25–34. [CrossRef]
36. Lombi, E.; Mclaughlin, M.J.; Johnston, C.; Armstrong, R.D.; Holloway, R.E. Mobility and lability of phosphorus from granular and fluid monoammonium phosphate differs in a calcareous soil. *Soil Sci. Soc. Am. J.* **2004**, *68*, 682–689. [CrossRef]

37. Silva, R.C. Eficiência Agronômica de Fertilizantes Fosfatados Com Solubilidade Variada [Agronomic Efficiencies of Phosphate Fertilizers with Variable Solubility]. Ph.D. Thesis, Luiz de Queiroz College of Agriculture—University of São Paulo, Piracicaba, Brazil, 2013. (In Portuguese).
38. Nascimento, C.A.C.; Pagliari, P.H.; Faria, L.A.; Vitti, G.C. Phosphorus mobility and behavior in soils treated with calcium, ammonium and magnesium phosphates. *Soil Sci. Soc. Am. J.* **2018**, *82*, 622–663. [CrossRef]
39. Cerozi, B.S.; Fitzsimmons, K. The effect of pH on phosphorus availability and speciation in an aquaponics nutrient solution. *Bioresour. Technol.* **2016**, *219*, 778–781. [CrossRef]
40. Golden, D.C.; Stewart, R.B.; Tillman, R.W.; White, R.E. Partially acidulated reactive phosphate rock (PAPR) fertilizer and its reactions in soil—II. Mineralogy and morphology of the reaction products. *Fertil. Res.* **1991**, *28*, 281–293. [CrossRef]
41. Williams, C.H. Reactions of surface applied superphosphate with soil II. Movement of the phosphorus and sulphur into the soil. *Aust. J. Soil Res.* **1971**, *9*, 95–106. [CrossRef]
42. Chesworth, W.; Van Straaten, P.; Smith, P.; Sadura, S. Solubility of apatite in clay and zeolite bearing systems: Application to agriculture. *Appl. Clay Sci.* **1987**, *2*, 291–297. [CrossRef]
43. Avila, M.A.P. Influência do Silício Sobre a Difusão do Fósforo no Solo e na Eficiência Agronômica de Fertilizantes Fosfatados Granulados [Influence of Silicon on Phosphorus Diffusion in the Soil and on Agronomic Efficiency of Granulated Phosphate Fertilizers]. Master's Thesis, Center of Nuclear Energy in Agriculture—University of São Paulo, Piracicaba, Brazil, 2016. (In Portuguese).
44. Degryse, F.; Baird, R.; Da Silva, R.C.; Mclaughlin, M.J. Dissolution rate and agronomic effectiveness of struvite fertilizers – effect of soil pH, granulation and base excess. *Plant Soil* **2017**, *410*, 139–152. [CrossRef]
45. Bouldin, D.R.; Dement, J.D.; Sample, E.C. Interaction between dicalcium and monoammonium phosphates granulated together. *J. Agric. Food Chem.* **1960**, *8*, 470–474. [CrossRef]
46. Benbi, D.K.; Gilkes, R.J. The movement into soil of P from superphosphate grains and its availability to plants. *Fertil. Res.* **1987**, *12*, 21–36. [CrossRef]
47. Gatiboni, L.C.; Kaminski, J.; Rheinheimer, D.S.; Flores, J.P.C. Biodisponibilidade de formas de fósforo acumuladas em solo sob sistema plantio direto [Bioavailability of forms of phosphorus accumulated in soil under a direct planting system]. *Rev. Bras. Cienc. Solo* **2007**, *31*, 691–699. (In Potuguese) [CrossRef]
48. Pavinato, P.S.; Merlin, A.; Rosolem, C.A. Phosphorus fractions in Brazilian Cerrado soils as affected by tillage. *Soil Tillage Res.* **2009**, *105*, 149–155. [CrossRef]
49. Tiecher, T.; Rheinheimer, D.S.; Kaminski, J.; Calegari, A. Forms of inorganic phosphorus in soil under different long-term soil tillage systems and winter crops. *Rev. Bras. Cienc. Solo* **2012**, *36*, 271–281. [CrossRef]
50. Coelho, M.J.A.; Aguiar, A.C.F.; Sena, V.G.L.; Moura, E.G. Utilization and fate of phosphorus of different sources applied to cohesive soil of Amazonian periphery. *Sci. Agric.* **2017**, *74*, 242–249. [CrossRef]
51. Shanableh, A.M.; Elsergany, M.M. Removal of phosphate from water using six Al-, Fe-, and Al-Fe-modified bentonite adsorbents. *J. Environ. Sci. Health A* **2013**, *48*, 223–231. [CrossRef] [PubMed]
52. Bolan, N.S. A critical review on the role of mycorrhizal fungi in the uptake of phosphorus by plants. *Plant Soil* **1991**, *134*, 189–207. [CrossRef]
53. Soltangheisi, A.; Moraes, M.T.; Cherubin, M.R.; Alvarez, D.O.; Souza, L.F.; Bieluczyk, W.; Navroski, D.; Teles, A.P.B.; Pavinato, P.S.; Martinelli, L.A.; et al. Forest conversion to pasture affects soil phosphorus dynamics and nutritional status in Brazilian Amazon. *Soil Tillage Res.* **2019**, *194*, 104330. [CrossRef]
54. Redel, Y.D.; Rubio, R.; Rouanet, J.L.; Borie, F. Phosphorus bioavailability affected by tillage and crop rotation on a Chilean volcanic derived Ultisol. *Geoderma* **2007**, *139*, 388–396. [CrossRef]
55. Rodrigues, M.; Pavinato, P.S.; Withers, P.J.A.; Teles, A.P.B.; Herrera, W.F.B. Legacy phosphorus and no tillage agriculture in tropical oxisols of the Brazilian savanna. *Sci. Total Environ.* **2016**, *542*, 1050–1061. [CrossRef]
56. Teles, A.P.B.; Rodrigues, M.; Herrera, W.F.B.; Soltangheisi, A.; Sartor, L.R.; Withers, P.J.A.; Pavinato, P.S. Do cover crops change the lability of phosphorus in a clayey subtropical soil under different phosphate fertilizers? *Soil Use Manag.* **2017**, *33*, 34–44. [CrossRef]
57. Khasawneh, F.E.; Doll, E.C. The use of phosphate rock for direct application to soils. *Adv. Agron.* **1978**, *30*, 159–206.
58. Chien, S.H.; Menon, R.G. Factors affecting the agronomic effectiveness of phosphate rock for direct application. *Fertil. Res.* **1995**, *41*, 227–234. [CrossRef]
59. Rajan, S.S.S.; Brown, M.W.; Boyes, M.K.; Upsdell, M.P. Extractable phosphorus to predict agronomic effectiveness of ground and unground phosphate rocks. *Fertil. Res.* **1992**, *32*, 291–302. [CrossRef]

60. Horowitz, N.; Meurer, E.J. Eficiência agronômica de fosfatos naturais. In *Simpósio Sobre Fósforo na Agricultura Brasileira*; Potafos/Anda: Piracicaba, Brazil, 2003; CD-ROM.
61. Beura, K.; Padbhushan, R.; Pradhan, A.K.; Mandal, N. Partial acidulation of phosphate rock for enhanced phosphorus availability in alluvial soils of Bihar. *J. Nat. Appl. Sci.* **2016**, *8*, 1393–1397. [CrossRef]
62. Chien, S.H.; Prochnow, L.I.; Tu, S.; Snyder, C.S. Agronomic and environmental aspects of phosphate fertilizers varying in source and solubility: An update review. *Nutr. Cycl. Agroecosyst.* **2011**, *89*, 229–255. [CrossRef]
63. Hammond, L.L.; Chien, S.H.; Mokwunye, A.U. Agronomic Value of Unacidulated and Partially Acidulated Phosphate Rocks Indigenous to the Tropics. *Adv. Agron.* **1986**, *40*, 89–140.
64. Lewis, D.; Sale, P.W.; Johnson, D. Agronomic effectiveness of a partially acidulated reactive phosphate rock fertiliser. *Aust. J. Exp. Agric.* **1997**, *37*, 985–993. [CrossRef]
65. Owusu-Bennoah, E.; Zapata, F.; Fardeau, J.C. Comparison of greenhouse and ^{32}P isotopic laboratory methods for evaluating the agronomic effectiveness of natural and modified rock phosphates in some acid soils of Ghana. *Nutr. Cycl. Agroecosyst.* **2002**, *63*, 1–12. [CrossRef]
66. Rodriguez, R.; Herrera, J. Field evaluation of partially acidulated phosphate rocks in a Ferralsol from Cuba. *Nutr. Cycl. Agroecosyst.* **2002**, *63*, 21–26. [CrossRef]
67. Mizane, A.; Rehamnia, R. Study of some parameters to obtain the P_2O_5 water- soluble from partially acidulated phosphate rocks (PAPRs) by sulfuric acid. *Phosphorus Res. Bull.* **2012**, *27*, 18–22. [CrossRef]
68. Nkebiwe, P.M.; Weinmann, M.; Bar-Tal, A.; Müller, T. Fertilizer placement to improve crop nutrient acquisition and yield: A review and meta-analysis. *Field Crops Res.* **2016**, *196*, 389–401. [CrossRef]

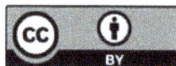

© 2020 by the authors. Licensee MDPI, Basel, Switzerland. This article is an open access article distributed under the terms and conditions of the Creative Commons Attribution (CC BY) license (http://creativecommons.org/licenses/by/4.0/).

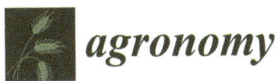

Article

Silicon Modulates the Production and Composition of Phenols in Barley under Aluminum Stress

Isis Vega [1,2], Cornelia Rumpel [3], Antonieta Ruíz [4], María de la Luz Mora [2,4], Daniel F. Calderini [5] and Paula Cartes [2,4,*]

1. Doctoral Program in Science of Natural Resources, Universidad de La Frontera, Avenida Francisco Salazar 01145, P.O. Box 54-D, Temuco, Chile; i.vega01@ufromail.cl
2. Center of Plant–Soil Interaction and Natural Resources Biotechnology, Scientific and Technological Bioresource Nucleus (BIOREN-UFRO), Universidad de La Frontera, Avenida Francisco Salazar 01145, P.O. Box 54-D, Temuco, Chile; mariluz.mora@ufrontera.cl
3. CNRS, Institute of Ecology and Environmental Sciences, (IEES, UMR 7618, UPMC-CNRS-INRA-IRD-UPEC), Bâtiment EGER, Aile P, 78850 Thiverval-Grignon, France; cornelia.rumpel@inra.fr
4. Departamento de Ciencias Químicas y Recursos Naturales, Facultad de Ingeniería y Ciencias, Universidad de La Frontera, Avenida Francisco Salazar 01145, P.O. Box 54-D, Temuco, Chile; maria.ruiz@ufrontera.cl
5. Institute of Plant Production and Protection, Universidad Austral de Chile, Campus Isla Teja, Valdivia 14101, Chile; danielcalderini@uach.cl
* Correspondence: paula.cartes@ufrontera.cl

Received: 7 July 2020; Accepted: 31 July 2020; Published: 5 August 2020

Abstract: Silicon (Si) exerts beneficial effects in mitigating aluminum (Al) toxicity in different plant species. These include attenuating oxidative damage and improving structural strengthening as a result of the increased production of secondary metabolites such as phenols. The aim of this research was to evaluate the effect of Si on phenol production and composition in two barley cultivars under Al stress. Our conceptual approach included a hydroponic experiment with an Al-tolerant (Sebastian) and an Al-sensitive (Scarlett) barley cultivar treated with two Al doses (0 or 0.2 mM of Al) and two Si doses (0 or 2 mM) for 21 days. Chemical, biochemical and growth parameters were assayed after harvest. Our results indicated that the Al and Si concentration decreased in both cultivars when Al and Si were added in combination. Silicon increased the antioxidant activity and soluble phenol concentration, but reduced lipid peroxidation irrespective of the Al dose. Both barley cultivars showed changes in culm creep rate, flavonoids and flavones concentration, lignin accumulation and altered lignin composition in Si and Al treatments. We concluded that Si fertilization could increase the resistance of barley to Al toxicity by regulating the metabolism of phenolic compounds with antioxidant and structural functions.

Keywords: aluminum toxicity; antioxidant; barley; lignin; phenols; silicon

1. Introduction

Silicon (Si) is a beneficial element that improves the growth, development and yield of plants subjected to different stresses [1–3]. However, the beneficial effects of Si depend on the capacity of plants to take up Si from the growth media, and transport it to the plant tissues [4]. To date, numerous studies have indicated that Si uptake and accumulation in plants are modulated by different influx and efflux transporters [5–8]. Most of the Si taken up by plants is deposited in the cell walls, where it increases mechanical strength [9,10].

In recent years, it has been suggested that Si can alter the secondary metabolism of plants [2,11–14]. In this regard, Si appears to stimulate the production of phenols in plants subjected to salinity, drought, temperature stress, UV radiation, cadmium, chromium [2], manganese [15], aluminum [16,17], nickel [11], soil acidity [18] and biotic [12,19,20] stresses. There is some evidence showing that the positive effects of Si on phenol metabolism in plants growing in stressful environments is due to (i) the regulation of the gene expression or activity of key enzymes in the phenylpropanoid pathway [21,22], (ii) the enhancement of total phenol production [17,23], and/or (iii) the formation of complexes involving lignin and carbohydrates [24,25] or Si-polyphenol in the cell wall [15]. However, there is still no information about the impact of Si on the production and composition of phenolic compounds with either antioxidant capacity or structural action.

Barley is one of the most cultivated cereals around the world due to the high nutritional value of its grains, which provide complex carbohydrates, proteins, minerals, fiber and antioxidants, including phenols [26]. The main phenolic compounds in barley grains belong to the group of flavonoids (cyanidin-3-glucoside, petunidin-3-glucoside, delphinidin-3-glucoside) and phenolic acids (ferulic acid, p-coumaric acid, vanillic acid, sinapic acid), which benefit human health by reducing the risk of various diseases such as cancer and coronary heart diseases [27,28]. However, in acid soils, barley growth is limited due to its high sensitivity to Al^{3+}, which reduces both the yield and quality of the grains. In this context, some reports have demonstrated an improvement in the Al tolerance of barley following Si addition [17,29,30].

For various other plant species, it has been suggested that Si attenuates Al phytotoxicity by means of (i) increasing the pH in the growth media, (ii) the formation of aluminosilicate complexes, (iii) enhancement of the chlorophyll and carotenoids content in plant tissues (iv) the stimulation of antioxidant enzyme activities and production of antioxidant compounds, and (vi) the exudation of phenolic compounds with Al chelation ability by plant roots [7,8,18,31–33].

Nevertheless, to the best of our knowledge only a few reports have described the effects of Si on the phenolic metabolism of barley subjected to Al stress. Moreover, the influence of Si on the phenolic metabolism of barley cultivars with contrasting Al tolerance has rarely been studied [17]. Therefore, the general objective of this research was to evaluate the effect of Si on phenol production and composition in tolerant and sensitive barley cultivars under Al stress. To address this objective, we carried out a hydroponic experiment with both types of cultivars grown under Al toxicity with and without Si addition and investigated the barley growth and the antioxidant as well as the structural phenol composition. We hypothesized that Si addition would improve barley's resistance to Al stress due to enhanced phenol production.

2. Materials and Methods

2.1. Plant Material and Growth Conditions

Seeds of the barley cultivars Sebastian (Al-tolerant) and Scarlet (Al-sensitive) were germinated (10 days) on filter paper moistened with deionized water. After germination, 48 seedlings of each barley cultivar were transferred to plastic containers filled with 8 L of nutrient solution [34], and grown for 15 days under controlled conditions. Thereafter, Al and Si were applied in combination according to the following treatments: −Al/−Si (0 mM Al and 0 mM Si; control), +Al/−Si (0.2 mM Al and 0 mM Si), −Al/+Si (0 mM Al and 2 mM Si), +Al/+Si (0.2 mM Al and 2 mM Si). These treatments were selected from our previous kinetic study concerning the effect of Si on barley under Al stress [17]. The nutrient solutions were replaced every 5 days, and the pH was adjusted (HCl or NaOH) daily to 4.5. For the experiment, barley cultivars were arranged in a factorial design with three replicates per treatment. Plants were harvested 21 days after the initiation of the experimental treatments and subjected to chemical and biochemical analyses.

2.2. Plant Growth Traits and Chemical Analyses

2.2.1. Growth Traits

Plant tissues (shoots and roots) were dried (65 °C for 48 h) to determine the dry weight (DW). Barley growth was determined by measuring the length of the longest root and the shoot of 10 plants randomly selected from each plastic container.

2.2.2. Aluminum and Si Concentration in Barley

The Al concentration in barley tissue (shoots and roots) was determined with the method described by Sadzawka et al. [35]. Briefly, dried samples were heated at 500 °C for 8 h, and treated with 2 M hydrochloric acid. The Al concentration was quantified by flame atomic absorption spectrophotometry (FAAS) at 324.7 nm. For Si concentration, dried shoots and roots (0.1 g) were digested with 5 mL of nitric acid (HNO_3) at 70 °C for 5 h. Thereafter, 1 mL of hydrofluoric acid (HF, 40%) and 10 mL of deionized water were added, and left overnight. The next day, the solutions were treated with 5 mL boric acid (H_3BO_3, 2% w/v), and the solution was made up to 25 mL by adding distilled water. Silicon concentration of the digested samples was determined by FAAS at 251.6 nm as described in Pavlovic et al. [36].

2.3. Biochemical Analyses

2.3.1. Total Soluble Phenols in Plants

Total soluble phenols were determined in root and shoot samples according to the Slinkard and Singleton method [37] using Folin–Ciocalteu reagent. The standard curve was calculated using chlorogenic acid as standard, and the absorbance was measured spectrophotometrically at 765 nm.

2.3.2. Identification and Quantification of Phenolic Compounds in Barley

Barley roots and shoots (0.1 g) were milled with liquid nitrogen and macerated in methanol as described by Slinkard and Singleton [37]. Phenolic compounds were determined by high performance liquid chromatography with a diode array detector (HPLC-DAD) using a Shimadzu HPLC system (Tokyo, Japan) with a LC-20AT quaternary pump, a DGU-20A5R degassing unit, a CTO-20A oven, a SIL-20a automatic injector and an SPD-M20A UV-Vis diode spectrophotometer. Data were analyzed using Lab solutions (Shimadzu, Duisburg, Germany) for DAD analysis. Identification was performed by LC-MSD Trap VL, model G2445C VL with electrospray ionization (ESI-MS/MS) detectors (Agilent, Waldbronn, Germany); control and data analyses were carried out by the Agilent ChemStation (version B.01.03) data processing station and Agilent LC-MS Trap Software (version 1.3, Santa Clara, CA, USA). The chromatographic separation method (HPLC-DAD) for the determination of phenolic compounds used a Kromasil ClassicShell-2.5-C_{18} (4.6 × 100 mm, 2.5 µm) column and a C_{18} precolumn (Novapak; Waters, Milford, MA, USA; 22 × 3.9 mm, 4 µm) as reported by Santander et al. [38]. The samples were injected using water:acetonitrile:formic acid (92:3:5 v/v/v) and water:acetonitrile:formic acid (45:50:5 v/v/v) as A and B mobile phases, respectively, with an elution gradient between 6% and 50% B over 30 min at 0.55 mL min^{-1} and 40 °C. Quantification was carried out by external calibration using chlorogenic acid for the roots and apigenin for the shoots as standards at 320 nm.

2.3.3. Antioxidant Capacity in Barley Plants

The antioxidant capacity of the roots and shoots was analyzed by the method described by Chinnici et al. [39] using DPPH (2,2-diphenyl-1-picrylhydrazyl) radical, and Trolox as standard. The absorbance of samples was measured in spectrophotometer at 515 nm.

2.3.4. Lipid Peroxidation Assay

Lipid peroxidation was assayed on fresh root and shoot samples by following the thiobarbituric acid reactive substances (TBARS) procedure reported by Du and Bramlage [40]. The absorbance of the samples was registered spectrophotometrically at 532, 600 and 440 nm.

2.4. Plant Stretching

The creep rate of culm was measured as an index of plant stretching. The extension of the first 5 cm of culm was measured with a constant load extensometer as described by Perini et al. [41]. Briefly, the fresh culms were scraped with carborundum to break the cuticle and then were placed in hot water for 15 min. Subsequently, the tissue was inserted between two clamps under a constant tension of 10 g per 30 min. The extension was measured through the movement of the upper clamp, detected by an electronic sensor and recorded in a microcomputer. All extension tests reported here were repeated at least three times for each sample.

2.5. Lignin Accumulation and Composition in Plants

To visualize the lignin distribution in the plant tissues, fresh roots and leaf sections were stained with Safranine O, and analyzed by Laser Scanning Confocal Microscopy (CLSM; Olympus FV1000, Arquimed, Tokyo, Japan) at λ emission/excitation of 543/590 nm according to the method described by Sant' Anna et al. [42]. The images were processed using Image Processing software (software FV10-ASW v0.200c; Arquimed).

A quantitative analysis of the total lignin composition (calculated as the sum of monomers vanillyl [V], syringyl [S] and cinnamyl [C]) was carried out by means of the alkaline cupric oxide (CuO) oxidation method proposed by Kögel and Bochter [43]. Briefly, 0.05 g of roots or shoots were oxidized in teflon vials for 2 h under N_2. Thereafter, the CuO oxidation products were purified by acidification and solid phase extraction using a C_{18} inverted column. Samples were derivatized by the addition of BSTFA (N, O-Bis (trimethylsilyl) trifluoroacetamide) before being analyzed by gas chromatography. For the separation and quantification of the monomers (V, S and C), a HP 6890 gas chromatograph (Agilent Technologies, Santa Clara, CA, USA) equipped with a SGE BPX-5 column and a flame ionization detector (GC/FID) was used. Phenylacetic acid was used as an internal standard for quantification.

2.6. Data Analysis

Experimental data were checked for normality by the Shapiro-Wilk test and for homogeneity of variance by the Levene test. Statistical differences of means (95% significance level) were analyzed using two-way (cultivar and treatment) analyses of variance (two-way ANOVA). Post hoc tests were performed with a Tukey-test to determine the explanatory variables independently when the ANOVA detected significant differences. For each data set, the standard deviation (SD) was also determined. In addition, the relationship between two response variables was analyzed through Pearson correlation at a significance level of 5%.

3. Results

3.1. Plant Growth and Concentrations of Al and Si

3.1.1. Plant Growth Traits

The interaction between cultivar and treatment had a significant effect on the growth traits of roots, but dry weight (DW) and length of shoots were not significantly affected by the interaction (Table 1). Aluminum toxicity led to a significant reduction in DW and the tissue length of the plants. For the Al-tolerant Sebastian cultivar, the DW of the shoots and roots decreased by about 30% when grown under Al toxicity (Table 1). Greater reductions were recorded for the Al-sensitive Scarlett cultivar ranging from 36% for shoots to 52% for roots. However, DW was enhanced in Sebastian (roots) and Scarlett (roots and shoots) when Al and Si were supplied together. The root length of Sebastian was greater than that of Scarlett, and both cultivars showed strong diminution of root length under +Al/−Si compared to the control treatment (−Al/−Si; Table 1). In plants growing under Al supply, the addition of 2 mM Si improved root length by 10% (Sebastian) and 17% (Scarlett).

Table 1. Dry weight (DW) and length of roots and shoots of barley cultivars (Sebastian and Scarlett). Treatments were 0 or 0.2 mM Al, combined with 0 or 2 mM Si. Values represent the mean of three replicates per treatment ± SD.

Cultivar	Treatment		Shoot DW (g pot^{-1})	Root DW (g pot^{-1})	Shoot Length (cm)	Root Length (cm)
	Al (mM)	Si (mM)				
Sebastian	0	0	3.99 ± 0.07 a	1.47 ± 0.10 a	50.2 ± 1.3 b	27.4 ± 1.3 Aa
	0.2	0	2.83 ± 0.31 b	1.05 ± 0.05 b	47.6 ± 3.1 c	19.4 ± 1.4 Ac
	0	2	4.17 ± 0.48 a	1.42 ± 0.16 a	52.4 ± 0.6 a	27.1 ± 0.9 a
	0.2	2	3.19 ± 0.23 b	1.14 ± 0.07 a	49.5 ± 1.1 b	21.3 ± 1.2 Ab
Scarlett	0	0	3.51 ± 0.50 a	1.24 ± 0.25 a	49.2 ± 2.3 a	23.5 ± 0.2 Ba
	0.2	0	2.25 ± 0.05 b	0.59 ± 0.10 b	45.5 ± 0.3 a	14.4 ± 1.4 Bb
	0	2	3.44 ± 0.06 a	1.18 ± 0.12 a	48.3 ± 1.2 a	22.8 ± 0.8 a
	0.2	2	3.00 ± 0.19 a	1.03 ± 0.98 a	46.1 ± 0.7 a	16.8 ± 1.6 Bb
Cultivar			*	n.s	***	***
Treatment			***	***	**	***
Cultivar × Treatment			n.s	**	n.s	***

Different letters indicate statistically significant differences ($p \leq 0.05$) among treatments. The lower case letters represent significant differences between treatments for one barley cultivar. The upper case letters indicate significant differences between barley cultivars for the same treatment. When uppercase letters do not appear, no significant differences between the same treatment in different cultivars were found. The significance of the interaction between cultivar and treatment was determined through the p-values: n.s, not significant; * $p \leq 0.05$; ** $p \leq 0.01$; *** $p \leq 0.001$.

3.1.2. Aluminum and Si Concentration

We observed that the interaction between cultivar and treatment had a significant effect on the Al and Si concentration in shoots and roots (Table 2). Roots of barley treated with 0.2 mM Al accumulated 5232 ± 417 mg of Al kg^{-1} DW for the Sebastian cultivar and 5285 ± 167 mg Al kg^{-1} DW for the Scarlett cultivar. Sebastian shoots showed 3153 ± 417 mg Al kg^{-1} DW and 4876 ± 581 mg Al kg^{-1} DW was recorded for Scarlett shoots. However, Si addition decreased the Al concentration in roots by 45% (Sebastian) and 68% (Scarlett), while the Al reduction in shoots was 49% (Sebastian) and 42% (Scarlett) as compared to the Al treatment without Si addition (Table 2). On the other hand, the Si concentration in plant tissues increased when plants were exposed to 2 mM of Si as compared to the control (Table 2). However, shoot Si concentration decreased with Al supply in both barley cultivars. Thus, Al addition reduced Si concentration in the shoots by 47% (Sebastian) and 37% (Scarlett), and by 55% (Sebastian) and 13% (Scarlett) in the roots.

Table 2. Aluminum and silicon concentrations in roots and shoots of the two barley cultivars (Sebastian and Scarlett). Treatments were 0 or 0.2 mM Al, combined with 0 or 2 mM Si. Values represent the mean of three replicates per treatment ± SD.

Cultivars	Treatment		Shoot Al (mg kg^{-1} DW)	Root Al (mg kg^{-1} DW)	Shoot Si (g kg^{-1} DW)	Root Si (g kg^{-1} DW)
	Al (mM)	Si (mM)				
Sebastian	0	0	99.32 ± 13 c	126.39 ± 13 c	1.09 ± 0.29 c	0.11 ± 0.04 c
	0.2	0	3153.70 ± 417 Ba	5232.41 ± 417 Aa	1.12 ± 0.24 c	0.24 ± 0.11 c
	0	2	99.77 ± 19 c	115.63 ± 19 c	11.00 ± 0.33 Aa	8.21 ± 0.64 a
	0.2	2	1609.15 ± 506 Bb	2869.36 ± 506 Ab	5.84 ± 0.34 b	3.70 ± 0.67 Bb
Scarlett	0	0	99.20 ± 65 c	116.74 ± 199 c	0.17 ± 0.11 c	1.10 ± 0.07 c
	0.2	0	4876.53 ± 581 Aa	5285.11 ± 167 Bb	0.25 ± 0.17 c	1.30 ± 0.25 c
	0	2	92.99 ± 42 c	120.15 ± 104 c	8.10 ± 0.53 a	7.30 ± 0.28 Aa
	0.2	2	2808.81 ± 334 Ab	1695.54 ± 185 Bb	5.10 ± 0.11 Ab	6.40 ± 0.25 b

Table 2. Cont.

Cultivars	Treatment		Shoot Al (mg kg^{-1} DW)	Root Al (mg kg^{-1} DW)	Shoot Si (g kg^{-1} DW)	Root Si (g kg^{-1} DW)
	Al (mM)	Si (mM)				
Cultivar			***	***	***	***
Treatment			***	***	***	***
Cultivar × Treatment			***	***	***	***

Different letters indicate statistically significant differences ($p \leq 0.05$) among treatments. The lower case letters represent significant differences between treatments for one barley cultivar. The upper case letters indicate significant differences between barley cultivars for the same treatment. When uppercase letters do not appear, no significant differences between the same treatment in different cultivars were found. The significance of the interaction between cultivar and treatment was determined through the p-values: n.s, not significant; * $p \leq 0.05$; ** $p \leq 0.01$; *** $p \leq 0.001$.

3.2. The Effect of Al and Si on Phenol Production and Antioxidant Performance

3.2.1. Total Soluble Phenols and Phenolic Profile

In general, the phenol concentration in plant tissues was affected by the interaction between the barley cultivar and Al/Si treatment (Figure 1A,B). Silicon addition did not alter the total phenol concentration in the Sebastian shoots (Figure 1A). However, when plants were exposed to 0.2 mM Al, lower concentrations of soluble phenols were recorded. Conversely, Sebastian roots showed an increase in phenols when Si was applied (Figure 1B). On the other hand, for Scarlett shoots, the highest phenol concentrations were observed in the +Al/−Si treatment (Figure 1A). Similarly, total phenols increased by 24% in Scarlet as a consequence of Si addition to the growth media, and it increased by 57% in the +Al/+Si treatment (Figure 1B).

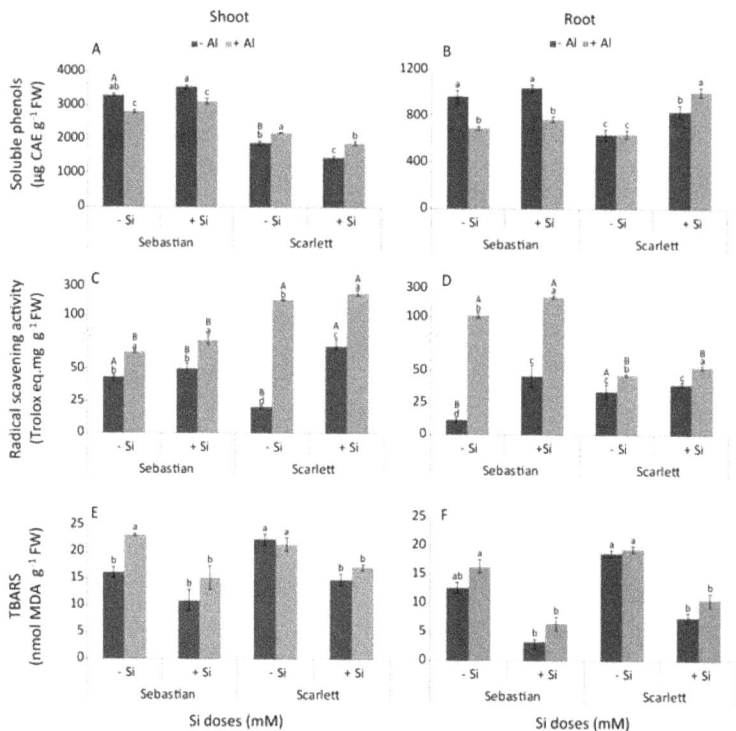

Figure 1. Total phenols (**A,B**), free radical scavenging activity (**C,D**) and lipid peroxidation (**E,F**) in

shoots and roots of barley cultivars. Treatments were 0 or 0.2 mM Al, combined with 0 or 2 mM Si. Different letters indicate statistically significant differences ($p \leq 0.05$) among treatments. The lower case letters represent significant differences between treatments for same barley cultivar. The upper case letters indicate significant differences between barley cultivars for the same treatment. When uppercase letters do not appear, no significant differences between the same treatment were found for different cultivars.

Seven flavonoids (flavone-glucosides) were identified in barley shoots (Table 3), but only four compounds reached quantifiable levels: (1) isoorientin-7-O-glucoside (lutonarin), (2) apigenin-pentoxide-hexoside isomer 1, (3) isovitexin-7-O-[6-sinapoyl]-glucoside, and (4) isovitexin-7-O-[6-feruloyl]-glucoside (Figure 2C). Caffeoylquinic acid isomer, a phenolic acid belonging to the chlorogenic acid family, was detected in barley roots (Table 3 and Figure 2A).

Table 3. Identification of phenolics from barley extracts by using HPLC–DAD–ESI-MS/MS.

Tr (min)	Tentative Identification	λ max (nm)	[M − H]⁻	Products-Ions
Roots				
6.4	Caffeoylquinic acid isomer (Chlorogenic acid)	306	353.1	263.1; 219.1
Shoots				
10.8	Isoorientin-7-O-glucoside (Lutonarin)	349	609	447.0; 377.0
18.1	Apigenin-pentoxide-hexoside isomer 1	336	593.3	502.8; 472.8; 430.8; 310.9
22.9	Apigenin- pentoxide-hexoside isomer 2	338	563.9	544.8; 472.9; 442.9; 383
30.3	Isoorientin-7-O-[6-sinapoyl]-glucoside	342	815.6	446.9; 327.2; 299.1
31.1	Isoorientin-7-O-[6-feruloyl]-glucoside	338	785.6	446.9; 327.1
34.5	Isovitexin-7-O-[6-sinapoyl]-glucoside	319	799.6	430.4; 311.0; 283
35.8	Isovitexin-7-O-[6-feruloyl]-glucoside	333	769.6	430.8; 311.0

The interaction between cultivar and treatment also had a significant effect on lutonarin, apigenin-pentoxide-hexoside and isovitexin-7-O-[6-sinapoyl]-glucoside concentrations (Figure 2D–F), but isovitexin-7-O-[6-feruloyl]-glucoside concentration was not affected by the interaction (Figure 2G). There were no differences in the lutonarin concentration in the shoots of Scarlett among treatments (Figure 2D). However, it decreased in all treatments for Sebastian shoots with respect to the control (Figure 2D). Similarly, apigenin-pentoxide-hexoside and isovitexin-7-O-[6-sinapoyl]-glucoside decreased in the shoots of both cultivars with the application of Si alone or in combination with Al (Figure 2E,F). Moreover, isovitexin-7-O-[6-feruloyl]-glucoside significantly increased in Scarlett shoots when the plants were exposed to the Al treatment (Figure 2G). In contrast, Sebastian plants treated with Si showed a decrease in the concentration of this phenol, irrespective of Al addition (Figure 2G).

In addition, we observed that the interaction between cultivar and treatment significantly affected the caffeoylquinic acid isomer (CQA) concentration. In the roots, a higher concentration of CQA was found for Sebastian compared to Scarlett in all treatments (Figure 2B). Sebastian showed a decrease in its concentration compared to control when plants were treated with Si and Al alone or in combination. Scarlett did not show any difference in the CQA concentration among the different treatments.

3.2.2. Radical Scavenging Activity

The interaction between cultivar and treatment significantly affected radical scavenging activity in shoots and roots (Figure 1C,D). In fact, radical scavenging activity in plant tissues of both cultivars increased following the addition of 0.2 mM Al compared to the control. A further increase was found in roots and shoots of barley cultivars simultaneously supplied with Al and Si. For Sebastian, the highest antioxidant capacity was observed in the roots (Figure 1D) of plants treated with Al and Si, showing a 22-fold increase as compared to the control. For Scarlett, the highest antioxidant capacity was also observed in shoots (Figure 1C) and roots (Figure 1D) as a consequence of the simultaneous addition of Si and Al, with a 13-fold and 1.7-fold increase, respectively, as compared to the control.

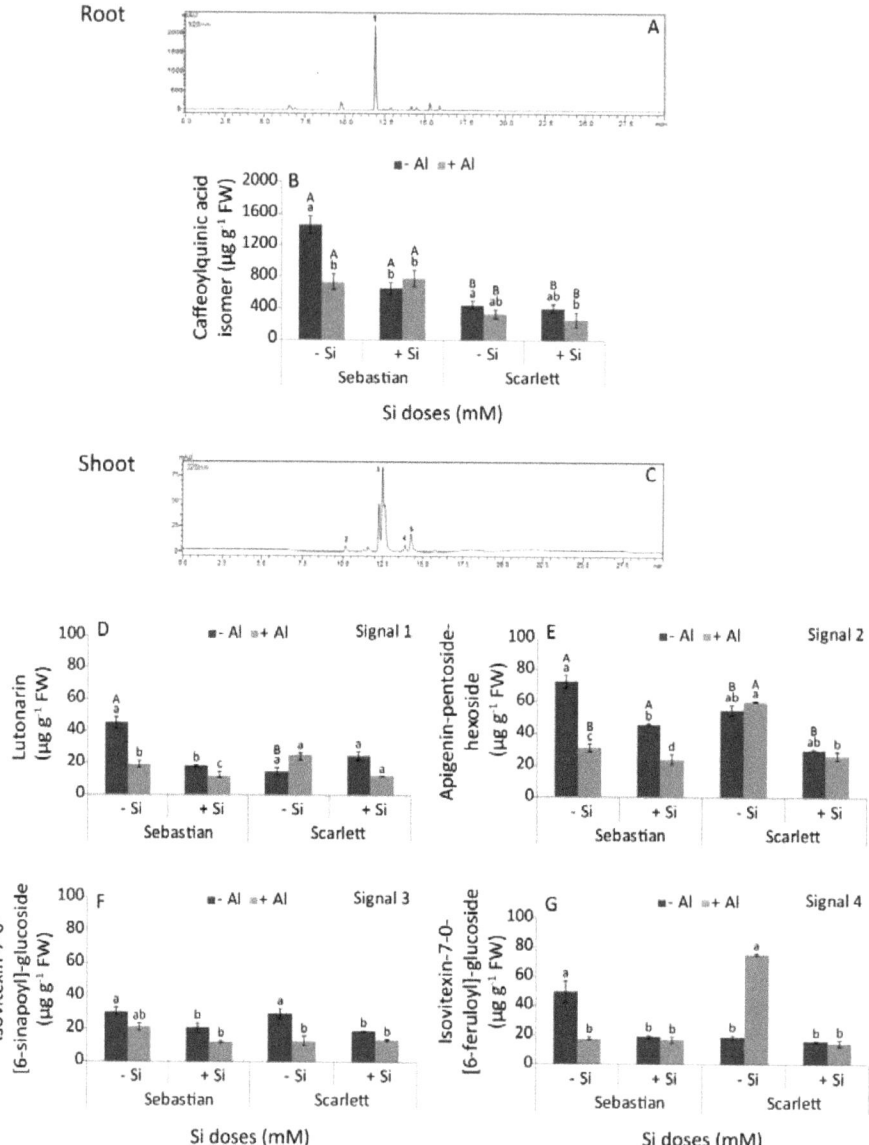

Figure 2. HPLC-DAD chromatograms (**A,C**) and individual phenolic concentration in shoots (**D–G**) and roots (**B**) of barley cultivars. Treatments were 0 or 0.2 mM Al, combined with 0 or 2 mM Si. Phenolic concentration values represent the mean of three replicates per treatment ± SD. Different letters indicate statistically significant differences ($p \leq 0.05$) among treatments. The lower case letters represent significant differences between treatments for the same barley cultivar. The upper case letters indicate significant differences between barley cultivars for the same treatment. When uppercase letters do not appear, no significant differences between the same treatment in different cultivars were found.

3.2.3. Oxidative Damage

Lipid peroxidation was not significantly affected by the interaction between cultivar and treatment, but a significant effect of Al/Si treatments on oxidative damage was observed. Barley cultivars showed an increase in lipid peroxidation as a result of the application of 0.2 mM Al. For Sebastian this increase was about 44% in shoots and 29% in roots, whereas for Scarlett the oxidative damage increased by 28% in shoots and 57% in roots in Al-treated plants (Figure 1E,F). By contrast, lipid peroxidation decreased in Sebastian shoots (Figure 1E) when Si was applied alone (38%) or in combination with Al (35%). Likewise, in roots, this reduction was about 75% and 60%, respectively (Figure 1F). Similarly, a reduction in lipid peroxidation was observed in Scarlett following Si addition (29% in shoots and 60% in roots) compared to control. Moreover, plants supplied with 0.2 mM Al and 2 mM Si showed a reduction in lipid peroxidation of about 37% in shoots and 68% in roots, compared to plants exposed to 0.2 mM Al (Figure 1E,F).

3.3. Silicon Influence on Plant Structure

3.3.1. Plant Stretching

We measured hypocotyl stretching by using an extensometer to evaluate cell wall creep in culms of plants cultivated under the different experimental treatments. Barley culm stretching was significantly influenced by the interaction between cultivar and treatment (Figure 3). For both cultivars, when Al was applied alone, greater stretching was evidenced compared to the control. However, Si addition decreased the stretching independent of added Al, thus improving the strength of the tissues.

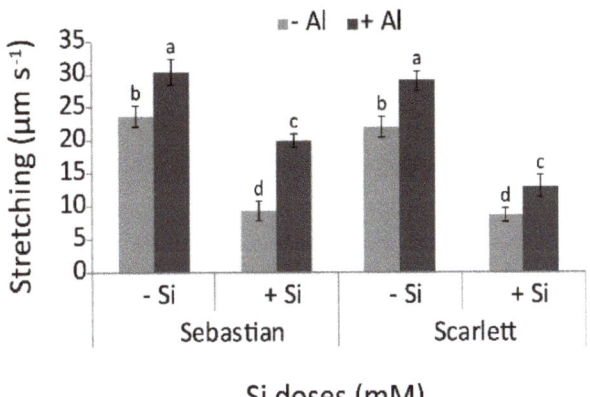

Figure 3. Stretching culm of the two barley cultivars in all treatments (0 or 0.2 mM Al, combined with 0 or 2 mM Si). Values represent the mean of three replicates per treatment ± SD. Different letters indicate statistically significant differences ($p \leq 0.05$) among treatments. The lower case letters represent significant differences between treatments for the same barley cultivar. The upper case letters indicate significant differences between barley cultivars for the same treatment. When uppercase letters do not appear, no significant differences between the same treatment in different cultivars were found.

3.3.2. Lignin Content and Composition

Sebastian and Scarlett shoots and roots showed greater lignin accumulation when Al or Si was applied (Figure 4). The highest accumulation was observed in both cultivars under the +Al/+Si treatment.

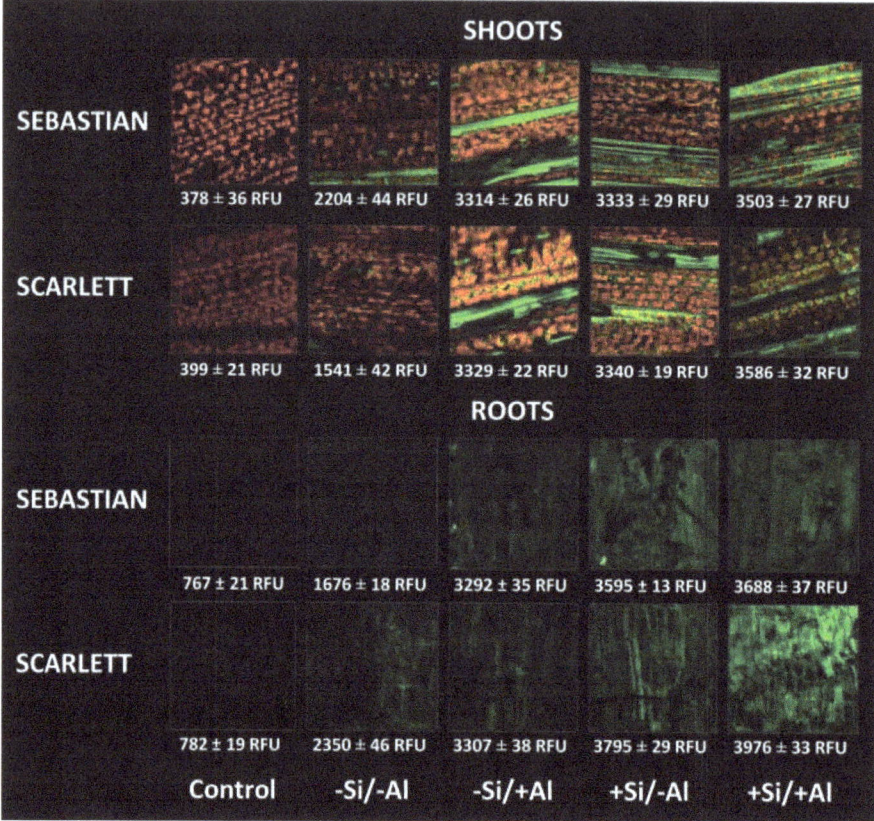

Figure 4. Visualization of lignin contents (green color) in barley roots and shoots of Sebastian and Scarlett cultivars, harvested after 21 days. Treatments were 0 or 0.2 mM Al, combined with 0 or 2 mM Si. The detection of safranine fluorescence was expressed as relative fluorescence unit (RFU). Values represent the mean of three replicates per treatment ± SD.

The effect of Al and Si on the total lignin calculated as the sum of monomers vanillyl (V), syringyl (S) and cinnamyl (C) and its composition were determined. The interaction between cultivar and treatment had a significant effect on lignin monomers and total lignin concentration of shoots and roots. Accordingly, Sebastian shoots showed an increase in cinnamyl and total lignin concentration (Figure 5A) as a consequence of Al addition. In the roots, the lignin concentration was reduced in the +Al/+Si treatment (Figure 6A). For Scarlett, increased concentrations of vanillyl phenols (shoots), cinnamyl phenols (roots) and total lignin (roots) were recorded in the +Al/+Si treatment compared to control (Figures 5B and 6B).

Sebastian shoots showed an increased cinnamyl:vanillyl (C/V) ratio when Al was supplied (Figure 5C), whereas the syringyl:vanillyl (S/V) ratio of roots exhibited higher values for the +Al/+Si treatment (Figure 6C). In contrast, the C/V (shoots) and S/V (roots) ratios of Scarlett were enhanced by 2 mM Si. Moreover, the C/V ratio of shoots was reduced when 0.2 mM Al and 2 mM Si were added, whereas it was increased in roots (Figures 5D and 6D). The acid to aldehyde ratio of vanillin in Sebastian shoots was enhanced by Si supply, irrespective of the Al dose (Figure 5E). Similarly, Scarlett roots in the +Al/−Si treatment increased the acid to aldehyde ratio of vanillin (Figure 6F). Conversely, plants treated with −Al/+Si reduced the acid to aldehyde ratio of syringyl (Figure 6F).

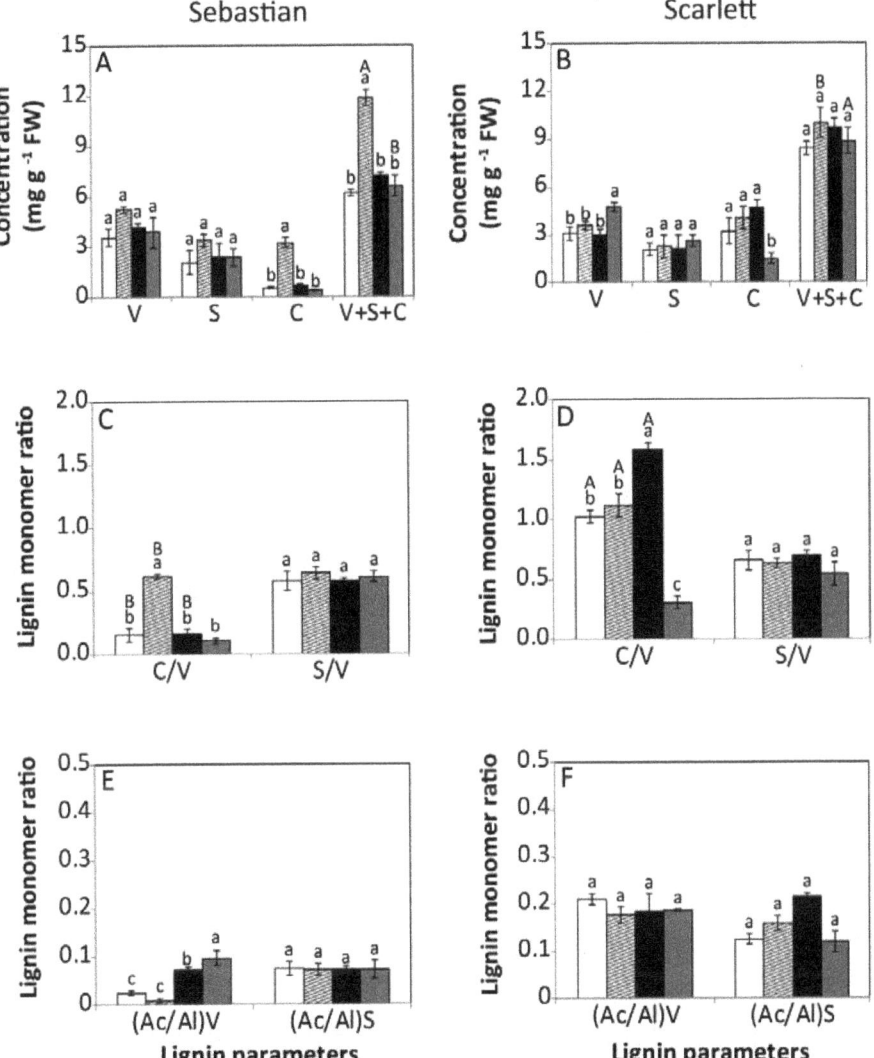

Figure 5. Lignin parameters of the shoots of Sebastian and Scarlett barley cultivars. The main lignin groups (**A**,**B**), comprising vanillyl [V], syringyl [S] and cinnamyl [C] phenols, and total lignin concentration [S + V + C]; their ratios (**C**,**D**); and acid to aldehyde ratios (**E**,**F**) of vanillyl [(Ac/Al)v] and syringyl [(Ac/Al)s]. Treatments were 0 or 0.2 mM Al, combined with 0 or 2 mM Si. Values represent the mean of three replicates per treatment ± SD. Different letters indicate statistically significant differences ($p \leq 0.05$) among treatments. The lower case letters represent significant differences between treatments for the same barley cultivar. The upper case letters indicate significant differences between barley cultivars for the same treatment. When uppercase letters do not appear, no significant differences between the same treatment in different cultivars were found.

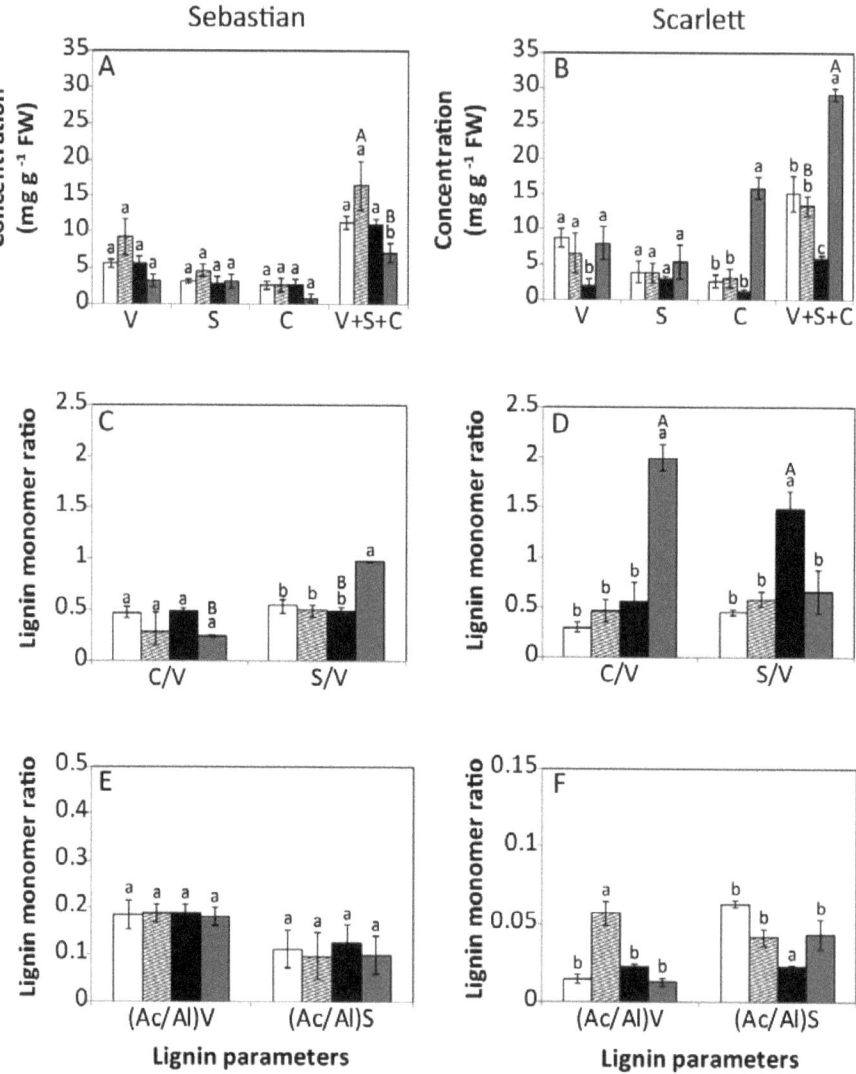

Figure 6. Lignin parameters of the roots of Sebastian and Scarlett barley cultivars. The main lignin groups (**A,B**), comprising vanillyl [V], syringyl [S] and cinnamyl [C] phenols, and total lignin concentration [S + V + C]; their ratios (**C,D**); and acid to aldehyde ratios (**E,F**) of vanillyl [(Ac/Al)v], and syringyl [(Ac/Al)s]. Treatments were 0 or 0.2 mM Al, combined with Si (0 or 2 mM). Values represent the mean of three replicates per treatment ± SD. Different letters indicate statistically significant differences ($p \leq 0.05$) among treatments. The lower case letters represent significant differences between treatments for the same barley cultivar. The upper case letters indicate significant differences between barley cultivars for the same treatment. When uppercase letters do not appear, no significant differences between the same treatment in different cultivars were found.

4. Discussion

It is well known that the effects of Al on plant growth vary markedly among plant species and cultivars [44]. In this respect, the Scarlett cultivar was more sensitive to Al than the Sebastian cultivar, and showed a higher Al concentration in the roots and shoots and a much lower plant dry weight (DW) than Sebastian (Tables 1 and 2). These findings agree with the greater Al-tolerance of Sebastian, and with earlier research showing different Al sensitivity for both barley cultivars in the short-term [17]. On the other hand, Si supply increased root DW in Sebastian and Scarlett cultivars. Nevertheless, both Si and Al concentrations were reduced in plant tissues when Al and Si were added simultaneously. Thus, our findings confirmed the improvement in plant growth and Al detoxification in plant tissues due to Si addition, which is in agreement with similar studies of other plant species [8,18,33,45,46].

In previous investigations, Si resulted in an improvement in the antioxidant system of plants subjected to abiotic stresses [1–3,11,12,14,47]. Under Si supply, different biochemical responses during Al exposure such as an increment in antioxidant compounds (e.g. phenols compounds, vitamins) and enzyme activities have been reported [30,48–51]. We observed an increase in both soluble phenol concentration and free radical scavenging activity in roots exposed to the +Al/+Si treatment (Figure 1B,D). This increase was accompanied by a reduction in lipid peroxidation (Figure 1F), which was more evident in the Al-sensitive (Scarlett) than in the Al-tolerant (Sebastian) cultivar. These responses could be at least partially associated with either the mitigation of Al stress through Al chelation by flavonoids at the cell wall level [16,52] or the incorporation of soluble phenols into the lignin biosynthetic pathway as demonstrated by the increase in lignin content under Al supply (Figure 4).

Additionally, we identified caffeoylquinic acid isomer (CQA), which belongs to the group of chlorogenic acids, in the roots of both barley cultivars (Figure 2A). In this context, chlorogenic acids function as intermediates in the lignin biosynthesis pathway, and they are regarded as powerful antioxidant compounds [53]. In all treatments, a higher CQA concentration was found in Sebastian roots as compared to those of Scarlett (Figure 2B). Nevertheless, Sebastian showed a reduction in CQA concentration compared to the control when plants were treated with either Si or Al alone or in combination, whereas in Scarlett the decrease in CQA was only found in the +Al/+Si treatment. Since chlorogenic acids are one of the main building blocks of lignin, the decrease of CQA due to the combined application of Si and Al might be associated with the greater accumulation of lignin in the roots (Figure 4).

The phenolic compounds identified in shoots belong to the group of flavonoids, specifically flavone-glucosides (i.e., compounds (1) to (7) mentioned above). Briefly, lutonarin, apigenin derivate (apigenin-pentoxide-hexoside) and saponarin derivatives (isovitexin-7-O-[6-sinapoyl]-glucoside, isovitexin-7-O-[6-feruloyl]-glucoside) were identified and quantified (Figure 2C). These compounds were similar to those already described for barley shoots [54,55]. In our study, the concentration of lutonarin and apigenin-pentoxide-hexoside was decreased in Sebastian shoots in all treatments compared to control, but no changes in lutonarin were observed in Scarlett (Figure 2D,E). However, the concentration of isovitexin-7-O-[6-feruloyl]-glucoside was increased 2.7-fold by Al addition (Figure 2G). Despite the reduction in flavones as a result of Al or Si addition, high antioxidant activity by flavonoids such as saponarin and lutonarin has been reported in barley shoots [56].

On the other hand, increased lignin accumulation in shoots following Al and Si supply was observed for both cultivars (Figure 4). In fact, a reduction in culm stretching after Si addition in barley plants confirmed there was an improvement in lignin accumulation in shoots irrespective of Al addition (Figure 3). In the Al-sensitive cultivar (Scarlett) total lignin concentration in roots, quantified as the sum of the monomers (V + C + S), was improved by Si addition under Al stress. This increase is in agreement with the higher intensity of safranine staining (Figure 4), and supports previous findings showing that Si has a mitigating effect due to increased production of lignin under stressful conditions [19,22,57]. Such an effect may be associated with either increased hydrogen peroxide production or peroxidase activity in cell walls [58,59]. Likewise, it has been demonstrated that Si increases the activities of enzymes such as peroxidase, polyphenol oxidase, and phenylalanine ammonia lyase, which are involved in the lignin biosynthesis pathway [18,60].

Moreover, differences in lignin composition have been observed under stress conditions [61–65], but little is known about the role that lignin with different compositions might exert in vascular plants [66]. While the monomer composition allows us to distinguish the origin of vegetation (i.e., angiosperms or gymnosperms), C/V and S/V ratios could be used as indicators of the origin and degradability of lignin [67,68]. Thus, the range of individual monomers (V, C, S) obtained here (Figure 5A,B and Figure 6A,B) agree with those reported in grasses [69]. In Scarlett roots, increased C/V and S/V ratios were observed in plants treated with Si, irrespective of the Al addition (Figure 6D). A similar trend in the S/V ratio in Sebastian roots was found due to the combined application of 0.2 mM Al and 2 mM Si (Figure 6C). In addition, Si decreased the acid to aldehyde ratio of V in Scarlett roots (Figure 6F). Higher proportions of C and S units indicate lower lignin stability and may influence biogeochemical cycling differently after it is returned to soil. Further studies under field conditions are needed to confirm this hypothesis.

Hence, Si fertilization in barley can be envisaged as a key strategy for counteracting Al toxicity. Changes in soluble phenols and lignin production/composition mediated by Si appear to be involved in improving the performance of barley cultivars, since an enhancement in root growth and plant antioxidant ability was observed when Si was supplied to Al stressed plants. Some hypotheses have been proposed to explain the possible linkage between Si and phenol metabolism. For example, Williams [70] proposed that OH groups of phenols are condensed with Si(OH) in biological systems, and Inanaga et al. [24] suggested that Si may be associated with lignin-carbohydrate complexes in the wall of epidermal cells. Silicon might also be involved in signal transduction pathways, thus inducing lignin production [21]. Despite the evidence regarding the impact of Si supply on the production of antioxidant or structural phenolic compounds, the mechanisms implicated in the modulation of phenolic metabolism by Si need to be investigated further.

Author Contributions: Data curation, I.V.; Formal analysis, I.V., C.R., A.R. and D.F.C.; Funding acquisition, P.C.; Methodology, I.V.; Supervision, P.C.; Visualization, I.V.; Writing—original draft, I.V.; Writing—review & editing, I.V., C.R., A.R., D.F.C., M.d.l.L.M. and P.C. All authors have read and agreed to the published version of the manuscript.

Funding: This research was funded by FONDECYT projects 1161326 and 1201257.

Acknowledgments: The authors gratefully acknowledge the Institute of Ecology and Environmental Sciences of Paris, Institute of Plant Production and Protection of Universidad Austral de Chile, University of Castilla-La Mancha, Spain, Centro de Investigación en Micorrizas y Sustentabilidad Agroambiental and Scientific and Technological Bioresource Nucleus of Universidad de La Frontera, for providing access to specialized equipment used in phenolics, lignin and plant stretching analyses. The authors also thank the Maltexco company for contributing the barley seeds used in this research and Dirección de Investigación of Universidad de La Frontera. CR acknowledges the MEC-CONICYT project 80180025.

Conflicts of Interest: The authors declare no conflict of interest.

References

1. Liang, Y.; Wong, J.W.C.; Wei, L. Silicon-mediated enhancement of cadmium tolerance in maize (*Zea mays* L.) grown in cadmium contaminated soil. *Chemosphere* **2005**, *58*, 475–483. [CrossRef] [PubMed]
2. Kim, Y.H.; Khan, A.L.; Waqas, M.; Lee, I.J. Silicon regulates antioxidant activities of crop plants under abiotic-induced oxidative stress: A review. *Front. Plant Sci.* **2017**, *8*, 510. [CrossRef] [PubMed]
3. Wang, M.; Gao, L.; Dong, S.; Sun, Y.; Shen, Q.; Guo, S. Role of silicon on plant–pathogen interactions. *Front. Plant Sci.* **2017**, *8*, 701. [CrossRef] [PubMed]
4. Ma, J.F.; Yamaji, N. Silicon uptake and accumulation in higher plants. *Trends Plant Sci.* **2006**, *11*, 392–397. [CrossRef]
5. Ma, J.F.; Tamai, K.; Yamaji, N.; Mitani, N.; Konishi, S.; Katsuhara, M.; Yano, M. A silicon transporter in rice. *Nature* **2006**, *440*, 688–691. [CrossRef]

6. Ma, J.F.; Yamaji, N.; Mitani, N.; Tamai, K.; Konishi, S.; Fujiwara, T. An efflux transporter of silicon in rice. *Nature* **2007**, *448*, 209–212. [CrossRef]
7. Pontigo, S.; Ribera, A.; Gianfreda, L.; Mora, M.D.L.L.; Nikoli, M.; Cartes, P. Silicon in vascular plants: Uptake, transport and its influence on mineral stress under acidic conditions. *Planta* **2015**, *242*, 23–37. [CrossRef]
8. Pontigo, S.; Godoy, K.; Jiménez, H.; Gutiérrez-Moraga, A.; Mora, M.L.; Cartes, P. Silicon-mediated alleviation of aluminum toxicity by modulatin of Al/Si uptake and antioxidant performance in ryegrass plants. *Front. Plant Sci.* **2017**, *8*, 642. [CrossRef]
9. Guerriero, G.; Hausman, J.F.; Legay, S. Silicon and the Plant Extracellular Matrix. *Front. Plant Sci.* **2016**, *7*, 463. [CrossRef]
10. Luyckx, M.; Hausman, J.F.; Lutts, S.; Guerriero, G. Silicon and Plants: Current Knowledge and Technological Perspectives. *Front. Plant Sci.* **2017**, *8*, 411. [CrossRef]
11. Abd_Allah, E.F.; Hashem, A.; Alam, P.; Ahmad, P. Silicon alleviates nickel-induced oxidative stress by regulating antioxidant defense and glyoxalase systems in mustard plants. *J. Plant Growth Regul.* **2019**, *38*, 1260–1273. [CrossRef]
12. Lukacova, Z.; Svubova, R.; Janikovicova, S.; Volajova, Z.; Lux, A. Tobacco plants (*Nicotiana benthamiana*) were influenced by silicon and were not infected by dodder (*Cuscuta europaea*). *Plant Physiol. Biochem.* **2019**, *139*, 179–190. [CrossRef] [PubMed]
13. Schaller, J.; Heimes, R.; Ma, J.F.; Meunier, J.D.; Shao, J.F.; Fujii-Kashino, M.; Knorr, K.H. Silicon accumulation in rice plant aboveground biomass affects leaf carbon quality. *Plant Soil.* **2019**, *444*, 399–407. [CrossRef]
14. Ahanger, M.A.; Bhat, J.A.; Siddiqui, M.H.; Rinklebe, J.; Ahmad, P. Silicon and secondary metabolites integration in plants: A Significant association in stress tolerance. *J. Exp. Bot.* **2020**. [CrossRef] [PubMed]
15. Maksimović, J.; Bogdanović, J.; Maksimović, V.; Nikolic, M. Silicon modulates the metabolism and utilization of phenolic compounds in cucumber (*Cucumis sativus* L.) grown at excess manganese. *J. Soil Sci. Plant Nutr.* **2007**, *170*, 739–744. [CrossRef]
16. Kidd, P.S.; Llugany, M.; Poschenrieder, C.H.; Gunse, B.; Barcelo, J. The role of root exudates in aluminium resistance and silicon-induced amelioration of aluminium toxicity in three varieties of maize (*Zea mays* L.). *J. Exp. Bot.* **2001**, *52*, 1339–1352. [CrossRef]
17. Vega, I.; Nikolic, M.; Pontigo, S.; Godoy, K.; Mora, M.D.L.L.; Cartes, P. Silicon improves the production of high antioxidant or structural phenolic compounds in barley cultivars under aluminum stress. *Agronomy* **2019**, *9*, 388. [CrossRef]
18. Ribera-Fonseca, A.; Rumpel, C.; Mora, M.L.; Nikolic, M.; Cartes, P. Sodium silicate and calcium silicate differentially affect silicon and aluminium uptake, antioxidant performance and phenolics metabolism of ryegrass in an acid Andisol. *Crop. Pasture Sci.* **2018**, *69*, 205–215. [CrossRef]
19. Filha, M.X.; Rodrigues, F.A.; Domiciano, G.P.; Oliveira, H.V.; Silveira, P.R.; Moreira, W.R. Wheat resistance to leaf blast mediated by silicon. *Australas. Plant Pathol.* **2011**, *40*, 28–38. [CrossRef]
20. Shetty, R.; Fretté, X.; Jensen, B.; Shetty, N.P.; Jensen, J.D.; Jørgensen, H.J.L.; Christensen, L.P. Silicon-induced changes in antifungal phenolic acids, flavonoids, and key phenylpropanoid pathway genes during the interaction between miniature roses and the biotrophic pathogen *Podosphaera pannosa*. *Plant Physiol.* **2011**, *157*, 2194–2205. [CrossRef]
21. Fleck, A.T.; Nye, T.; Repenning, C.; Stahl, F.; Zahn, M.; Schenk, M.K. Silicon enhances suberization and lignification in roots of rice (*Oryza sativa*). *J. Exp. Bot.* **2010**, *62*, 2001–2011. [CrossRef] [PubMed]
22. Hussain, S.; Shuxian, L.; Mumtaz, M.; Shafiq, I.; Iqbal, N.; Brestic, M.; Bing, C. Foliar application of silicon improves stem strength under low light stress by regulating lignin biosynthesis genes in soybean (*Glycine max* (L.) Merr.). *J. Hazard. Mater.* **2020**, 123256. [CrossRef]
23. Shahnaz, G.; Shekoofeh, E.; Kourosh, D.; Moohamadbagher, B. Interactive effects of silicon and aluminum on the malondialdehyde (MDA), proline, protein and phenolic compounds in *Borago officinalis* L. *J. Med. Plant Res.* **2011**, *5*, 5818–5827.
24. Inanaga, S.; Okasaka, A.; Tanaka, S. Does silicon exist in association with organic compounds in rice plant? *J. Soil Sci.* **1995**, *41*, 111–117. [CrossRef]
25. Watteau, F.; Villemin, G. Ultrastructural study of the biogeochemical cycle of silicon in the soil and litter of a temperate forest. *Eur. J. Soil Sci.* **2001**, *52*, 385–396. [CrossRef]
26. Baik, B.K.; Ullrich, S.E. Barley for food: Characteristics, improvement, and renewed interest. *J. Cereal Sci.* **2008**, *48*, 233–242. [CrossRef]

27. Lahouar, L.; El Arem, A.; Ghrairi, F.; Chahdoura, H.; Salem, H.B.; El Felah, M.; Achour, L. Phytochemical content and antioxidant properties of diverse varieties of whole barley (*Hordeum vulgare* L.) grown in Tunisia. *Food Chem.* **2014**, *145*, 578–583. [CrossRef]
28. Stuper-Szablewska, K.; Perkowski, J. Phenolic acids in cereal grain: Occurrence, biosynthesis, metabolism and role in living organisms. *Crit. Rev. Food Sci.* **2019**, *59*, 664–675. [CrossRef]
29. Hammond, K.E.; Evans, D.E.; Hodson, M.J. Aluminium/silicon interactions in barley (*Hordeum vulgare* L.) seedlings. *Plant Soil* **1995**, *173*, 89–95. [CrossRef]
30. Balakhnina, T.I.; Matichenkov, V.V.; Wlodarczyk, T.; Borkowska, A.; Nosalewicz, M.; Fomina, I.R. Effects of silicon on growth processes and adaptive potential of barley plants under optimal soil watering and flooding. *Plant Growth Regul.* **2012**, *67*, 35–43. [CrossRef]
31. Cocker, K.M.; Evans, D.E.; Hodson, M.J. The amelioration of aluminium toxicity by silicon in higher plants: Solution chemistry or an in planta mechanism? *Physiol. Plant.* **1998**, *104*, 608–614. [CrossRef]
32. Khandekar, S.; Leisner, S. Soluble silicon modulates expression of Arabidopsis thaliana genes involved in copper stress. *J. Plant Physiol.* **2011**, *168*, 699–705. [CrossRef] [PubMed]
33. Dorneles, A.O.S.; Pereira, A.S.; Sasso, V.M.; Possebom, G.; Tarouco, C.P.; Schorr, M.R.W.; Tabaldi, L.A. Aluminum stress tolerance in potato genotypes grown with silicon. *Bragantia* **2019**. [CrossRef]
34. Taylor, G.J.; Foy, C.D. Effects of aluminum on the growth and element composition of 20 winter cultivars of *Triticum aestivum* L. (wheat) grown in solution culture. *J. Plant Nutr.* **1985**, *8*, 811–824. [CrossRef]
35. Sadzawka, A.; Carrasco, M.; Demane, R.; Flores, H.; Grez, R.; Mora, M.L.; Neaman, A. Métodos de análisis de tejidos vegetales. *Serie Actas INIA* **2007**, *40*, 140.
36. Pavlovic, J.; Samardzic, J.; Maksimović, V.; Timotijevic, G.; Stevic, N.; Laursen, K.H.; Nikolic, M. Silicon alleviates iron deficiency in cucumber by promoting mobilization of iron in the root apoplast. *N. Phytol.* **2013**, *198*, 1096–1107. [CrossRef]
37. Slinkard, K.; Singleton, V.L. Total phenol analysis: Automation and comparison with manual methods. *Am. J. Enol. Vitic.* **1977**, *28*, 49–55.
38. Santander, C.; Ruiz, A.; García, S.; Aroca, R.; Cumming, J.; Cornejo, P. Efficiency of two arbuscular mycorrhizal fungal inocula to improve saline stress tolerance in lettuce plants by changes of antioxidant defense mechanisms. *J. Sci. Food Agric.* **2020**, *100*, 1577–1587. [CrossRef]
39. Chinnici, F.; Bendini, A.; Gaiani, A.; Riponi, C. Radical scavenging activities of peels and pulps from cv. Golden Delicious apples as related to their phenolic composition. *J Agric. Food Chem.* **2004**, *52*, 4684–4689. [CrossRef]
40. Du, Z.; Bramlage, W.J. Modified thiobarbituric acid assay for measuring lipid oxidation in sugar-rich plant tissue extracts. *J Agric. Food Chem.* **1992**, *40*, 1566–1570. [CrossRef]
41. Perini, M.A.; Sin, I.N.; Martinez, G.A.; Civello, P.M. Measurement of expansin activity and plant cell wall creep by using a commercial texture analyzer. *Electron J. Biotechnol.* **2017**, *26*, 12–19. [CrossRef]
42. Sant'Anna, V.; Gurak, P.D.; Marczak, L.D.F.; Tessaro, I.C. Tracking bioactive compounds with colour changes in foods–A review. *Dyes Pigments* **2013**, *98*, 601–608. [CrossRef]
43. Kögel, I.; Bochter, R. Characterization of lignin in forest humus layers by high-performance liquid chromatography of cupric oxide oxidation products. *Soil Biol. Biochem.* **1985**, *17*, 637–640. [CrossRef]
44. Singh, S.; Tripathi, D.K.; Singh, S.; Sharma, S.; Dubey, N.K.; Chauhan, D.K.; Vaculík, M. Toxicity of aluminium on various levels of plant cells and organism: A review. *Environ. Exp. Bot.* **2017**, *137*, 177–193. [CrossRef]
45. De Freitas, L.B.; Fernandes, D.M.; Maia, S.C.M.; Fernandes, A.M. Effects of silicon on aluminum toxicity in upland rice plants. *Plant Soil.* **2017**, *420*, 263–275. [CrossRef]
46. De Jesus, L.R.; Batista, B.L.; da Silva Lobato, A.K. Silicon reduces aluminum accumulation and mitigates toxic effects in cowpea plants. *Acta Physiol. Plant.* **2017**, *39*, 138. [CrossRef]
47. Vaculík, M.; Lukačová, Z.; Bokor, B.; Martinka, M.; Tripathi, D.K.; Lux, A. Alleviation mechanisms of metal (loid) stress in plants by silicon: A review. *J. Exp. Bot.* **2020**. [CrossRef]
48. Zhang, Y.M.; Li, Y.; Chen, W.F.; Wang, E.T.; Tian, C.F.; Li, Q.Q.; Chen, W.X. Biodiversity and biogeography of rhizobia associated with soybean plants grown in the North China Plain. *Appl. Environ. Microbiol.* **2011**, *77*, 6331–6342. [CrossRef]
49. Zhu, Z.; Wei, G.; Li, J.; Qian, Q.; Yu, J. Silicon alleviates salt stress and increases antioxidant enzymes activity in leaves of salt-stressed cucumber (*Cucumis sativus* L.). *Plant Sci.* **2004**, *167*, 527–533. [CrossRef]

50. Farooq, M.A.; Ali, S.; Hameed, A.; Ishaque, W.; Mahmood, K.; Iqbal, Z. Alleviation of cadmium toxicity by silicon is related to elevated photosynthesis, antioxidant enzymes; suppressed cadmium uptake and oxidative stress in cotton. *Ecotoxicol. Environ. Saf.* **2013**, *96*, 242–249. [CrossRef]
51. Farooq, M.A.; Saqib, Z.A.; Akhtar, J.; Bakhat, H.F.; Pasala, R.K.; Dietz, K.J. Protective role of silicon (Si) against combined stress of salinity and boron (B) toxicity by improving antioxidant enzymes activity in rice. *Silicon* **2019**, *11*, 1–5. [CrossRef]
52. Wang, Y.; Stass, A.; Horst, W.J. Apoplastic binding of aluminum is involved in silicon-induced amelioration of aluminum toxicity in maize. *Plant Physiol.* **2004**, *136*, 3762–3770. [CrossRef] [PubMed]
53. Silva, N.; Mazzafera, P.; Cesarino, I. Should I stay or should I go: Are chlorogenic acids mobilized towards lignin biosynthesis? *Phytochemistry* **2019**, *166*, 112063. [CrossRef] [PubMed]
54. Ferreres, F.; Andrade, P.B.; Valentao, P.; Gil-Izquierdo, A. Further knowledge on barley (*Hordeum vulgare* L.) leaves O-glycosyl-C-glycosyl flavones by liquid chromatography-UV diode–array detection-electrospray ionisation mass spectrometry. *J. Chromatogr. A* **2008**, *1182*, 56–64. [CrossRef] [PubMed]
55. Piasecka, A.; Jedrzejczak-Rey, N.; Bednarek, P. Secondary metabolites in plant innate immunity: Conserved function of divergent chemicals. *N. Phytol.* **2015**, *206*, 948–964. [CrossRef] [PubMed]
56. Kamiyama, M.; Shibamoto, T. Flavonoids with potent antioxidant activity found in young green barley leaves. *J. Agric. Food Chem.* **2012**, *60*, 6260–6267. [CrossRef]
57. Zhang, J.L.; Shi, H. Physiological and molecular mechanisms of plant salt tolerance. *Photosynth. Res.* **2013**, *115*, 1–22. [CrossRef]
58. Yang, Y.F.; Liang, Y.C.; Lou, Y.S.; Sun, W.C. Influences of silicon on peroxidase, superoxide dismutase activity and lignin content in leaves of wheat *Tritium aestivum* L. and its relation to resistance to powdery mildew. *Sci. Agric. Sin.* **2003**, *36*, 813–817.
59. Ma, J.F.; Yamaji, N.; Mitani, N. Transport of silicon from roots to panicles in plants. *Proc. Jpn. Acad. Ser. B Phys. Biol. Sci.* **2011**, *87*, 377–385. [CrossRef]
60. Cai, X.N.; Davis, E.J.; Ballif, J.; Liang, M.X.; Bushman, E.; Haroldsen, V.; Torabinejad, J.; Wu, Y.J. Mutant identification and characterization of the laccase gene family in Arabidopsis. *J. Exp. Bot.* **2006**, *57*, 2563–2569. [CrossRef]
61. Betz, G.A.; Knappe, C.; Lapierre, C.; Olbrich, M.; Welzl, G.; Langebartels, C.; Ernst, D. Ozone affects shikimate pathway transcripts and monomeric lignin composition in European beech (*Fagus sylvatica* L.). *Eur. J. For. Res.* **2009**, *128*, 109–116. [CrossRef]
62. Cabané, M.; Pireaux, J.C.; Léger, E.; Weber, E.; Dizengremel, P.; Pollet, B.; Lapierre, C. Condensed lignins are synthesized in poplar leaves exposed to ozone. *Plant Physiol.* **2004**, *134*, 586–594. [CrossRef] [PubMed]
63. Finger-Teixeira, A.; Ferrarese, M.D.L.L.; Soares, A.R.; da Silva, D.; Ferrarese-Filho, O. Cadmium-induced lignification restricts soybean root growth. *Ecotoxicol. Environ. Saf.* **2010**, *73*, 1959–1964. [CrossRef] [PubMed]
64. Frankenstein, C.; Schmitt, U.; Koch, G. Topochemical studies on modified lignin distribution in the xylem of poplar (*Populus* spp.) after wounding. *Ann. Bot.* **2006**, *97*, 195–204. [CrossRef] [PubMed]
65. Pitre, F.; Cooke, J.; Mackay, J. Short-term effects of nitrogen availability on wood 1056 formation and fibre properties in hybrid poplar. *Trees Struct. Funct.* **2007**, *1057*, 249–259. [CrossRef]
66. Liu, Q.; Luo, L.; Zheng, L. Lignins: Biosynthesis and biological functions in plants. *Int. J. Mol. Sci.* **2018**, *19*, 335. [CrossRef]
67. Thevenot, M.; Dignac, M.F.; Rumpel, C. Fate of lignins in soils: A review. *Soil Biol. Biochem.* **2010**, *42*, 1200–1211. [CrossRef]
68. Abiven, S.; Heim, A.; Schmidt, M.W. Lignin content and chemical characteristics in maize and wheat vary between plant organs and growth stages: Consequences for assessing lignin dynamics in soil. *Plant Soil* **2011**, *343*, 369–378. [CrossRef]
69. Otto, A.; Shunthirasingham, C.; Simpson, M.J. A comparison of plant and microbial biomarkers in grassland soils from the Prairie Ecozone of Canada. *Org. Geochem.* **2005**, *36*, 425–448. [CrossRef]
70. Williams, R.J.P. Introduction to Silicon Chemistry and Biochemistry. In *Silicon Biochemistry*; John Wiley & Sons: Hoboken, NJ, USA, 1986; pp. 24–29.

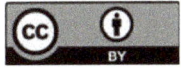

© 2020 by the authors. Licensee MDPI, Basel, Switzerland. This article is an open access article distributed under the terms and conditions of the Creative Commons Attribution (CC BY) license (http://creativecommons.org/licenses/by/4.0/).

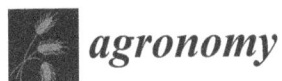

Article

Improved Growth and Yield Response of Jew's Mallow (*Corchorus olitorius* L.) Plants through Biofertilization under Semi-Arid Climate Conditions in Egypt

Ahmed Fathy Yousef [1,2,†], Mohamed Ahmed Youssef [3,†], Muhammad Moaaz Ali [1], Muhammed Mustapha Ibrahim [1,4], Yong Xu [5,6,*] and Rosario Paolo Mauro [7,*]

1. College of Horticulture, Fujian Agriculture and Forestry University, Fuzhou 350002, China; ahmedfathy201161@yahoo.com (A.F.Y.); muhammadmoaazali@yahoo.com (M.M.A.); scholarmusty@yahoo.com (M.M.I.)
2. Department of Horticulture, College of Agriculture, University of Al-Azhar (branch Assiut), Assiut 71524, Egypt
3. Department of Soils and Water, College of Agriculture, University of Al-Azhar (branch Assiut), Assiut 71524, Egypt; Dr_mayoussef@azhar.edu.eg
4. Department of Soil Science, University of Agriculture Makurdi, Makurdi 972211, Nigeria
5. College of Mechanical and Electronic Engineering, Fujian Agriculture and Forestry University, Fuzhou 350002, China
6. Institute of Machine Learning and Intelligent Science, Fujian University of Technology, 33 Xuefu South Road, Fuzhou 350118, China
7. Dipartimento di Agricoltura, Alimentazione e Ambiente (Di3A) Via Valdisavoia, Università degli Studi di Catania, 5-95123 Catania, Italy
* Correspondence: y.xu@fafu.edu.cn (Y.X.); rosario.mauro@unict.it (R.P.M.); Tel.: +86-591-8378-9374 (Y.X.); +39-095-4783314 (R.P.M.)
† Both authors contributed equally to this work.

Received: 17 October 2020; Accepted: 13 November 2020; Published: 16 November 2020

Abstract: This study was conducted to comparatively assess the effects of fertilization typology (organic, inorganic, and biofertilization) on the growth, yield, and compositional profile of Jew's mallow. The experiment was carried out over two growing seasons, under semi-arid climate conditions on silty loam soil. We adopted three fertilization strategies: (1) inorganic NPK fertilizer (146, 74, and 57 kg ha^{-1} for N, P_2O_5, and K_2O, respectively), (2) farmyard manure (36 m^3 ha^{-1}), and (3) a biofertilizer (a set of mixed cultures of *Bacillus* spp., *Candida* spp., and *Trichoderma* spp. at 36 L ha^{-1}). Treatment combinations were control (without fertilization, T_1), NPK fertilizer (T_2), farmyard manure (FYM, T_3), biofertilizer (T_4), NPK+biofertilizer (T_5), and FYM+biofertilizer (T_6). The T_5 treatment maximized both plant and leaf biomass (up to 31.6 and 8.0 t ha^{-1}, respectively), plant height (68.5 cm), leaf area (370 cm m^{-2}), leaf protein content (18.7%), as well as N, P, and K concentration in leaves (2.99, 0.88, and 2.01 mg 100 g^{-1}, respectively). The leaves' weight incidence was lower in T_5 treatment (36.7%) as compared to the unfertilized plants (T_1). The results revealed that the combined application of inorganic NPK plus biofertilizer is most beneficial to increase growth, yield, and nutrient accumulation in Jew's mallow plants.

Keywords: leafy vegetable; mineral nutrients; soil structure; chlorophyll content; cation exchange capacity

1. Introduction

Over the years, mineral fertilizers have helped agriculture enhance crop productivity to meet the ever-increasing demand for food. However, the overutilization of inorganic fertilizers poses a negative impact on the environment and soil functioning and fertility [1]. Moreover, it leads to the high cost of crop production. Therefore, many researchers have tried to restore soil fertility through the use of organic materials of plant or/and animal origin, in the forms of organic fertilizers. Organic fertilization involves the use of naturally occurring material that includes animal manures and agricultural residues [2]. These materials have been proposed to boost the supply of inorganic nutrients, which can bridge fertilizer demand due to economic and environmental reasons [3]. Organic manure increases the status of soil nutrients via the gradual release of minerals to the soil as well as enhancing its physical, biological, and chemical properties [4,5]. Also, organic manure has been shown to improve the agronomic performances of many crops [6].

Biofertilizers are substances containing living organisms and organic materials that can be utilized to increase soil nutrients availability and promote plant growth and productivity. They are also considered an eco-friendly way toward sustainable agriculture because they do not cause pollution [7,8]. Biofertilizers have become a preferable alternative or supplement to organic and inorganic fertilizers. Therefore, to increase soil productivity, the utilization of biofertilizers has become increasingly important, because they help in stimulating plant growth hormones, thereby enhancing nutrients uptake and increasing tolerance towards several abiotic stressors too [9]. Biofertilizers can be applied to seeds, soils, rhizosphere, or plant surfaces. Moreover, they are less costly and sometimes more effective as compared to inorganic fertilizers [10–12] Jew's mallow (*Corchorus olitorious* L.) belongs to the Malvaceae (Tiliacea) family and classed in the genera of about 40–100 species of the flowering plants [13]. It is also known as jute mallow in English and called Mulukhiyah in Egypt. The leaves are edible either fresh, dried, or frozen by many Egyptians because it is a quite cheap vegetable and forms part of the national Egyptian dishes [8]. It is one of the popular tropical green leafy vegetables of great importance in most countries in the Middle East and Latin America [14], Africa, and Asia [15].

Jew's mallow is a source of income for smallholders and poor families in Egypt, farmers cultivate Jew's mallow in many marginal areas. They use their seeds, which consequently result in genetic diversity in Jew's mallow distribution in Egypt [16]. Recently, Jew's mallow, which is a neglected and underutilized crop species (NUS), has received great international recognition because of its role in providing food and nutrition security and income opportunities among smallholder farmers. Moreover, NUS can be utilized to adapt agriculture and food systems to climate change [17]. Jew's mallow plays an important role in humans nutrition because its leaves contain an average 13–15% dry matter, 4.7 mg vitamin A, 259–266 mg Ca, 250–261 Mg, 4.5–8 mg Fe, 4.8–6 g protein, 92 µg foliates, 105 mg ascorbic acid, 1.5 mg nicotinamide, 0.9 g folic acid, 0.7 g oil, 5 g carbohydrate, and 1–5 g fiber per 100 g of edible leaves [13,18]. Additionally, the seeds of *C. olitorius* can be integrated into livestock feeds and human diets [19].

Jew's mallow performs well in marginal areas, even without the addition of organic and/or inorganic fertilizers, as well as under fertilized conditions, especially with application of N [20]. In this regard, Olaniyi and Ajibola [21] found that the use of N, P, and K fertilization significantly increased plant height, fresh shoots biomass, number of leaves, and dry matter content of Jew's mallow above the control (no fertilization). Thus, it is concluded that the yields and growth of the crop could significantly be improved by soil application of N, P, and K fertilizers at the optimum rate of 45, 30, and 20 kg ha^{-1}, respectively. Also, Aisha, et al. [22] found that application of 70% (100, 100, and 80 kg ha^{-1} NPK, respectively) of inorganic fertilizer recommended rate on spinach plants gave rise to the longest harvest period, the highest total weight of leaves and its various organs and improve leaves nutritional values, including N, P, K, and protein contents. However, using biofertilizers in Jew's mallow cultivation has not received adequate attention, whether singly or in integrated use with organic and inorganic fertilizers. Similarly, the effects of these combinations on the nutrient uptake require proper understanding and documentation, which is still lacking in the reported literature.

Therefore, this study aimed to assess the bio-agronomical response of Jew's mallow to the combined soil incorporation of organic, inorganic and biofertilization, so checking the possibility to obtain a more sustainable fertilization technique for the crop.

2. Materials and Methods

2.1. Experimental Site

A two-year field experiment was carried out under semi-arid climate conditions on silty loam soil at the Research Farm of the College of Agriculture, Al-Azhar University, Assiut branch. The location is (27°12′16.67″ N; 31°09′36.86″ E) in Assiut governorate, Egypt. Table 1 shows some physical and chemical properties of the soil at the experimental site, collected at a depth of 0–30 cm and analyzed as described by [23].

Table 1. Some physical and chemical properties of the experimental soil in 2017 and 2018.

Parameter		Value	
		2017	2018
Particle Size Dist.	Sand (%)	20.0	18.3
	Silt (%)	56.5	59.6
	Clay (%)	23.5	22.1
Texture grade		Silty loam	Silty loam
pH Susp. (1:2.5)		8.22	8.28
E.C (dSm^{-1}) soil past		0.487	0.336
O.M (%)		1.98	1.91
Total CaCO$_3$ %		1.48	1.42
Cations (cmol.kg^{-1} soil)			
Ca^{++}		8.54	6.89
Mg^{++}		13.56	10.43
Na^{+}		22.72	18.07
K^{+}		3.32	2.12
Anions (cmol.kg^{-1} soil)			
HCO$_3^-$		6.54	4.87
Cl$^-$		20.52	16.65
SO$_4^=$		2.84	2.15

Each value represents a mean of three replicates. E.C: electrical conductivity; O.M: organic matter.

2.2. Experimental Design and Treatments

Treatments were laid out using a randomized blocks design with three replications. Each plot unit included a totally flat area of 10.5 m^2. The seeds of Jew's mallow were sprinkled on 25 March 2017 and 2 April 2018 for each season, respectively. The irrigation of experimental units was immersed-way once per 10 days, as per local custom. Weeds were removed manually at 20 and 40 days after sowing (DAS) in both growing seasons, before irrigation was affected. The treatments application comprised three fertilization types (alone or in combinations), namely an organic fertilization (farmyard manure, FYM), an inorganic NPK fertilization, and a biofertilizer. The organic fertilizer was obtained from the animal Production Farm, College of Agriculture, Al-Azhar University, Assiut, and was incorporated into the soil during plowing at the recommended dose of 36 m^3 ha^{-1}. Its chemical composition was reported by Silva [24] and presented here in Table 2. For the inorganic fertilization, the recommended P$_2$O$_5$ dose of 74 kg ha^{-1} (as Ca super phosphate) was incorporated into the soil during plowing, while 146 kg ha^{-1} (as urea) and 57 kg ha^{-1} K$_2$O (as potassium sulfate) were divided in two equal applications at 10 and 20 DAS, as commonly used for growing Jew's mallow plants, recommended by the Ministry of Agriculture [25]. The liquid biofertilizer (T.S) contains of molasse as organic material carrier of microorganisms, and a set of mixed cultures of *Bacillus circulans*, *B. poylmyxa*, *B. megatherium*,

Candida spp., and Trichoderma spp., whose amount in terms of living cells was $>0.5 \times 10^9$ cfu ml^{-1}, $>2 \times 10^7$ cfu ml^{-1}, $>1.5 \times 10^9$ cfu ml^{-1}, $>1.5 \times 10^7$ cfu ml^{-1} and $>0.5 \times 10^6$ cfu ml^{-1}, respectively. The biofertilizer was added at 36 L ha^{-1} with irrigation in three equal doses at 20, 30 and 40 DAS. The biofertilizer was obtained from the directorate of Agriculture in Assiut. Overall, the trials comprised an unfertilized control (T_1), inorganic NPK fertilization (T_2), farmyard manure (FYM) (T_3), biofertilizer (T_4), inorganic NPK+biofertilizer (T_5), and FYM+biofertilizer (T_6).

Table 2. Chemical composition of farmyard manure used in the experiments on dry weight basis.

Characteristic	Values	Characteristics	Values
Total-N %	1.87	pH (1:5) Susp.	8.43
Total-P %	1.12	EC (dSm^{-1}) (1:5)	4.030
Total-K %	2.06	C/N Ratio	12:1
Organic-C %	22.91	Organic matter %	40.43

EC: Electrical Conductivity.

2.3. Data Collection

Data were collected using plant samples from 0.5 m^2 in the middle of each experimental unit. Plant height was taken from the base of the rhizome to the top of the plant using a ruler. The fresh biomass of total plants, fresh weight of leaves, and dry weight of leaves was weighed using an electronic balance (0.01 g). Fresh biomass of total plants and fresh weight of leaves were put in paper bags and transferred to a drying oven at 70 °C until constant weight to obtain the dry weight. Leaf area was estimated as described by Pandey and Singh [26], whereas leaf weight incidence, expressed on a percentage basis, was calculated by using the following Equation (1).

$$\text{Leaves dressing (\%)} = \frac{\text{leaves dry weight (g)}}{\text{plant dry weight (g)}} \times 100 \qquad (1)$$

Harvesting was done in the two seasons at 28-May and 5-Jun, respectively. The following soil properties were determined after harvest: cation exchange capacity (CEC) and organic-C, determined according to Clark, et al. [27]. The soil bulk density was calculated by using Equation (2).

$$\text{Soil bulk density} = \frac{\text{Dry wieght of bulk sample (g)}}{\text{the volume of soil core (cm3)}} \qquad (2)$$

Leaf samples from each experimental unit during two seasons were collected, the fifth leaf from the top of 20 plants after 65 DAS (the first season) and 62 DAS (second season), and washed three times with distilled water, before chemical analysis. N-content in leaves was determined using the Kjeldahl procedure according to Motsara and Roy [28]. P-content in leaves was determined by the colorimeter method (ammonium molybdate) using a JENWAY 6305 UV/Visible Spectrophotometer at 643 nm (OD643) [28]. K-content in leaves was determined photometrically using a Flame Photometer (BWB Model BWB-XP, 5 Channel) as described by Motsara and Roy [28]. Protein content in leaves (expressed on a percentage basis) was calculated as N content (%) X 6.25. Leaf chlorophyll content was determined using a mobile chlorophyll meter (SPAD-502-m Konica Minolta, Inc., Tokyo, Japan). Before taking the readings, the performance of the chlorophyll meter was calibrated according to the manufacturer' instructions. At the measurement date, 6 readings from each replicate were taken at 65 DAS (the first season) and 62 DAS (second season), using the youngest fully expanded leaves.

2.4. Statistical Analysis

All data collected were subjected to one-way analysis of variance (ANOVA) using SPSS statistical software package version 16.0 (SPSS Inc., Chicago, IL, USA). Significantly different means were separated using Duncan's multiple range test at the $p \leq 0.05$ level of probability [29]. Mean values were presented as mean ± SD.

2.5. Weather Condition during the Experiment

During the first year of experiment (2017), the average mean temperature was 26.3 °C, with a gradual increase from 3 April (17.3 °C) to 15 May (29.7 °C), whereas average minimum and maximum temperatures fluctuated between 11–28.4 °C and 24.6–40.8 °C, respectively. The average relative humidity varied between 20% and 60%, with the lowest value recorded at 20 April and the highest one at 13 April (Figure 1). During the second year of experiment (2018), the average mean temperature was 28.6 °C, with a gradual increase from 20.8 °C to 31.5 °C, whereas average minimum and maximum temperatures fluctuated between 12–28 °C and 20.8–46 °C, respectively. The average relative humidity varied between 16% and 58%, with the lowest value recorded at 6 May and the highest one at 6 April (Figure 1).

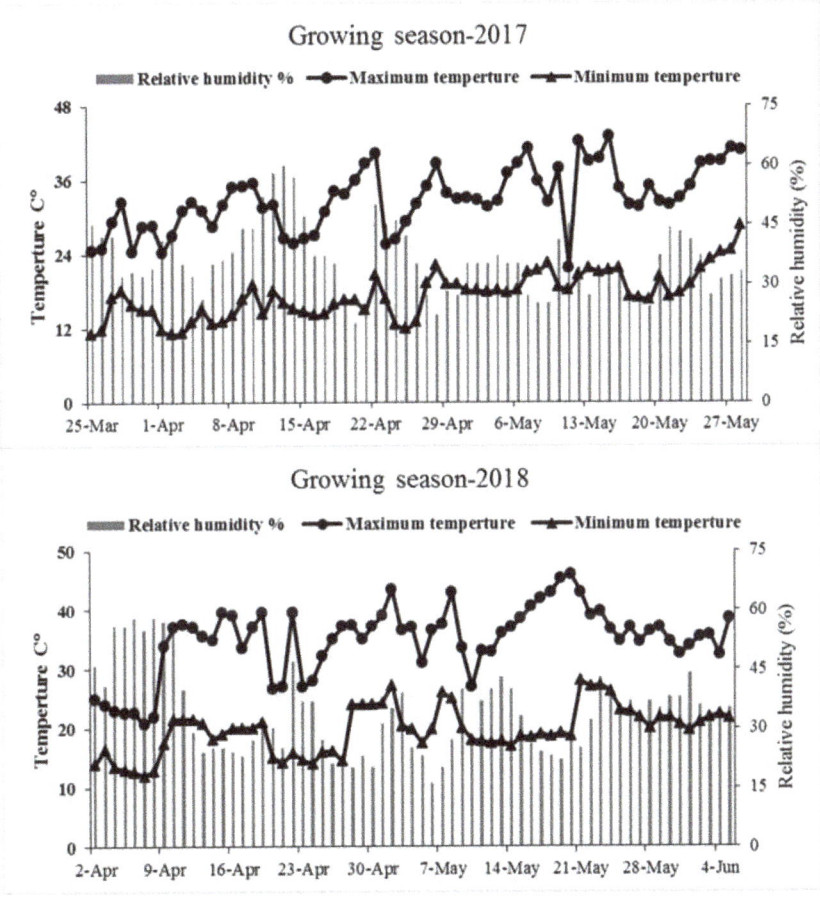

Figure 1. Weather conditions during the two growing periods of Jew's mellow cultivation.

3. Results

3.1. Growth Variables

Tables 3–5 show the effect of organic, inorganic, and biofertilizers supplementations on the growth and yield of Jew's mallow plants. The results showed no significant difference in the plants height under T_2, T_3, T_5, and T_6, but they were higher than those under the other treatments in the mean of both growing seasons (Table 3). There were statistically significant differences between the treatments, where the maximum fresh plants weight, leaves fresh weight, plant dry weight, leaves dry weight, and leaves area (3.16 kg.m^{-2}, 797.88 g.m^{-2}, 646.79 g.m^{-2}, 223.35 g.m^{-2}, and 369.5 cm^2.m^{-2}, respectively) were showed by the plants treated with NPK with biofertilizers (T_5), and that of without fertilization, T_1 treatment gave the lowest values (Tables 3 and 4) in the mean of both growing seasons.

The highest leaves weight incidence was observed in plants treated with biofertilizer (T_4) having non-significant difference among FYM+biofertilizer (T_6), NPK fertilizer (T_2), and T_1 during first growing season, while in second growing season the plants treated with T_1 showed significant highest values (Table 5). There was no significant difference in dry matter content of plants under all the treatments except T_1, but T_4 was higher than other treatments in the first season, while in the second season, there was no significant difference in dry matter contents of plants in T_1, T_4, T_5, and T_6 treatments, but T_4 was highest compared to other treatments in the mean of both growing seasons.

3.2. Compositional Variables

As shown in Tables 3–5, the accumulation of protein in Jew's mallow plants in both seasons was the significantly highest under NPK with biofertilizers (T_5). Data presented in Table 6 shows that the average accumulation of N, P, and K in leaves were under T_5 higher than other treatments in both growing seasons, while T_1 gave the least N, P, and K accumulation.

Table 3. Effect of organic, inorganic, and biofertilizers on plant growth characteristics (plant height, plant fresh weight, and leaves fresh weight) of Jew's mallow (*Corchorus olitorius* L.) plants.

	Plant Height (cm)			Plant Fresh Weight (kg m^{-2})			Leaves Fresh Weight (g m^{-2})		
	2017	2018	Means	2017	2018	Means	2017	2018	Means
T_1	34.33 ± 2.31 ^{c}	25.67 ± 3.51 ^{b}	30.00 ^{c}	1.33 ± 0.10 ^{e}	1.02 ± 0.06 ^{c}	1.18 ^{e}	478.81 ± 29.25 ^{c}	348.22 ± 11.57 ^{e}	413.52 ^{e}
T_2	78.33 ± 2.60 ^{a}	50.67 ± 9.45 ^{a}	64.50 ^{a}	2.13 ± 0.04 ^{c}	1.86 ± 0.15 ^{c}	2.00 ^{c}	655.71 ± 78.74 ^{b}	503.07 ± 12.03 ^{c}	579.39 ^{c}
T_3	75.67 ± 4.51 ^{a}	49.67 ± 5.69 ^{a}	62.67 ^{a}	2.52 ± 0.09 ^{b}	2.26 ± 0.11 ^{b}	2.39 ^{b}	748.79 ± 58.24 ^{b}	592.33 ± 15.25 ^{b}	670.56 ^{b}
T_4	51.33 ± 4.04 ^{b}	45.33 ± 2.52 ^{a}	48.33 ^{b}	1.64 ± 0.22 ^{d}	1.25 ± 0.14 ^{d}	1.45 ^{d}	543.38 ± 54.65 ^{c}	433.03 ± 15.47 ^{d}	488.21 ^{d}
T_5	84.33 ± 4.16 ^{a}	52.67 ± 3.51 ^{a}	68.50 ^{a}	3.57 ± 0.05 ^{a}	2.74 ± 0.14 ^{a}	3.16 ^{a}	897.79 ± 17.21 ^{a}	697.97 ± 14.64 ^{a}	797.88 ^{a}
T_6	82.33 ± 8.33 ^{a}	51.67 ± 2.08 ^{a}	67.00 ^{a}	1.71 ± 0.16 ^{d}	1.41 ± 0.02 ^{d}	1.56 ^{d}	549.79 ± 55.22 ^{c}	427.75 ± 4.6 ^{d}	488.77 ^{d}
Means	67.72 ^{a}	45.95 ^{b}		2.15 ^{a}	1.76 ^{b}		645.71 ^{a}	500.40 ^{b}	

Values are means of three replicates; different letters in the same column indicate significant differences according to Duncan's multiple range test at $p \leq 0.05$. Where without fertilization (T_1), NPK fertilizer (T_2), farmyard manure (T_3), biofertilizer (T_5), NPK+biofertilizer (T_4), and Farmyard manure +biofertilizer (T_6).

Table 4. Effect of organic, inorganic, and biofertilizers on plant growth characteristics (plant dry yield, leaves dry yield, and leaf area) of Jew's mallow (*Corchorus olitorius* L.) plants.

Treatment	Plant Dry Weight (g m^{-2})			Leaves Dry Weight (g m^{-2})			Leaf Area (cm^2 m^{-2})		
	2017	2018	Means	2017	2018	Means	2017	2018	Means
T_1	274.92 ± 6.02 ^{e}	138.78 ± 6.22 ^{c}	206.85 ^{e}	112.20 ± 11.05 ^{c}	95.20 ± 13.39 ^{d}	103.7 ^{d}	219.50 ± 2.38 ^{f}	199.56 ± 10.18 ^{e}	209.53 ^{f}
T_2	416.96 ± 9.12 ^{c}	326.56 ± 22.70 ^{c}	317.76 ^{c}	184.94 ± 17.77 ^{b}	123.84 ± 5.03 ^{c}	154.39 ^{c}	321.79 ± 1.79 ^{c}	290.26 ± 1.32 ^{c}	306.025 ^{c}
T_3	560.85 ± 10.44 ^{b}	398.65 ± 10.17 ^{b}	479.75 ^{b}	198.14 ± 7.05 ^{b}	155.91 ± 9.20 ^{b}	177.03 ^{b}	336.65 ± 5.93 ^{b}	308.25 ± 8.66 ^{b}	322.45 ^{b}
T_4	328.60 ± 42.73 ^{d}	272.47 ± 17.12 ^{d}	300.54 ^{d}	167.28 ± 29.13 ^{b}	120.99 ± 1.59 ^{c}	144.14 ^{c}	247.83 ± 4.22 ^{e}	205.36 ± 7.48 ^{de}	226.59 ^{e}
T_5	713.36 ± 27.96 ^{a}	580.22 ± 23.39 ^{a}	646.79 ^{a}	240.42 ± 15.81 ^{a}	206.29 ± 7.00 ^{a}	223.35 ^{a}	392.15 ± 7.78 ^{a}	346.85 ± 9.28 ^{a}	369.5 ^{a}
T_6	311.85 ± 26.62 ^{de}	256.33 ± 10.90 ^{d}	284.09 ^{d}	154.20 ± 41.25 ^{b}	119.75 ± 4.16 ^{c}	136.97 ^{c}	257.86 ± 5.79 ^{d}	217.15 ± 3.91 ^{d}	237.50 ^{d}
Means	434.42 ^{a}	286.11 ^{b}		176.20 ^{a}	136.99 ^{b}		295.96 ^{a}	261.24 ^{b}	

Values are means of three replicates; different letters in the same column indicate significant differences according to Duncan's multiple range test at $p \leq 0.05$. Where without fertilization (T_1), NPK fertilizer (T_2), farmyard manure (T_3), biofertilizer (T_5), NPK+biofertilizer (T_4), and Farmyard manure +biofertilizer (T_6).

Table 5. Effect of organic, inorganic, and biofertilizers on plant growth characteristics and chemical contents (leaves weight incidence, dry matter content, and protein) of Jew's mallow (*Corchorus olitorius* L.) plants.

Treatment	Leaves Weight Incidence (%)			Dry Matter Content %			Protein (%)		
	2017	2018	Means	2017	2018	Means	2017	2018	Means
T₁	40.78 ± 3.37 ᵃ⁻ᶜ	68.63 ± 5.55 ᵃ	54.71 ᵃ	23.6 ± 3.76 ᵇ	27.27 ± 2.90 ᵃ⁻ᶜ	25.44 ᵈ	8.00 ± 0.25 ᶠ	7.27 ± 0.28 ᶠ	7.64 ᶠ
T₂	44.34 ± 3.97 ᵃ⁻ᶜ	38 ± 1.21 ᶜᵈ	41.17 ᵇᶜ	28.3 ± 1.31 ᵃᵇ	24.63 ± 1.20 ᶜ	26.47 ᶜ	17.67 ± 0.38 ᵇ	16.44 ± 0.23 ᵇ	17.06 ᵇ
T₃	35.35 ± 1.91 ᵇᶜ	39.11 ± 2.21 ᵇ⁻ᵈ	37.23 ᶜ	26.5 ± 1.18 ᵃᵇ	26.33 ± 1.70 ᵇᶜ	26.42 ᶜ	14.19 ± 0.35 ᵈ	13.71 ± 0.22 ᵈ	13.95 ᵈ
T₄	52.02 ± 14.35 ᵃ	44.5 ± 2.30 ᵇᶜ	48.26 ᵃᵇ	31.0 ± 5.85 ᵃ	27.97 ± 1.01 ᵃᵇ	29.49 ᵃ	12.02 ± 0.29 ᵉ	10.56 ± 0.33 ᵉ	11.29 ᵉ
T₅	33.68 ± 0.89 ᶜ	35.61 ± 2.40 ᵈ	34.65 ᶜ	26.8 ± 1.24 ᵃᵇ	29.57 ± 1.34 ᵃ	28.19 ᵇ	19.00 ± 0.44 ᵃ	18.31 ± 0.29 ᵃ	18.66 ᵃ
T₆	48.99 ± 9.01 ᵃᵇ	46.78 ± 2.69 ᵇ	47.89 ᵃᵇ	27.8 ± 5.28 ᵃᵇ	27.99 ± 0.85 ᵃᵇ	27.90 ᵇ	15.83 ± 0.29 ᶜ	14.69 ± 0.25 ᶜ	15.26 ᶜ
Means	42.53 ᵃ	45.44 ᵃ		27.33 ᵃ	27.29 ᵃ		14.45 ᵃ	13.50 ᵇ	

Values are means of three replicates; different letters in the same column indicate significant differences according to Duncan's multiple range test at $p \leq 0.05$. Where without fertilization (T₁), NPK fertilizer (T₂), farmyard manure (T₃), biofertilizer (T₄), NPK+biofertilizer (T₅), and Farmyard manure +biofertilizer (T₆).

Table 6. Effect of organic, inorganic, and biofertilizers on compositional variables (N-Content, P-Content, and K-Content) of Jew's mallow (*Corchorus olitorius* L.) plants.

Treatment	N-Content in Leaves (mg 100g⁻¹)			P-Content in Leaves (mg 100g⁻¹)			K-Content in Leaves (mg 100g⁻¹)		
	2017	2018	Means	2017	2018	Means	2017	2018	Means
T₁	1.28 ± 0.04 ᶠ	1.16 ± 0.05 ᶠ	1.22 ᶠ	0.35 ± 0.04 ᶠ	0.31 ± 0.04 ᵉ	0.33 ᶠ	1.15 ± 0.05 ᶠ	1.03 ± 0.02 ᶠ	1.09 ᶠ
T₂	2.83 ± 0.06 ᵇ	2.63 ± 0.04 ᵇ	2.73 ᵇ	0.85 ± 0.06 ᵇ	0.70 ± 0.02 ᵇ	0.78 ᵇ	1.91 ± 0.03 ᵇ	1.75 ± 0.04 ᵇ	1.83 ᵇ
T₃	2.27 ± 0.06 ᵈ	2.19 ± 0.04	2.23 ᵈ	0.57 ± 0.02 ᵈ	0.41 ± 0.02 ᵈ	0.49 ᵈ	1.62 ± 0.04 ᵈ	1.44 ± 0.04 ᵈ	1.53 ᵈ
T₄	1.92 ± 0.05 ᵉ	1.69 ± 0.05 ᵉ	1.81 ᵉ	0.45 ± 0.03 ᵉ	0.36 ± 0.02 ᵈᵉ	0.41 ᵉ	1.41 ± 0.03 ᵉ	1.32 ± 0.03 ᵉ	1.37 ᵉ
T₅	3.04 ± 0.07 ᵃ	2.93 ± 0.05 ᵃ	2.99 ᵃ	0.95 ± 0.04 ᵃ	0.81 ± 0.05 ᵃ	0.88 ᵃ	2.09 ± 0.05 ᵃ	1.93 ± 0.03 ᵃ	2.01 ᵃ
T₆	2.53 ± 0.05 ᶜ	2.35 ± 0.04 ᶜ	2.44 ᶜ	0.75 ± 0.03 ᶜ	0.61 ± 0.03 ᶜ	0.68 ᶜ	1.75 ± 0.03 ᶜ	1.60 ± 0.03 ᶜ	1.68 ᶜ
Means	2.31 ᵃ	2.16 ᵇ		0.65 ᵃ	0.53 ᵇ		1.66 ᵃ	1.60 ᵇ	

Values are means of three replicates; different letters in the same column indicate significant differences according to Duncan's multiple range test at $p \leq 0.05$. Where without fertilization (T₁), NPK fertilizer (T₂), farmyard manure (T₃), biofertilizer (T₄), NPK+biofertilizer (T₅), and Farmyard manure +biofertilizer (T₆).

The average leaf chlorophyll content the first season was higher than in the second season in all variants, where the highest value of leaf chlorophyll content 41.21 mg g^{-1} was obtained in T$_5$, while the lowest one (29.47 mg g^{-1}) was recorded in T$_1$ (Figure 2).

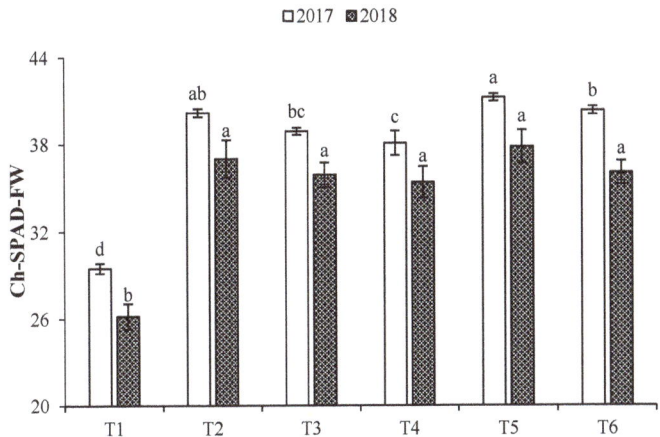

Figure 2. Effect of organic, inorganic, and biofertilizers on leaf chlorophyll content of Jew's mallow (*Corchorus olitorius* L.). Each column represents the mean of three replicates; different letters on similar columns indicate significant differences using Duncan's multiple range test at $p \leq 0.05$.

3.3. Soil Properties at the End of the Experimental Period

The result of soil properties after harvesting Jew's mallow plant showed that the soil was variably influenced by the different treatments. The average values for the soil organic-C (%) contents were influenced by the individual treatments. The highest value for soil organic-C, as shown in Figure 3a, was observed in T$_3$ in both of seasons and in T$_6$ in the 2018 season, while the lowest values were recorded in T$_1$ and T$_2$. As shown in Figure 3b, the application of organic manure with biofertilizers significantly enhanced the CEC value. The highest average values CEC were noticed in T$_6$ (17.98 cmol kg^{-1}), and T$_3$ (17.93 cmol kg^{-1}) which were statistically undifferentiated. The lowest value (15.72 and 16.01 cmol kg^{-1}) were obtained in control (T$_1$) and NPK fertilizer (T$_2$), respectively. The treatment effects on the average soil bulk density for two seasons are presented in Figure 3c. These treatments (T$_3$–T$_6$) had positive and significant effects on soil bulk density. The bulk density was reduced in the T$_3$–T$_6$ treatments (1.39 g cm^{-3}, on average) and showed statistically lower values than obtained in the control (1.46 g cm^{-3}).

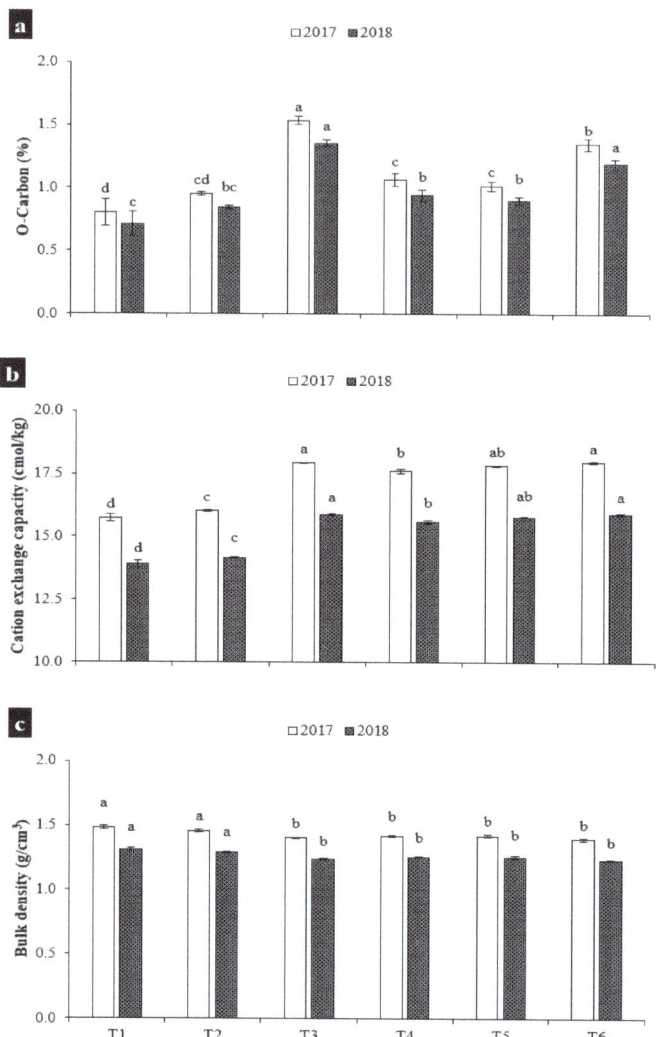

Figure 3. Effect of organic, inorganic, and biofertilizers on the soil properties [O-carbon (**a**), cation exchange capacity (**b**) and bulk density (**c**)] on which Jew's mallow (*Corchorus olitorius* L.) was grown. Each column represents the mean of three replicates; different letters on similar columns indicate significant differences using Duncan's multiple range test at $p \leq 0.05$.

4. Discussion

4.1. Growth Variables

The positive effects of NPK with biofertilizers (T_5) on growth variables may have been due to the efficiency of the microorganism in the biofertilizer in immobilizing N for a longer time in the form of NH_4^+, which helped in the nutrient uptake by the plant [30]. According to Alori and Babalola [31], a biofertilizer is a living organisms that is added into the soil as inoculant that helps to provide certain nutrients for crop growth. Furthermore, these positive effects may be related to the increased availability of nutrients provided by mineral fertilization, which also served as an energy source for the microbial community [32]. Similar to our findings, Al-Zabee and Al-Maliki [32] reported that the combination of mycorrhizal fungi, algae, and yeast with a higher rate of chemical fertilization (120 kg N, 60 kg P, and 200 kg K per hectare) was beneficial to soil microbial metabolism and potato yield. Besides, Asmamaw, et al. [33] reported that the application of dry cyanobacterial biofertilizer could serve as an auxiliary N source to inorganic fertilizer for pepper, maize, and kale production. It was also noted that the use of biofertilizers in combination with chemical N fertilizers increased growth, productivity, and chemical compositions of the dill plant (Anethum graveolens L.) compared to the untreated control, where the highest values of plant growth were recorded when biofertilizer was used in combination to 97.6 kg.ha^{-1} N [34]. Observations have also shown that the most effective treatment for growth characteristics of barley cultivars (Giza-128 and Giza-129) under newly reclaimed sandy soil was 178.57 kg N ha^{-1} + Yeast [35]. Moreover, Sen, et al. [36] reported that the combined use of 100% of the recommended dose [714.3 kg.ha^{-1} ammonium sulfate (20.5% N), 476.2 kg ha^{-1} calcium superphosphate (15.5% P_2O_5), and 119.05 kg ha^{-1} potassium sulfate (48% k_2O)] of inorganic fertilizers with biofertilizer was optimal for increasing oil yield (33.22 mg g^{-1}) of cumin black (Nigella sativa L.). The co-application of biofertilizers like Azospirillum and Phosphobacteria spp. and inorganic fertilizers had a significant effect on the growth variables of cucumber (Cucumis sativus L.) [37]. Application of biofertilizer at 300–400 kg ha^{-1} dose combined with inorganic fertilizer at 75% of crop requirement dose was the best combination for increasing NPK nutrient uptake for rice crop and weight of milled dry rice. Marlina, et al. [38] recommended the use of dry cyanobacterial biofertilizer which serve as a supplementary N source in place of inorganic fertilizer for rice production in inception soil of lowland swamp area.

4.2. Compositional Variables

The data in Tables 5 and 6 indicated differences in the average proportion of protein, N, P, and K content in leaves among treatments. The NPK with biofertilizers (T_5) treatment significantly increased these variables in both seasons. The results presented by Hellal, Mahfouz and Hassan [34] showed that the highest NPK-accumulation were recorded after the combination of biofertilizer with 476.2 kg ha^{-1} ammonium sulphate (20.5% N) in the Dill plant. The pronounced positive effect on protein, N, P, and K in leaves resulting from T_5 addition may be attributed to the increased uptake of N by plants, and thus, the biosynthesis of protein was increased. Moreover, Tisdale et al. [39] reported that the addition of N in combination with adequate P tended to increase K-uptake by plants. They also showed that K concentration may be high in the NH_4^+-nourished plants as it is adsorbed by soil colloids, so it does not get leached from the soil. This gave the plant a greater chance of taking up N, and thus some nutrients, to build the dry matter. Also, data in Figure 2 for leaf chlorophyll content supported the results of Hellal, Mahfouz and Hassan [34], where it was observed that the highest values of chlorophyll content were recorded where biofertilizer was used in combination to 97.6 kg ha^{-1} N in the dill plant. Moreover, Sen, Choudhuri, Chatterjee and Jana [36] reported that the combination of 100% of the recommended dose of inorganic fertilizers with biofertilizer increased the leaf chlorophyll content (13.18 mg.g^{-1}) in cumin black (Nigella sativa L.) in the eastern Himalayan region of West Bengal. Moreover, Youssef, et al. [40] reported that the combined application of organic manures and biofertilizer (EM) had a synergistic effect on the total chlorophyll content of plants.

4.3. Soil Properties at the End of the Experimental Period

The combined application of the biofertilizer with the organic or the inorganic fertilizer was beneficial for the physical and chemical properties of soil and were important for the quality and productivity of the soil. The application of organic fertilizer in T_3 and its combination with biofertilizer in T_6 increased the soil organic-C content of the soil at the end of experimental period by 91.25 % and 68.75%, respectively, over the control treatment (without fertilization T_1). This organic fertilizer in the soil can increase the soil organic-C due to higher soil organic matter added from organic fertilizer. This serves as nutrient sources for plants and improves physical, chemical, and biological properties of the soil through improved structure and stable aggregates. This is because organic matrices are a natural chelating material with high moisture retention capacity [41,42]. These results are in agreement with Nesgea, et al. [43], who reported that the application of organic fertilizer increased the soil organic-C content after harvest by up to 65%.

As for the cation exchange capacity of the soil, our results showed that the application of organic fertilizer with biofertilizer increased in CEC of the soil after crop harvest, which were statistically undifferentiated with T_3 and T_5. The increased CEC might be attributed to the addition of organic fertilizer with the biofertilizer, which might have helped in releasing more nutrients into the soil. This could be an indication of increased exchange sites on the surface of the soil colloids. In line with this result, Tana and Woldesenbet [44] reported that CEC significantly increased with increasing organic fertilizer (15 ton ha^{-1}) with inorganic fertilizer.

The data in Figure 3c indicated that there were no differences between treatments (T_3, T_4, T_5, and T_6), but the highest average reduction in soil bulk density was recorded in farmyard manure +biofertilizer (T_6). Soil bulk density was reduced after the combined use of organic manure with biofertilizer (T_6) compared to soil amended with only inorganic fertilizer (T_3). This could be due to improved soil aggregation as a result of decreased soil bulk density. Several studies have shown that the appropriate addition of combined biofertilizers, inorganic and organic, improved soil porosity and decreased its bulk density. Our results are in harmony with Khan, et al. [45] who reported that organic fertilizer improved soil organic matter content and decreased soil bulk density.

5. Conclusions

Biofertilizers play a significant role in improving soil structure, and inorganic fertilizers are important due to their ability to provide essential nutrients, resulting in the better growth and productivity of crops. The results of the present study, conducted on a silty loam soil and in semi-arid climate conditions, revealed that the Jew's mallow plants treated with the combined application of biofertilizer and NPK fertilizer showed maximum growth and productivity among all other treatments. Although the current study unfolded the performance ability of a neglected crop under the application of different kinds of fertilizers, there is a further need to understand the molecular mechanism behind it and to improve the fertilization techniques and material according to the need for crops.

Author Contributions: M.A.Y. and A.F.Y. equally contributed in experimentation and draft preparation; M.M.A. and M.M.I. helped in data analysis and editing; Y.X. reviewed and editing; R.P.M. helped in draft preparation and revised the manuscript. All authors have read and agreed to the published version of the manuscript.

Funding: This research received no external funding.

Acknowledgments: Thanks to all field technicians at College of Agriculture, Al-Azhar University branch Assiut, Egypt and College of Horticulture, Fujian Agriculture and Forestry University, Fuzhou, China.

Conflicts of Interest: The authors declare no conflict of interest.

References

1. Ierna, A.; Mauro, R.P.; Mauromicale, G. Improved yield and nutrient efficiency in two globe artichoke genotypes by balancing nitrogen and phosphorus supply. *Agron. Sustain. Dev.* **2012**, *32*, 773–780. [CrossRef]
2. Kumar, P.; Pandey, S.; Singh, B.; Singh, S.; Kumar, D. Influence of source and time of potassium application on potato growth, yield, economics and crisp quality. *Potato Res.* **2007**, *50*, 1–13. [CrossRef]
3. Adeniyan, O.; Ojeniyi, S. Effect of poultry manure, NPK 15-15-15 and combination of their reduced levels on maize growth and soil chemical properties. *Niger. J. Soil Sci.* **2005**, *15*, 34–41.
4. Bot, A.; Benites, J. *The Importance of Soil Organic Matter: Key to Drought-Resistant Soil and Sustained Food Production*; Food and Agriculture Organization of the United Nations: Rome, Italy, 2005.
5. Baghdadi, A.; Halim, R.A.; Ghasemzadeh, A.; Ramlan, M.F.; Sakimin, S.Z. Impact of organic and inorganic fertilizers on the yield and quality of silage corn intercropped with soybean. *PeerJ* **2018**, *6*, e5280. [CrossRef] [PubMed]

6. Adebayo, O.; Akoun, J. Effect of organic manure and spacing on the yield and yield components of *Amaranthus cruentus*. In Proceedings of the 20th Annual Conference of Horticultural Society of Nigeria Held at National Horticultural Research Institute (NIHORT) Auditorium Ibadan, Ibadan, Nigeria, 14–17 May 2002; pp. 30–32.
7. Cocking, E.C. Helping plants get more nitrogen from the air. *Eur. Rev.* **2000**, *8*, 193–200. [CrossRef]
8. Shariati, S.; Alikhani, H.A.; Pourbabaei, A. Application of vermicompost as a carrier of phosphate solubilizing bacteria (*Pseudomonas fluorescens*) in increase growth parameters of maize. *Int. J. Agron. Plant Prod.* **2013**, *4*, 2010–2017.
9. Bargaz, A.; Lyamlouli, K.; Chtouki, M.; Zeroual, Y.; Dhiba, D. Soil microbial resources for improving fertilizers efficiency in an integrated plant nutrient management system. *Front. Microbiol.* **2018**, *9*, 1606. [CrossRef]
10. Mazher, A.; Abdel-Aziz, N.; El-Dabh, R.; El-Khateeb, M.; Abd El-Badaie, A. Effect of bio fertilization on growth and constituents of *Moringa oleifera* Lam. Plants. *Middle East J. Agric. Res.* **2014**, *3*, 793–798.
11. Rajasekaran, S.; Sundaramoorthy, P. Effect of FYM, N, P fertilizers and biofertilizers on germination and growth of paddy (*Oryza sativa* L). *Int. Lett. Nat. Sci.* **2015**, *8*, 59–65.
12. Youssef, M.A. Impact of bio-fertilizers on growth and yield of *Moringa oleifera* Lam. Plants Al-Azhar. *J. Agric. Res.* **2016**, *26*, 127–138.
13. Grubben, G.L.H.; Denton, O.A. *Plant Resources of Tropical Africa 2. Vegetables*; PROTA Foundation: Wageningen, The Netherlands, 2004.
14. Odofin, A.; Oladiran, J.; Oladipo, J.; Wuya, E. Determination of evapotranspiration and crop coefficients for bush okra (*Corchorus olitorius*) in a sub-humid area of Nigeria. *Afr. J. Agric. Res.* **2011**, *6*, 3949–3953.
15. Nwangburuka, C.; Olawuyi, O.; Oyekale, K.; Ogunwenmo, K.; Denton, O.; Nwankwo, E. Growth and yield response of Corchorus olitorius in the treatment of *Arbuscular mycorrhizae* (AM), Poultry manure (PM), Combination of AM-PM and Inorganic Fertilizer (NPK). *Adv. Appl. Sci. Res.* **2012**, *3*, 1466–1471.
16. Youssef, A.F.; Younes, N.A.; Youssef, M. Genetic diversity in Corchorus olitorius L. revealed by morphophysiological and molecular analyses. *Mol. Biol. Rep.* **2019**, *46*, 2933–2940. [PubMed]
17. Mabhaudhi, T.; Chimonyo, V.G.; Chibarabada, T.P.; Modi, A.T. Developing a roadmap for improving neglected and underutilized crops: A case study of South Africa. *Front. Plant Sci.* **2017**, *8*, 2143. [PubMed]
18. Ghoneim, I.; El-Araby, S. Effect of organic manure source and biofertilizer type on growth, productivity and chemical composition of Jew's Mallow (*Corchorus Olitorious* L.) plants. *J Agric. Env. Sci. Alex. Univ. Egypt* **2003**, *2*, 88–105.
19. Isuosuo, C.; Akaneme, F.; Abu, N. Nutritional evaluation of the seeds of *Corchorus olitorius*: A neglected and underutilized species in Nigeria. *Pak. J. Nutr.* **2019**, *18*, 692–703.
20. Ogunrinde, A.; Fasinmirin, J. Soil moisture distribution pattern and yield of jute mallow (*Corchorus olitorius*) under three different soil fertility management. *COLERM Proc.* **2012**, *2*, 372–380.
21. Olaniyi, J.; Ajibola, A. Growth and yield performance of Corchorus olitorius varieties as affected by nitrogen and phosphorus fertilizers application. *Am.-Eurasian J. Sustain. Agric.* **2008**, *2*, 234–241.
22. Aisha, H.A.; Hafez, M.M.; Asmaa, R.M.; Shafeek, M. Effect of Bio and chemical fertilizers on growth, yield and chemical properties of spinach plant (*Spinacia oleracea* L.). *Middle East J. Agric. Res.* **2013**, *2*, 16–20.
23. Page, A.L.; Miller, R.H.; Keeney, D.R. *Methods of Soil Analysis*; American Society of Agronomy: Madison, WI, USA, 1982.
24. Silva, F.C.D. *Manual de Análises Químicas de Solos, Plantas e Fertilizantes*; Embrapa Informação Tecnológica: Rio de Janeiro, Brazil, 2009.
25. Hassan, A.A. *Post Harvest Technology and Physiology of Fruit Vegetables (In Arabic)*; Al-Dar Al-Arabiah Lil Nashr Wa Al-Tawsia: Cairo, Egypt, 2011.
26. Pandey, S.; Singh, H. A simple, cost-effective method for leaf area estimation. *J. Bot.* **2011**, *2011*, 1–6.
27. Clark, M.S.; Horwath, W.R.; Shennan, C.; Scow, K.M. Changes in soil chemical properties resulting from organic and low-input farming practices. *Agron. J.* **1998**, *90*, 662–671. [CrossRef]
28. Motsara, M.; Roy, R.N. *Guide to Laboratory Establishment for Plant Nutrient Analysis*; Food and Agriculture Organization of the United Nations Rome: Rome, Italy, 2008.
29. Duncan, D.B. Multiple range and multiple F tests. *J Biom.* **1955**, *11*, 1–42. [CrossRef]
30. Di, H.; Cameron, K.J.S.U. Effects of the nitrification inhibitor dicyandiamide on potassium, magnesium and calcium leaching in grazed grassland. *Soil Use Manag.* **2004**, *20*, 2–7. [CrossRef]

31. Alori, E.T.; Babalola, O.O. Microbial inoculants for improving crop quality and human health in Africa. *Front. Microbiol.* **2018**, *9*, 2213. [CrossRef] [PubMed]
32. Al-Zabee, M.R.; Al-Maliki, S.M. Effect of biofertilizers and chemical fertilizers on soil biological properties and potato yield. *Euphrates J. Agric. Sci.* **2019**, *11*, 1–13.
33. Asmamaw, M.; Wolde, G.; Yohannes, M.; Yigrem, S.; Woldemeskel, E.; Chala, A.; Davis, J.G. Comparison of cyanobacterial bio-fertilizer with urea on three crops and two soils of Ethiopia. *Afr. J. Agric. Res.* **2019**, *14*, 588–596.
34. Hellal, F.; Mahfouz, S.; Hassan, F. Partial substitution of mineral nitrogen fertilizer by bio-fertilizer on (*Anethum graveolens* L.) plant. *Agri. Biol. J. N. Am.* **2011**, *4*, 652–660.
35. Ahmed, A.G.; Hassanein, M.; Zaki, N.M. Performance of two barley cultivars as affected by nitrogen and bio-fertilizer under newly reclaimed lands. *Middle East J.* **2019**, *8*, 684–691.
36. Sen, A.; Choudhuri, P.; Chatterjee, R.; Jana, J. Influence of inorganic nutrient, organic nutrient and bio-fertilizer on growth, yield and quality of cumin black (*Nigella sativa* L.) in eastern Himalayan region of West Bengal. *J. Pharmacogn. Phytochem.* **2018**, *7*, 2571–2575.
37. Kumar, M.; Kathayat, K.; Singh, S.K.; Singh, L.; Singh, T. Influence of bio-fertilizers application on growth, yield and quality attributes of cucumber (*Cucumis sativus* L.): A review. *Plant Arch.* **2018**, *18*, 2329–2334.
38. Marlina, N.; Gofar, N.; Subakti, A.H.P.K.; Rohim, A.M. Improvement of rice growth and productivity through balance application of inorganic fertilizer and biofertilizer in inceptisol soil of lowland swamp area. *AGRIVITA J. Agric. Sci.* **2014**, *36*, 48–56. [CrossRef]
39. Tisdale, S.L.; Nelson, W.L.; Beaton, J.D. *Soil Fertility and Fertilizers*; Collier Macmillan Publishers: London, UK, 1985.
40. Youssef, M.A.; Elgharably, G.A.; Mahmoud, S.M.; Hegab, S. Impact of combined organic manures, Chemical fertilizer and Effective Microorganisms on growth and yield of Marjoram plants under drip and flood irrigation systems. *Assiut J. Agric. Sec.* **2010**, *41*, 91–105.
41. Bhattacharya, C.B.; Sen, S.; Korschun, D. Using corporate social responsibility to win the war for talent. *MIT Sloan Manag. Rev.* **2010**, *49*, 37–44.
42. Fageria, N.; Filho, M.B.; Moreira, A.; Guimarães, C. Foliar fertilization of crop plants. *J. Plant Nutr.* **2009**, *32*, 1044–1064. [CrossRef]
43. Nesgea, S.; Gebrekidan, H.; Sharma, J.; Berhe, T. Effects of nitrogen and phosphorus fertilizer application on yield attributes, grain yield and quality of rain fed rice (NERICA-3) in Gambella, Southwestern Ethiopia. *East Afr. J. Sci.* **2012**, *6*, 91–104.
44. Tana, T.; Woldesenbet, M. Effect of combined application of organic and mineral nitrogen and phosphorus fertilizer on soil physico-chemical properties and grain yield of food barley (*Hordeum vulgare* L.) in Kaffa Zone, South-western Ethiopia. *Momona Ethiopian J. Sci.* **2017**, *9*, 242–261. [CrossRef]
45. Khan, N.I.; Malik, A.U.; Umer, F.; Bodla, M.I. Effect of tillage and farm yard manure on physical properties of soil. *Int. Res. J. Plant Sci.* **2010**, *1*, 75–82.

Publisher's Note: MDPI stays neutral with regard to jurisdictional claims in published maps and institutional affiliations.

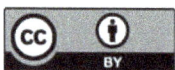

© 2020 by the authors. Licensee MDPI, Basel, Switzerland. This article is an open access article distributed under the terms and conditions of the Creative Commons Attribution (CC BY) license (http://creativecommons.org/licenses/by/4.0/).

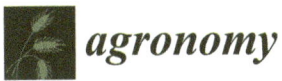

Article

Assessing the Potential of Jellyfish as an Organic Soil Amendment to Enhance Seed Germination and Seedling Establishment in Sand Dune Restoration

Iraj Emadodin *, Thorsten Reinsch, Raffaele-Romeo Ockens and Friedhelm Taube

Group Grass and Forage Science/Organic Agriculture, Institute for Crop Science and Plant Breeding, Christian-Albrechts-University, 24118 Kiel, Germany; treinsch@gfo.uni-kiel.de (T.R.); r.ockens@gmx.de (R.-R.O.); ftaube@gfo.uni-kiel.de (F.T.)
* Correspondence: iemadodin@gfo.uni-kiel.de

Received: 6 May 2020; Accepted: 16 June 2020; Published: 18 June 2020

Abstract: Worldwide, sandy coastlines are affected by extensive wind and water erosion. Both soil quality and periodic drought present major problems for sand dune restoration projects. Hence, soil amendments are needed to improve soil quality and enhance soil restoration efficiency. The jellyfish population has increased in some aquatic ecosystems and is often considered as a nuisance because of their negative impacts on marine ecosystem productivity as well as coastal attractiveness. Thus, development of new products derived from jellyfish biomass has received attention from researchers although utilization is still at a preliminary stage. Herein, our main objective was to test seed germination, seedling establishment, and seedling vitality of annual ryegrass (*Lolium multiflorum* L.) when supplied with organic soil amendment from two different jellyfish species (*Aurelia aurita* and *Cyanea capillata*) in comparison with an unfertilized control and mineral fertilizer treatment. We hypothesized that jellyfish dry matter as an organic soil amendment would improve seed germination and seedling establishment in sand dune environments. Germination and seedling growth experiments were conducted in the laboratory and greenhouse. The results indicate that jellyfish enhanced seedling growth and establishment in sand dune soil significantly ($p < 0.05$ and $p < 0.01$) under water scarcity conditions. Therefore, jellyfish may have potential for an auxiliary role in sand dune restoration projects in coastal areas in the future.

Keywords: seed germination; jellyfish; blue fertilizer; soil restoration; soil amendments; water use efficiency

1. Introduction

Human activities have damaged sandy beaches and coastal dunes. With further population growth, it is expected that human impacts on coastal ecosystems will only increase [1]. Furthermore, periodic environmental stress, including drought, is predicted to increase water scarcity problems worldwide. This creates additional and serious functional limitations for plant growth and also has significant adverse influences on crop yields [2,3]. Sand dune plants play an important role in dune stabilization and protect the adjacent coastal beaches from wind and water erosion but they are subjected to severe environmental stresses such as drought [4,5]. Therefore, organic soil amendments are important for ecological maintenance of the plants in sand dune restoration plans, especially in arid and semi-arid land where soils are under fragile conditions because of water scarcity and poor organic matter.

According to Donohue et al. [6], seed germination is a highly important stage in plant life cycles and factors affecting germination significantly impact subsequent seedling establishment, as well as plant environmental adaptation [7]. Seed germination is the initial process through which seeds develop into plants and it commences by the seed absorbing water under adequate temperature, which leads to the creation of a new plant [8]. According to Kildisheva et al. [9], taking seed germination into account in restoration planning is important to certify seed use efficiency and management. Seedling emergence is the most important phenological event that influences the success of plants [10] and it starts with seed germination. Seedling survival is also one of the most critical stages in plant growth and it is often adversely affected by drought and soil dryness [11]. According to Manz et al. [12] and Bewley et al. [13], water uptake by a seed includes three phases: first, the rapid initial uptake of water; second, a plateau phase (metabolic preparation for germination); and third, a further increase of water uptake. Therefore, soil moisture (available and adequate water) plays an important role in seed germination and seedling establishment.

Jellyfish, when supplied as an organic fertilizer, have a potential to promote seed germination, as reported by Emadodin et al. [14]. The term jellyfish as a group of marine invertebrates commonly refers to the medusae form of planktonic marine members of the class Scyphozoa or Cubozoa. Jellyfish populations have been a recurrent topic of debate over the past few decades, as mass aggregation (called blooms) of jellyfish are reported more frequently and have often been linked to human-induced environmental changes [15,16]. For example, blooms of some jellyfish species have been reported in the East Asian marginal seas [17], Red Sea [18], Mediterranean Sea, and Black Sea [19].

Positive effects from using jellyfish as inputs for agricultural production have been recorded by several researchers. Fukushi et al. [20] indicated the potential usefulness of two jellyfish species (*Aurelia aurita* and *Chrysaora melanaster*) as a source of fertilizer for vegetable production. Hossain et al. [21] introduced desalinated-dried jellyfishes (*Nemopilema nomurai* and *Aurelia aurita* from the Sea of Japan) as an alternative material to replace herbicides and chemical fertilizers in rice production. The possible use of jellyfish as pesticides was also investigated by Hussein et al. [22]. However, some jellyfish species may have different effects on plant growth processes due to their chemical components. Therefore, in this study, we evaluated the influences of two different jellyfish species (*Aurelia aurita* and *Cyanea capillata*) from the Baltic Sea Coast of Germany, on the early growth stages of annual ryegrass (*Lolium multiflorum* L.). It was hypothesized that the addition of jellyfish dry matter to the soil will enhance seed germination as well as seedling growth and establishment in sand dunes. This was considered to be particularly important in terms of soil restoration projects in dry lands where there is a need to establish new plant communities on degraded soil with very low productivity, as well as drought conditions. However, it should be emphasized that due to various ecological conditions and different species, several experiments (under greenhouse and field conditions) are required to investigate this hypothesis. Here, we report results from a petri plate germination experiment and a greenhouse pot experiment. The experiments are carried out, which is running under a European Union (EU) project entitled: Development of products from jellyfish biomass (Gojelly) with funding by the EU Horizon 2020 Research and Innovation Program.

2. Material and Methods

Two jellyfish species (*Aurelia aurita* and *Cyanea capillata*) were collected from two sites on the Baltic Sea Coast of Germany (54°25′ N, 10°10′ E and 54°47′ N, 9°84′ E) during summer of 2018 and 2019. The samples were put into plastic bags separately and stored at −20 °C before further processing. In this investigation, two drying methods including oven-dried and alcohol-dried methods have been conducted. Jellyfish were oven-dried at 50 °C until constant weight was reached. Alternatively, the alcohol-dried method of Pedersen et al. [23] was applied in which the fresh or frozen jellyfish were exposed to ethanol (70%) then after around one-hour the jellyfish were removed and put into distilled water. After about 30 min, jellyfish were taken out of the water and dried under room temperature (around 21 ± 1 °C).

The dry matter was homogenized in a ball mill (Retsch MM2000, Haan, Germany). The carbon and nitrogen content of the material was measured via dry combustion (Vario Max CN, Elementar Analysensysteme GmbH, Hanau, Germany).

For chemical analysis, 200 mg of dried and finely ground jellyfish material was digested with 10 mL 15.6 M HNO_3 (ROTIPURAN® Supra) at 190 °C for 45 min in 1800 W microwave oven (MARS 6, Xpress, CEM, Matthews, MC, USA). After digestion, the concentrations of Ca^{2+}, Cu^{2+}, Fe^{2+}, K^+, Mg^{2+}, Na^+, and Zn^{2+} were quantified with an atomic absorption spectrometer (AAS 5EA Thermo Electron S, Carl Zeiss, Jena, Germany). The citric acid extractable P was determined by using citric acid (2% v/v) and a jellyfish/solution ratio of 1:10. After shaking with an end-over-end shaker (Type RA 20, C. Gerhardt GmbH and Co. KG, Bonn, Germany) for 30 min, the citric acid extracts were filtered (MN 619 G$\frac{1}{4}$, Machery-Nagel GmbH and Co. KG, Düren, Germany). P concentrations in all extracts were determined photometrically with a continuous flow analyzer (Skalar Analytical B.V., Breda, The Netherlands) by using the modified molybdenum–ascorbic acid blue method. Results of the chemical analysis are given in Table 1.

Table 1. Some macro- and microelement compounds of jellyfishes (*Aurelia aurita* and *Cyanea capillata*).

Elements in Dry Matter	*Cyanea capillata* % per Dry Mass		*Aurelia aurita* % per Dry Mass	
	Alcohol Dried	Oven Dried	Alcohol Dried	Oven Dried
N	4.4	2.9	7.8	0.7
C	15.5	10.5	27.3	3.1
P	0.22	0.8	1.0	0.2
Ca	0.75	0.77	0.75	0.84
Mg	2	1.8	1.0	1.6
Na	17.8	19.5	9.2	33.4
K	0.16	1.2	0.44	0.96
Mn	<0.01	<0.01	<0.01	<0.01
Cu	<0.01	<0.01	<0.01	<0.01
Zn	0.01	0.02	0.04	<0.01
C:N	3.5	3.6	3.5	4.4

Seed of annual ryegrass (*Lolium multiflorum* L.) was used in this investigation. The soil used in this experiment was beach sand and this was collected from the Baltic Sea Coast of Germany (54°25′ N, 10°10′ E). Nitrogen and carbon contents of the soil were around 0.006% and 0.17%, respectively, with a C:N ratio around 28. Calcium ammonium nitrate (CAN) was used as a fertilizer treatment for comparison with jellyfish with regard to impacts on seed germination, seedling plant establishment and vitality. CAN is widely used as an inorganic fertilizer on grassland and other crops.

The pH and EC values of the jellyfish liquids that were provided for each treatment in pot experiment were the same as with a petri plate experiment. In order to test seed germination rate as well as seedling growth and establishment, a petri plate experiment and pot experiment were conducted as follows.

2.1. Petri Plate Experiment

The petri plate method was used to test germination rate. This method helps to monitor the processes of germination under a controlled environment. In pre-treatment the dry matter of *A. aurita*, *C. capillata* and calcium ammonium nitrate (CAN) was dissolved in distilled-water (0.5 g DM in 40 mL distilled water). Pure distilled water was also used as a control treatment. Filter paper was put in each petri plate (8.5 cm diameter) wetted by different aqueous solutions. In total, 20 annual ryegrass (*Lolium multiflorum* L.) seeds were placed in each petri plate. All plates were covered by plastic foil to mitigate evaporation and put in darkness at 21 ± 1 °C. The plates were controlled every day and observations (seed germination number and assessment of vitality) were recorded. The petri plate experiment was carried out with eight treatments and with four replications (Table 2). The pH and electronic conductivity (EC) of the different treatments were measured with a PC60 Premium Multi-Parameter tester (Apera instruments, Europa, GmbH; Table 3). Although the petri plate test is considered as a standard work for assessment of seed germination, it may not give an accurate prediction of seedling emergence in the field [24]. Therefore, a pot cultural experiment was also conducted in the greenhouse.

Table 2. Petri plate experiment treatments.

Nr.	Treatments	Abbreviation
1	Distilled water (Control)	Control
2	*Aurelia aurita* (Oven-dried)	Aur (Ov)
3	*Aurelia aurita* (Alcohol-dried)	Aur (Alc)
4	*Cyanea capillata* (Oven-dried)	Cya (Ov)
5	*Cyanea capillata* (Alcohol-dried)	Cya (Alc)
6	*Aurelia aurita* and *Cyanea capillata* (Oven-dried)	Aur + Cya (Ov)
7	*Aurelia aurita* and *Cyanea capillata* (Alcohol-dried)	Aur + Cya (Alc)
8	Calcium ammonium nitrate	CAN

Table 3. pH and electrical conductivity (EC) values of the treatments.

Treatments	pH	EC [µS/cm]
Control	6.1	0
Aurelia (Ov)	7.5	19.00
Aurelia (Alc)	7.42	5.06
Cyanea (Ov)	6.6	13.33
Cyanea (Alc)	6.83	2.89
Aur + Cya (Ov)	6.9	14.8
Aur + Cya (Alc)	7.2	4.23
CAN	7.15	15.21

2.2. Pot Experiment

This experiment was conducted in the greenhouse in summer 2019 at the University of Kiel. Plastic pots (around 11 cm top diameter, 6.5 cm bottom diameter, 10 cm height) were filled with 700 g of sand. In total, 20 uniform seeds of annual ryegrass (*Lolium multiflorum* L.) were placed in each pot and covered by 0.5 cm of sand material and irrigated with six different solutions (oven and alcohol dried materials from *Aurelia aurita* and *Cyanea capillata* and CAN (0.5 g DM in 40 mL distilled water) and 40 mL distilled water for control (Table 4). In order to reduce evaporation, the sand was covered by seagrass. The pot experiment was conducted in six treatments with four replications (Table 4). All treatments were irrigated three times (days 10, 15, and 17) during the experimental period, with 40 mL of tap water.

Table 4. Pot experiment treatments.

Nr.	Treatments	Abbreviation
1	Distilled water (Control)	Control
2	*Aurelia aurita* (Oven-dried)	Aur (Ov)
3	*Aurelia aurita* (Alcohol-dried)	Aur (Alc)
4	*Cyanea capillata* (Oven-dried)	Cya (Ov)
5	*Cyanea capillata* (Alcohol-dried)	Cya (Alc)
6	Calcium ammonium nitrate	CAN

2.3. Statistical Analysis

The petri plate test and the pot experiment were both conducted in a completely randomized design. The data were subjected to analysis of variance (ANOVA) and Welch's t-test as an adaptation of student's t-test [25]. The level of significance was declared at $p < 0.05$, $p < 0.01$ and $p < 0.001$.

3. Results

3.1. Petri Plate Experiment

Petri plate experimentation for testing germination rate and estimating seed viability is a standard practice [24]. In the petri plate experiment, the initial evidence of radicle protrusion (germination) appeared after two days. The germination rate was significantly less ($p < 0.05$; $p < 0.001$) than the control in Aur (Alc) and Aur + Cya (Alc) (Figure 1). Other treatments showed no indication of significant differences ($p > 0.05$) in germination rates relative to the control. Germination under the control (water) treatment started earlier than other treatments. However, after four days, germination rates under Cya (Ov) showed slightly more (2.5%) than control. All shoots under jellyfish treatments showed more vitality than water and chemical fertilizer treatments (according to the visual estimation).

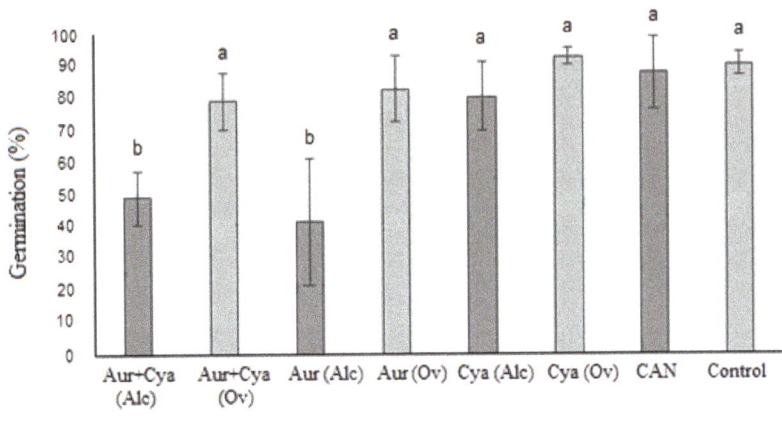

Figure 1. Total germination in percent depending on the different treatment applications in the petri plate experiment. The error bars represent the ± standard deviation. Welch test in two pairs only with control. Same letters indicate no significant differences with control.

3.2. Pot Experiment

In the pot experiment, the effect of jellyfish on seed germination and seedling growth varied with jellyfish species ($p < 0.05$). Seedling emergence occurred earliest in the control treatment, yet mortality increased sharply in the following days (Figure 2). Seedlings in the jellyfish treatment showed greater vitality with better establishment rate. The sprouts and seedlings had a stronger and greener appearance than those of the water (control) and chemical fertilizer treatments.

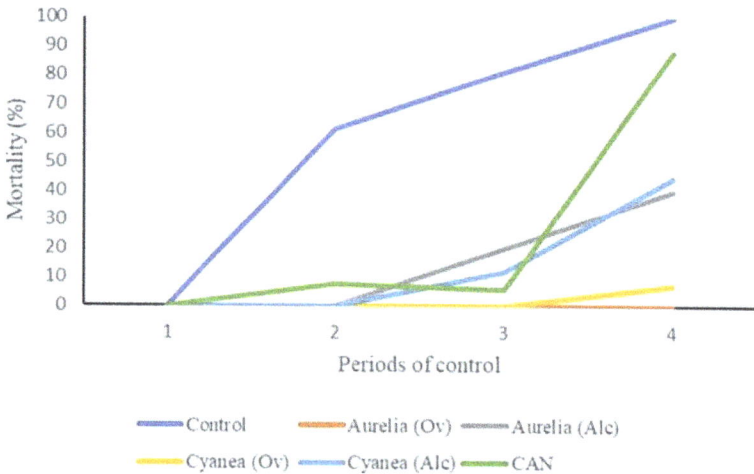

Figure 2. Mortality of seedlings (%) in the pot experiment during the first period of the control (two days).

Results of total germination and final seedling emergence, including surviving and non-surviving seedlings, for the different treatments at the end of the experiment confirmed there was less mortality and higher rates of seedling establishment in the Aur (Alc) and Aur (Ov) treatments (Figures 3 and 4). The results also indicated that the length of grass seedlings changed under different treatments significantly ($p < 0.05$ and $p < 0.01$, Figure 5). The maximum length of the grass seedlings recorded under the Aur (Alc) treatment was around 14 cm. Plant from Aur (Alc), Cya (Alc) and Cya (Ov) treatments were also significantly taller than control ($p < 0.05$; Figure 5).

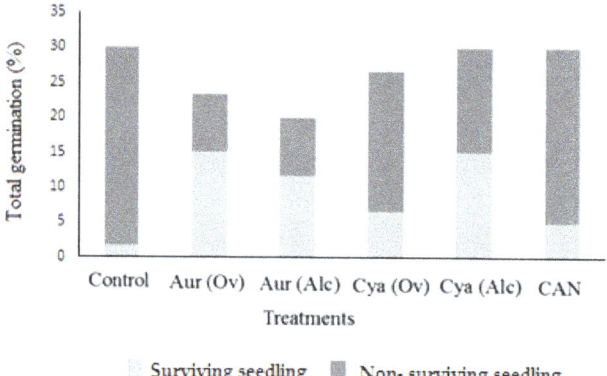

Figure 3. Total germination for final seedling emergence (including surviving and non-surviving seedlings) for each of the different treatments.

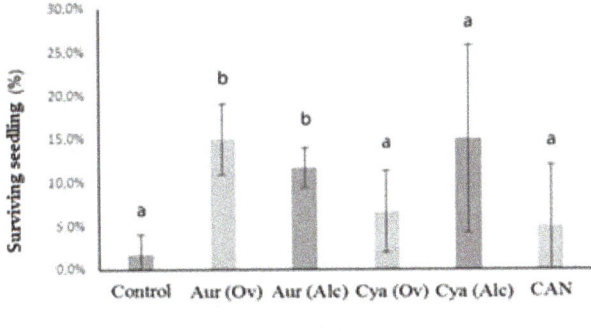

Figure 4. The proportion of surviving seedlings (as percent) among the different treatments in the pot experiment. Error bars represent the ± standard deviation. Welch test in two pairs only with control. Same letters indicate differences are non-significant with control.

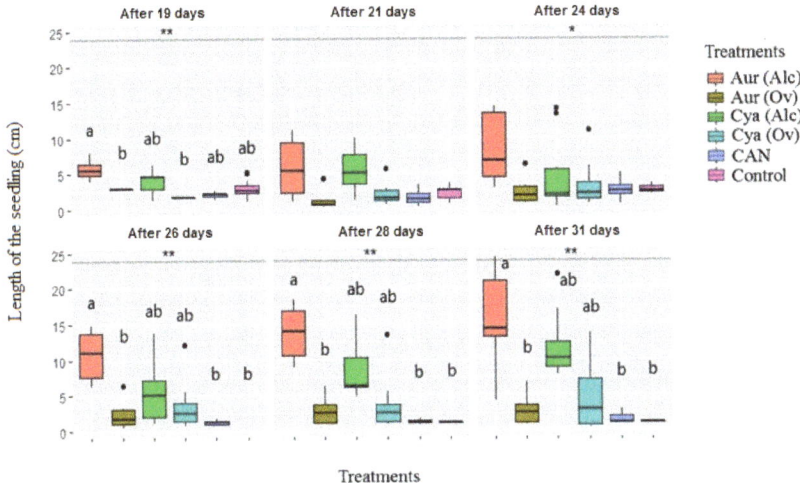

Figure 5. Average length of seedling (cm) under different treatments. Treatments followed by different letters according to Welch test significantly different at $p < 0.05$ and ANOVA test shows significantly different at * $p < 0.05$ and ** $p < 0.01$.

4. Discussion

In this investigation both of the jellyfish species *Aurelia aurita* and *Cyanea capillata* were considered as potential material for promoting seed germination. In the petri plate experiment, there were negative effects of Aur (Alc) and Aur + Cya (Alc) on germination, which may be related to the impacts of alcohol or the jelly form of Aur (Alc) liquid that may delay the time of germination. This effect did not occur in the pot experiment.

According to Bewley [8], the time for germination and post-germinative growth varies from several hours to many weeks, and it depends on the plant species and the germination conditions (Figure 6). Results from our investigation indicated that jellyfish amendments provided conditions that are likely to have caused a delay in germination in comparison with the control. However, evidence showed that in phase 3 (post-germinative growth), seedlings appeared to show greater vitality in treatments with the jellyfish amendments compared with the control. The delay in germination could be related to the salinity of jellyfish, which is indicated by high sodium concentrations in the jellyfish dry matter (Table 1). Delayed germination has been shown previously in many crops as a consequence of high salinity [26].

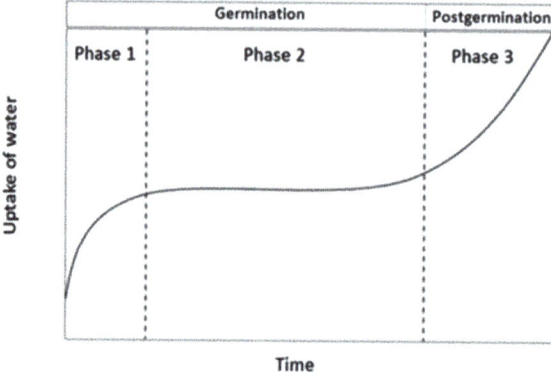

Figure 6. Germination and post-germinative growth divided into three phases regarding water uptake (adapted after Bewley [8]).

The electrical conductivity of alcohol dried jellyfish was shown in Table 3 to be less than other treatments. This could be related to the washing out of the ions by alcohol. The morphology of sprouts and seedlings under the jellyfish treatment shows greater vitality than in the control. This may be related to the presence of additional essential elements provided by jellyfish as well as enhancing soil water holding capacity. There is a good correlation between soil biological activities and soil water content [27]. Thus, there could be a key role for the use of jellyfish as an organic amendment in this context. The germination under control (water) treatment commenced earlier or proceeded faster to seedling emergence than other treatments. Therefore, it is assumed that jellyfish may affect germination by absorbing water and, if so, this may reduce the amount of water available for the seed in the initial stage of germination.

According to Smith and Doran [28], pH values from 5 to 8 represent the optimum range for most soil microorganisms. Hence the pH rates measured for different jellyfish liquids show no harmful effects in this case. The electrical conductivity was lower in treatments dried with alcohol. This may be attributed to different salinity levels and cation exchange capacities. According to Rawls et al. [29], soil organic matter content has impacts on soil structure as well as water adsorption properties. Thus, the application of jellyfish may also enhance soil water retention through enhancing soil organic carbon and collagen content, as well as provide some essential bio-, macro-, and microelements. According to Carter [30], using chemical fertilizer under conditions of low soil moisture content has harmful effects on seedling establishment. Our investigation also showed the same result. According to Killham [27], the most commonly used index to show resource quality is C:N ratio, and low C:N ratios indicate rapid rates of decomposition. The jellyfish used in this study also showed low C:N ratio = 3.5 (Table 1) in comparison with the green manures such as seagrass (C:N = 14) [16,31] that were also used as soil amendment materials.

5. Conclusions

Jellyfish generally did not reduce the germination rate and provided favorable conditions for seedling survival in sand dunes. However, the positive effects might depend on the species of jellyfish, drying process methods, natural environment (e.g., temperature), edaphic conditions, and plant types. In this study, a positive effect of *Aurelia aurita* was observed on seedling establishment of *Lolium multiflorum*, seedling length, and the vitality of seedlings under conditions of water scarcity.

In the context of this investigation, where there is a local surplus of jellyfish, it can be regarded as a local sustainable resource and its use can be considered an innovative organic soil amendment for sand dune restoration projects.

Author Contributions: Conceptualization, visualization, investigation, collected data, analyzed data, and writing original draft, I.E.; investigation, collected data, and analyzed data, R.-R.O.; project administration, investigation, reviewed and edited the manuscript, T.R.; supervision, reviewed and edited the manuscript, F.T. All authors have read and agreed to the published version of the manuscript.

Funding: This research was funded by European Union's Horizon 2020 research and innovation program (Grant agreement no. 774499).

Acknowledgments: The authors would like to thank anonymous reviewers for their constructive comments and suggestions. We also acknowledge financial support by DFG within the funding programme Open Access Publishing.

Conflicts of Interest: The authors declare no conflict of interest.

References

1. Lithgow, D.; Martinez, M.L.; Gallego-Fernandez, J.B.; Hesp, P.A.; Flores, P.; Gachuz, S.; Rodríguez-Revelo, N.; Jiménez-Orocio, O.; Mendoza-González, G.; Álvarez-Molina, L.L. Linking restoration ecology with coastal dune restoration. *Geomorphology* **2013**, *199*, 214–224. [CrossRef]
2. Torretta, V.; Katsoyiannis, I.; Collivignarelli, M.C.; Bertanza, G.; Xanthopoulou, M. Water reuse as a secure pathway to deal with water scarcity. *MATEC Web Conf.* **2020**, *305*, 1–6. [CrossRef]
3. Kim, J.H.; Lim, S.D.; Jang, C.S. Oryza sativa drought-, heat-, and salt-induced RING finger protein 1 (OsDHSRP1) negatively regulates abiotic stress-responsive gene expression. *Plant Mol. Biol.* **2020**. [CrossRef] [PubMed]
4. De Lillis, M.; Costanzo, L.; Bianco, P.M.; Tinelli, A. Sustainability of sand dune restoration along the coast of the Tyrrhenian sea. *J. Coast. Conserv.* **2004**, *10*, 93–100. [CrossRef]
5. Spano, C.; Balestri, M.; Bottega, S.; Grilli, I.; Forino, L.M.C.; Ciccarelli, D. Anthemis maritima L. in different coastal habitats: A tool to explore plant plasticity. *Estuar. Coast. Shelf Sci.* **2013**, *129*, 105–111. [CrossRef]
6. Donohue, K.; de Casas, R.R.; Burghardt, L.; Kovach, K.; Willis, C.G. Germination, postgermination adaptation, and species ecological ranges. *Annu. Rev. Ecol. Evol. Syst.* **2010**, *41*, 293–319. [CrossRef]
7. Yuan, X.; Wen, B. Seed germination response to high temperature and water stress in three invasive Asteraceae weeds from Xishuangbanna, SW China. *PLoS ONE* **2018**. [CrossRef]
8. Bewley, J.D. Seed germination and dormancy. *Plant Cell* **1997**, *9*, 1055–1066. [CrossRef]
9. Kildisheva, O.A.; Kingsley, W.; Dixon, K.W.; Silveira, F.A.O.; Chapman, T.; Sacco, A.D.; Mondoni, A.; Turner, S.R.; Cross, A.T. Dormancy and germination: Making every seed count in restoration. *Restor. Ecol.* **2020**. [CrossRef]
10. Forcella, F.; Benech, A.R.L.; Sanchez, R.; Ghersa, C.M. Modeling seedling emergence. *Field Crop. Res.* **2000**, *67*, 123–139. [CrossRef]
11. Padilla, F.M.; Pugnaire, F.I. Rooting depth and soil moisture control Mediterranean woody seedling survival during drought. *Funct. Ecol.* **2007**, *21*, 489–495. [CrossRef]
12. Manz, B.; Muller, K.; Kucera, B.; Volke, F.; Leubner-Metzger, G. Water uptake and distribution in germinating tobacco seeds investigated in vivo by nuclear magnetic resonance imaging. *Plant Physiol.* **2005**, *138*, 1538–1551. [CrossRef]
13. Bewley, J.D.; Bradford, K.J.; Hilhorst, H.W.M.; Nonogaki, H. *Seeds: Physiology of Development, Germination and Dormancy*; Springer: New York, NY, USA, 2013.
14. Emadodin, I.; Reinsch, T.; Taube, F. Potential of jellyfish as a seed germination promoter. *Jahrestag. Arbeitsgem. Grünl. Futterb.* 2019. Available online: https://www.lfl.bayern.de/mam/cms07/ipz/dateien/aggf_2019_emadodin_et_al.pdf (accessed on 6 May 2019).
15. Condon, R.H.; Steinberg, D.K.; del Giorgio, P.A.; Bouvier, T.C.; Bronk, D.A.; Graham, W.M.; Ducklow, H.W. Jellyfish blooms result in a major microbial respiratory sink of carbon in marine systems. *Proc. Natl. Acad. Sci. USA* **2011**, *108*, 10225–10230. [CrossRef] [PubMed]

16. Emadodin, I.; Reinsch, T.; Rotter, A.; Orlando-Bonaca, M.; Taube, F.; Javidpour, J. A perspective on the potential of using marine organic fertilizers for the sustainable management of coastal ecosystem services. *Environ. Sustain.* **2020**. [CrossRef]
17. Uye, S. Blooms of the giant jellyfish Nemopilema nomurai: A threat to the fisheries sustainability of the East Asian Marginal Seas. *Plankton Benthos Res.* **2008**, *3*, 125–131. [CrossRef]
18. Cruz-Rivera, E.; El-Regal, M.A. A bloom of an edible scyphozoan jellyfish in the Red Sea. *Mar. Biodivers.* **2015**, *46*, 515–519. [CrossRef]
19. Boero, F. *Review of jellyfish blooms in the Mediterranean and Black Sea*; Studies and Reviews; General Fisheries Commission for the Mediterranean; FAO: Rome, Italy, 2013; p. 53.
20. Fukushi, K.; Ishio, N.; Tsujimoto, J.; Yokota, K.; Hamatake, T.; Sogabe, H.; Toriya, K.; Nimomiya, T. Preliminary Study on the Potential usefulness of Jellyfish fertilizer. *J. Bull. Soc. Sea Water Sci.* **2003**, *2*, 209–217.
21. Hossain, S.T.; Sugimoto, H.; Asagi, N.; Araki, T.; Ueno, H.; Morokuma, M.; Kato, H. The use of desalinated-dried jellyfish and rice bran for controlling weeds and rice yield. *J. Org. Syst.* **2013**, *8*, 28–37.
22. Hussein, O.S.; Sayed, R.M.; Saleh, O.I. Uses of jellyfish in pre-sowing seeds treatment and pest control. *Am. J. Exp. Agric.* **2015**, *5*, 60–69. [CrossRef]
23. Pedersen, M.T.; Brewer, J.R.; Duelund, L.; Hansen, P.L. On the gastrophysics of jellyfish preparation. *Int. J. Gastron. Food Sci.* **2017**, *9*, 34–38. [CrossRef]
24. Esechie, H.A.; Al-Saidi, A.; Al-Khanjari, S. Effect of sodium chloride salinity on seedling emergence in chickpea. *J. Agron. Crop Sci.* **2002**, *188*, 155–160. [CrossRef]
25. Welch, B.L. The generalization of "Student's" problem when several different population variances are involved. *Biometrika* **1947**, *34*, 28–35. [PubMed]
26. Baath, G.S.; Shukla, M.K.; Bosland, P.W.; Steiner, R.L.; Walker, S.J. Irrigation water salinity influences at various growth stages of Capsicum annuum. *Agric. Water Manag.* **2017**, *179*, 246–253. [CrossRef]
27. Killham, K. *Soil Ecology*; Cambridge University Press: Cambridge, UK, 1994; p. 242.
28. Smith, J.L.; Doran, J.W. Measurement and use of pH and electrical conductivity for soil quality analysis. In *Methods for assessing Soil Quality*; Doran, J.W., Jones, A.J., Eds.; Soil Science Society of America Journal, SSSA: Madison, WI, USA, 1996; p. 49.
29. Rawls, W.J.; Pachepsky, Y.A.; Ritchie, J.C.; Sobecki, T.M.; Bloodworth, H. Effect of soil organic carbon on soil water retention. *Geoderma* **2003**, *116*, 61–76. [CrossRef]
30. Carter, O.G. The effect of chemical fertilizers on seedling establishment. *Aust. J. Exp. Agric. Anim. Husb.* **1967**, *7*, 174–180. [CrossRef]
31. Aulakh, M.; Khera, T.; Doran, J. Mineralization and denitrification in upland, nearly saturated and flooded subtropical soil II. Effect of organic manures varying in N content and C:N ratio. *Biol. Fertil. Soils* **2000**, *31*, 168–174. [CrossRef]

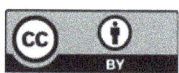

© 2020 by the authors. Licensee MDPI, Basel, Switzerland. This article is an open access article distributed under the terms and conditions of the Creative Commons Attribution (CC BY) license (http://creativecommons.org/licenses/by/4.0/).

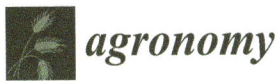

Communication

Suitability of Black Soldier Fly Frass as Soil Amendment and Implication for Organic Waste Hygienization

Thomas Klammsteiner [1,*], Veysel Turan [2], Marina Fernández-Delgado Juárez [1], Simon Oberegger [1] and Heribert Insam [1]

[1] Department of Microbiology, University of Innsbruck, Technikerstraße 25d, 6020 Innsbruck, Austria; marinafdj84@gmail.com (M.F.-D.J.); s.oberegger@student.uibk.ac.at (S.O.); heribert.insam@uibk.ac.at (H.I.)
[2] Department of Soil Science and Plant Nutrition, Bingöl University, Selahaddin-I Eyyubi, Üniversite Caddesi, 12000 Bingöl, Turkey; vturan@bingol.edu.tr
* Correspondence: thomas.klammsteiner@uibk.ac.at; Tel.: +43-512-507-51322

Received: 20 September 2020; Accepted: 14 October 2020; Published: 15 October 2020

Abstract: Because of its nutritious properties, the black soldier fly has emerged as one of the most popular species in advancing circular economy through the re-valorization of anthropogenic organic wastes to insect biomass. Black soldier fly frass accumulates as a major by-product in artificial rearing set-ups and harbors great potential to complement or replace commercial fertilizers. We applied frass from larvae raised on different diets in nitrogen-equivalent amounts as soil amendment, comparing it to NH_4NO_3 fertilizer as a control. While the soil properties did not reveal any difference between mineral fertilizer and frass, principal component analysis showed significant differences that are mainly attributed to nitrate and dissolved nitrogen contents. We did not find significant differences in the growth of perennial ryegrass between the treatments, indicating that frass serves as a rapidly acting fertilizer comparable to NH_4NO_3. While the abundance of coliform bacteria increased during frass maturation, after application to the soil, they were outcompeted by gram-negatives. We thus conclude that frass may serve as a valuable fertilizer and does not impair the hygienic properties of soils.

Keywords: animal feedstuff; circular economy; fertilizer; greenhouse; insect larva; organic waste

1. Introduction

In recent years, the use of saprobic insect larvae from the mealworm beetle (*Tenebrio molitor*), the black soldier fly (*Hermetia illucens*; BSF), or the house fly (*Musca domestica*) has attracted interest in the face of rising prices of animal feedstuff and accumulating amounts of waste [1,2]. In the European Union, green waste and food waste largely contribute to an annual amount of 118 to 138 million tons of organic wastes [3]. Especially BSF larvae (BSFL) have been shown to efficiently convert organic wastes into high quality fat and protein [4]. The economic potential and meaningful reintroduction of otherwise wasted nutrients into the biosphere via a circular economy enticed researchers, investors, and the public to contribute to a more efficient recycling of organic wastes by exploiting the potential of insect larvae on a large scale [5,6]. BSFL could also play a valuable role for smaller decentralized waste management systems operated by e.g., hobbyists or farmers in areas where the fly occurs naturally [7–9]. Additionally, the exploitation of BSF and its by-products could create an affordable opportunity for revenue generation by entrepreneurs and smallholder farmers in low-income countries [9–11]. The main by-product in the bioconversion of wastes into high quality protein for animal feedstuff is summarized as 'frass'. Frass in general describes insect excretions, but in a commercial context it often refers to a mixture of mainly insect feces, substrate residues, and shed exoskeletons. It is an inevitable side-stream during the mass-rearing of insects that can add up to 75% of the fed substrate [12] and is often merchandised as a fertilizing product. In recent years, an increasing number of studies started focusing on meaningful applications of insect frass [9,13–15], and the first large-scale field studies provided promising perspectives for its application in agriculture, especially in terms of plant nutrient availability [10,11,16].

The substrate used to grow insects affects the properties of the frass, since undegradable residues remain unused, while the digested fraction is modified by the gut microbiota when passing through the gastrointestinal tract [17,18]. Wang et al. [19] used frass from *T. molitor* for subsequent rearing of BSFL to exploit leftover nutrients that *T. molitor* could not take up or digest. In substrates carrying a high bioburden like human feces and manure, BSFL have shown to reduce pathogenic bacteria such as *Salmonella enterica* [20,21] and *Escherichia coli* [20,22], which is attributed to their production of antimicrobial peptides [23]. In the wild, frass from various insects can help to increase the chances of survival and reproduction by either deterring [24,25] or attracting [26,27] conspecifics. Frass can act as a vector for phytopathogenic microorganisms [28,29] and as a source of probiotic yeasts [30]. Its effect on the insects' environment can be observed in forests, where frass deposition goes hand in hand with insect canopy herbivory. It has been shown that frass has an impact on C and N dynamics, and has beneficial effects for tree growth by increasing soil total C, N, and NH_4^+, as well as microbial soil respiration [31,32]. In industrial environments, frass pyrolyzed to biochar has been successfully tested as a bioadsorbent for wastewater detoxification [33]. According to recent studies, frass' agriculturally and economically most meaningful potential could lie in its application as fertilizer [9,34].

In this study, we assessed the fertilizing potential of process residues (frass) from three generic diets degraded by BSFL. Two of the diets represent major streams of organic waste, namely grass-cuttings (GC) and fruit/vegetable (FV) mix, while the chicken feed (CF) control diet is a commonly used insect breeding substrate. We hypothesized that (I) microbial colonization increases with frass maturation and (II) frass may serve as a valuable alternative to mineral fertilizer by inducing beneficial effects on plant growth.

2. Materials and Methods

2.1. Black Soldier Fly Frass Collection

The frass was collected from a preparatory feeding experiment conducted at 27 °C, 60% relative humidity (Figures S1 and S2, Table 1). The chicken feed (CF; Grünes Legekorn Premium, Unser Lagerhaus, Klagenfurt, Austria) was processed with a Fidibus flour mill (Komo Mills, Hopfgarten, Austria) and mixed with water in a 40:60 ratio.

Table 1. Feeding experiment termination summary. The feeding experiment was terminated after a total of 23 days when more than 90% larvae from one treatment group transitioned to prepupal stage. Different lower-case letters indicate differences between treatments ($p \leq 0.05$) according to the Tukey's HSD test. (n = 4; average ± standard deviation; CF = Chicken feed diet, GC = Grass-cuttings diet, FW = Fruit/Vegetables diet).

	CF	GC	FV
Pupation rate [%]	55.2 ± 5.3 b	98.7 ± 2.0 c	22.4 ± 2.0 a
Prepupae fresh weight [mg]	198 ± 10	167 ± 11	165 ± 31
Prepupae dry weight [%]	32.6 ± 1.9	29.6 ± 1.9	32.2 ± 9.3
Prepupae water content [%]	67.4 ± 3.7	70.4 ± 5.6	67.8 ± 9.9
Prepupae organic content [%]	27.6 ± 1.6	26.5 ± 1.8	31.4 ± 8.4
Prepupae inorganic content [%]	5.1 ± 0.3 c	3.1 ± 0.2 b	0.9 ± 0.9 a
Frass residues [%]	43.7 ± 1.0 c	46.0 ± 1.5 b	28.5 ± 0.5 a

The fruit/vegetable mix (FV; cucumber, tomato, apple, orange, in ratio 0.5:1:1:1) and fresh grass-cutting diet (GC) were shredded and homogenized using a Total Nutrition Center blender

(Vitamix, Olmsted Township, United States). Feeding was done in organic content-equivalents (100, 250, and 370 mg larvae^{-1} day^{-1} for CF, GC, and FV). After termination of the feeding experiment, the black soldier fly frass (BSFF) from each treatment was collected in plastic bags and stored at room temperature until further use.2.2. Soil Preparation and Greenhouse Set Up

A greenhouse trial using soil collected from an agricultural site (47°15′54″ N, 11°20′20″ E; Table 2) was set up to evaluate the fertilizing effect of the BSFF on the soil. The neutral-to-slightly basic soil (pH 7.3 ± 0.4) had an electrical conductivity of 78.0 ± 2.7 µs cm^{-1} and a volatile solids content of 78.0 ± 26.6 g kg^{-1}. In addition to a P_{total} content of 823 ± 190 mg kg^{-1} ($P_{bioavailable}$ proportion 6.88 ± 1.28 mg kg^{-1}), elemental analysis determined a C/N ratio of 24 (40 g C_{total} kg^{-1}, 1.7 g N_{total} kg^{-1}). The soil classified as a calcaric Fluvisol (IUSS Working Group WRB, 2015) was sieved (Ø < 4 mm) and homogenously mixed with a vermiculite/sand blend (1:1; v:v) at a ratio 2:1 w:w (soil:blend).

Table 2. Characterization of the soil used for the greenhouse trial. Values expressed on a dry mass basis for n = 3 (average ± standard deviation). pH (pH CaCl$_2$), EC (Electrical conductivity), VS (Volatile solids), C_{tot} (Total carbon), N_{tot} (Total nitrogen), P_{tot} (Total phosphorous), P_{av} (Plant available P).

Parameter	Value
pH	7.3 ± 0.4
EC [µs cm^{-1}]	78.1 ± 2.7
VS [g kg^{-1}]	78.5 ± 26.6
C_{tot} [g kg^{-1}]	40
N_{tot} [g kg^{-1}]	1.7
P_{tot} [mg kg^{-1}]	823 ± 190
P_{av} [mg kg^{-1}]	6.88 ± 1.28

The four experimental treatments were performed in 500 mL pots: soil was mixed with (1) mineral fertilizer (which served as control); (2) GC BSFF; (3) FV BSFF; (4) and CF BSFF. The mineral fertilizer (NH$_4$NO$_3$) and the different types of BSFF (Table 3) were added in an amount of 40 mg N kg^{-1} soil, which is equivalent to 80 kg N ha^{-1}, considering the soil bulk density of 1 g cm^{-3} and a plough depth of 20 cm as described by Goberna et al. [35]. Thereby, all treatments received the same dose of total N.

Table 3. Main properties of the three different black soldier fly frass fractions (CF-F: Chicken feed frass; GC-F: Grass-cuttings frass; FV-F: Fruit/Vegetables frass). Values expressed on a dry mass basis for n = 3 (average ± standard deviation). Different lower-case letters indicate differences between treatments ($p \leq 0.05$) according to the Tukey´s HSD test. Different capital letters indicate significant differences between treatments ($p \leq 0.05$) according to the Mann–Whitney test. EC (Electrical conductivity), VS (Volatile solids), C_{tot} (Total carbon content), N_{tot} (Total nitrogen content).

	CF-F	GC-F	FV-F
pH	6.22 ± 0.14 C	5.40 ± 0.03 A	5.58 ± 0.01 B
EC [mS cm^{-1}]	5.67 ± 0.27 c	3.06 ± 0.03 b	2.36 ± 0.11 a
Dry matter [%]	90.9 ± 0.0	89.9 ± 0.0	90.4 ± 0.0
C_{tot} [g kg^{-1}]	479 ± 8 B	443 ± 6 A	488 ± 4 B
N_{tot} [g kg^{-1}]	25.9 ± 0.9 b	24.4 ± 0.2 b	18.3 ± 1.2 a
C:N ratio	18.5 ± 0.3 a	18.2 ± 0.4 a	26.6 ± 1.7 b
VS [g kg^{-1}]	910 ± 7 c	825 ± 9 a	873 ± 4 b

After an equilibration period of 16 h at 4 °C, pots were randomly placed in a greenhouse. Ryegrass (Lolium perenne; seed amount based on 30 kg seeds ha^{-1}) was sown and left to develop. During the incubation period of 28 days, at an average temperature of 20 °C with a light/darkness cycle of 10/14 h, the soil moisture was kept at field capacity (moisture of the soil after drainage by gravity). All treatments were applied in four replicates, resulting in a total of 16 pots in this study. After the incubation period, plants were removed from the pots, and soil samples were sieved (Ø < 2 mm) and immediately stored at +4 °C until analyses (Table 4).

Table 4. Physicochemical and biological properties of the control (C-S: NH_4NO_3) and the frass amended soils (CF-S: Chicken feed frass + soil; GC-S: Grass-cuttings frass + soil and FV-S: Fruit/Vegetables frass + soil). Values expressed on a dry mass basis for $n = 4$ (average ± standard deviation). Different lower-case letters indicate differences between treatments ($p \leq 0.05$) according to the Tukey's HSD test. Different capital letters indicate significant differences between treatments ($p \leq 0.05$) according to the Mann–Whitney test. EC (Electrical conductivity), VS (volatile solids), C_{tot} (Total carbon content), N_{tot} (Total nitrogen content), NH_4^+ (Ammonium content), NO_3^- (Nitrate content), DOC (Dissolved organic carbon), DC (Dissolved carbon), DN (Dissolved nitrogen), P_{av} (Plant available phosphorous content), P_{tot} (Total phosphorous content), BR (Basal respiration), qCO_2 (Metabolic quotient).

	C-S	CF-S	GC-S	FV-S
pH $CaCl_2$	7.53 ± 0.02 a	7.57 ± 0.01 ab	7.58 ± 0.03 b	7.58 ± 0.02 b
EC [µS cm^{-1}]	95.5 ± 1.8 B	79.8 ± 6.4 A	77.3 ± 2.9 A	81.5 ± 7.8 A
VS [g kg^{-1}]	37.3 ± 1.1	35.4 ± 1.3	38.4 ± 2.0	37.8 ± 2.1
C_{tot} [g kg^{-1}]	17.9 ± 3.2	21.7 ± 4.	22.5 ± 6.1	20.6 ± 5.2
N_{tot} [g kg^{-1}]	0.98 ± 0.35	0.99 ± 0.51	1.17 ± 0.39	0.98 ± 0.44
C:N ratio	20.3 ± 8.1	26.2 ± 11.7	21.0 ± 9.8	22.1 ± 9.0
NH_4^+ [mg kg^{-1}]	0.57 ± 0.13	0.58 ± 0.06	0.58 ± 0.08	0.61 ± 0.14
NO_3^- [mg kg^{-1}]	45.2 ± 4.1 b	15.4 ± 3.3 a	17.0 ± 3.5 a	12.1 ± 4.4 a
DOC [mg kg^{-1}]	48.3 ± 3.8	50.2 ± 1.5	48.5 ± 1.9	51.8 ± 1.3
DC [mg kg^{-1}]	95.6 ± 1.6 a	104.7 ± 1.4 b	103.5 ±4.0 b	112.1 ± 2.0 c
DN [mg kg^{-1}]	35.6 ± 3.9 C	17.0 ± 1.5 B	15.3 ± 1.8 AB	15.0 ± 0.6 A
P_{av} [mg kg^{-1}]	5.2 ± 0.4	6.1 ± 1.0	6.1 ± 1.4	5.8 ± 0.9
P_{tot} [mg kg^{-1}]	783 ± 46 ab	866 ± 35 b	757 ± 33 a	721 ± 45 a
P bioavailability [%]	67 ± 8	70 ± 12	81 ± 23	80 ± 12
BR [µg CO_2 g^{-1} dw h^{-1}]	5.6 ± 0.15	4.6 ± 1.5	6.7 ± 0.7	5.6 ± 0.5
C_{mic} [µg CO_2 g^{-1} dw soil]	416.1 ± 103.5	276.4 ± 38.7	279.0 ± 22.7	336.2 ± 16.1
qCO_2 [µg CO_2-C h^{-1}/µg^{-1} C mic]	14.7 ± 4.7	16.4 ± 4.3	24.5 ± 4.5	16.6 ± 1.4
Plant biomass [mg dw]	85 ± 7	80 ± 6	74 ± 4	75 ± 3

2.2. Frass and Soil Analyses

Frass and soil samples (10 g fresh weight) were placed into a glass Petri dish and oven-dried (105 °C) for 24 h to determine the content of total solids. Volatile organic solid (VS) content was determined from the weight loss following ignition in a muffle furnace (CWF 1000, Carbolite, Neuhausen, Germany) at 550 °C for 5 h. Total C and N contents were analyzed in dried samples using a CN analyzer (TruSpec CHN, LECO, St. Joseph, MI, USA). EC and pH were determined in distilled water and 0.01 M $CaCl_2$ extracts (1:2.5, w/v), respectively.

Soil inorganic nitrogen (NH_4^+ and NO_3^-) was determined in 0.0125 M $CaCl_2$ extracts as described by Kandeler [36,37]. Soil total P (P_{tot}) and plant available P (P_{av}) were determined as described by Illmer et al. [38]. To estimate dissolved organic carbon (DOC), dissolved carbon (DC), and dissolved nitrogen (DN), 10 g of field-moist soil were shaken in 40 mL distilled water, filtered, and immediately measured using a TOC-L analyzer (Shimadzu, Kyōto, Japan). Soil basal respiration (BR) and microbial biomass (C_{mic}) were measured according to Heinemeyer et al. [39]. The metabolic quotient (qCO_2) was calculated from BR and C_{mic} according to Anderson and Domsch [40]. At the end of the trial, aboveground plant biomass was determined by cutting plant shoots at the soil surface and drying them at 60 °C for 48 h. Samples were then re-weighted to determine the dry biomass.

2.3. Preparation of Media

For the assessment of the total cultivable bacterial colony forming units (CFUs), we used standard methods agar (0.5% peptone, 0.25% yeast extract, 0.1% glucose, 1.5% agar, pH adjusted to neutral). To determine the abundance of *Salmonella* sp., *E. coli*, coliforms, and other gram-negative bacteria,

XLT-4 and ChromoCult® coliform agar (Merck, Darmstadt, Germany) were prepared according to the enclosed recipe.

2.4. Pathogen Quantification/Assessment of Microbial Colonization in Frass and Soil

An amount of 2 g frass or soil sample was added to 18 mL sterile saline solution (0.95% NaCl) and placed on a rotation shaker at 200 rpm for 15 min. Samples were diluted to 10^{-2} and 10^{-3} for soil, and 10^{-5} and 10^{-6} for frass using sterile 0.95% NaCl. From each dilution, 50 µL was plated using the spread plate technique. Plates were then incubated at 37 °C for 24 h, and the CFUs were counted.

2.5. Statistical Analyses

The effect of the BSFF application on soil parameters was tested with a one-way analysis of variance (ANOVA). In case of significant F-values, a Tukey's HSD (honestly significant difference) post hoc test ($p < 0.05$) was performed. Prior to analysis, the homogeneity of the variances was tested (Levene's test), and data were also tested for normality. Non-normal data were subjected to non-parametric tests for several independent samples (Kruskal–Wallis test), and pairwise comparisons between treatments were performed using the Mann–Whitney U test ($p < 0.05$). Statistical analyses were performed using the SPSS v. 23.0 Software (IBM, Armonk, NY, USA). Principal component analysis was performed in R [41] using the vegan package [42]. Analysis of similarity (ANOSIM) on the physicochemical data (999 permutations) was also conducted with vegan. All graphical representations of data were created with ggplot2 [43].

3. Results and Discussion

3.1. Assessment of Microbial Load in Frass and Frass-Amended Soils

The high moisture content of substrates and air, as well as the pleasantly warm temperature common in insect breeding, favor microbial growth. While the type of diet is known to directly influence the BSFL gut microbiome [17,44], the excrements in turn may influence the microbiome in the frass. It is likely that by agitating and mixing their surrounding substrate with feces and their inherent microorganisms, the larvae have an impact on their habitat. Similar effects are known from the widely used earthworms (*Eisenia fetida*), which can stabilize organic wastes and introduce ammonia-oxidizing microorganisms, thereby boosting nitrification and increasing nitrate concentrations in the resulting vermicompost [45]. Other insect species inoculate the soil with excreted microorganisms and provide beneficial effects for its quality both in wild and artificial settings [46–48].

Before and after applying frass as soil amendment, the number of cultivable *E. coli*, coliform, and other gram-negative bacteria were assessed (Figure 1). While frass counted up to 10^9 CFU g^{-1}, the count in soil was down to 10^3–10^5 g^{-1}. With the nutrient media used in this study, untreated soil contained no cultivable *E. coli* or coliforms, and only low abundances of cultivable gram-negatives with 10^2 CFUs g^{-1}. In particular, frass from the CF treatment acted as a reservoir for coliforms with a CFU count of 1.9×10^9, thereby exceeding CFU counts recorded on larval surfaces (Figure S2). Gram-negative bacteria predominated the cultivable microbiota in frass-amended soil with highest CFU counts of up to 10^5 in soil treated with frass from a FV diet. High microbial load and dominance of coliforms in frass shifted to lower CFU numbers and predominantly gram-negative bacteria in the frass-soil mix, indicating that the autochthonous soil microbiota outcompeted allochthonous microorganisms introduced with frass [49–51].

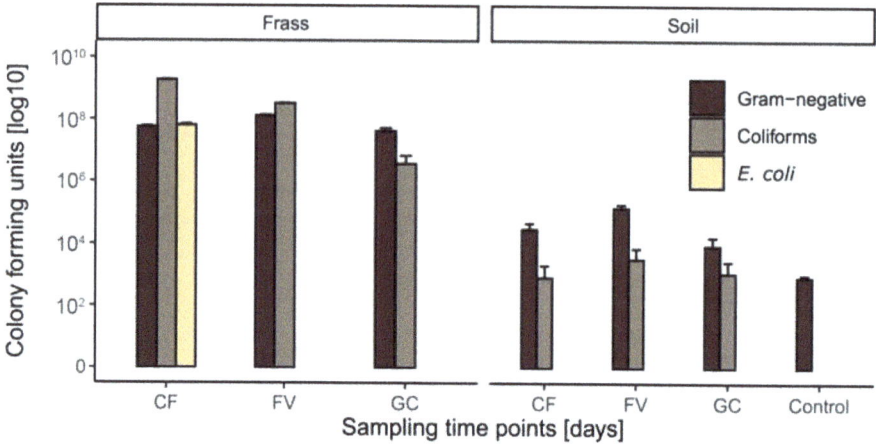

Figure 1. Colony forming units counted for gram-negative, coliform, and *Escherichia coli* from frass samples after collection from the feeding experiment and soil samples after having mixed the soil with frass ($n = 4$). CF = Chicken feed, FV = Fruit/vegetable mix, GC = Grass-cuttings.

3.2. Black Soldier Fly Frass Properties, Soil Quality and Plant Performance

The physicochemical properties of frass were influenced by the larval diet (Table 3). Especially CF frass was more alkaline, had a higher EC, and a higher content of VS. While total C contents were similar in all types of frass, FV frass showed a C:N-ratio of 26.6, compared to 18.5 and 18.2 in CF frass and GC frass, respectively. Similar C:N ratios as found in CF and GC frass have been reported by other studies that used brewery spent grains as larval substrate [11,16]. A C:N-ratio > 20 bears the risk of soil N immobilization, which may favor plants with a more efficient N exploitation attributed to their rhizobiome [46,52]. The addition of biochar to the larval waste conversion process might further improve the frass' N retention, while at the same time increasing larval biomass yield [10]. Moreover, larvae pass through six instars continuously shedding their exoskeleton. Chitin, an N-acetylglucosamine-based polymer $(C_8H_{13}O_5N)_n$, may influence not only the C:N ratio, but its degradation product chitosan may also provide underrated benefits for plant health and pathogen resistance [53,54]. The C:N ratio is one of the major parameters to consider when it comes to deciding whether frass should be used as soil amendment or as co-substrate in anaerobic digestion or composting [55,56]. Chitin utilization by insects is often associated with chitinolytic gut symbionts [57], which still needs to be further investigated in the context of BSF larvae. Chitin-containing fertilizers have previously been found to serve as splendid nitrogen sources [58].

Frass addition to the soil before planting *Lolium perenne* was adjusted on a basis of N-equivalence (80 kg N ha^{-1}; Tables 3 and 4). Soil amended with CF frass exhibited a higher P_{tot} content than the other frass-amended soils; however, P_{av} was not significantly different. Principal component analysis (Figure 2) highlighted the parameters that influenced the properties of the soil-frass mix the most, which was further confirmed by ANOSIM ($R = 0.5061$, $p < 0.001$). The three frass-amended soils clustered closely together, with P_{tot} and P_{av}, pH, DC, N_{tot}, C:N ratio, BR, and the qCO_2 being the most influential parameters for their similarity.

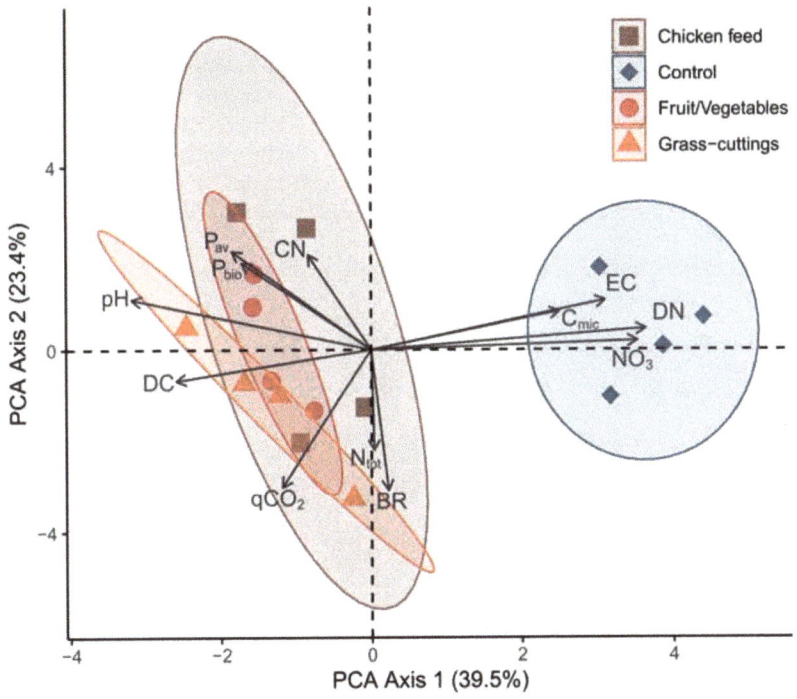

Figure 2. Principal component analysis of samples from control soil and soil mixed with the three different frass types. Data points represent replicates, and arrows show the most influential parameters for the spread of the data. NO_3 = Nitrate, DN = Dissolved nitrogen, CN = Carbon/Nitrogen ratio, P_{bio} = Phosphorus bioavailability, BR = Soil basal respiration, qCO_2 = Metabolic quotient, C_{mic} = Microbial biomass, N_{tot} = Total nitrogen, P_{av} = Plant available phosphorus, DC = Dissolved carbon, EC = Electric conductivity.

The qCO_2 describing the microbial soil respiration per unit C_{mic} is known to be tightly connected to the C:N ratio and increases when less N is available [59]. Higher qCO_2 can indicate stress or disturbances within the soil because, although C sources are readily available, microbial metabolism and substrate decomposition are limited by N [60]. NO_3 and DN, on the other hand, were the major drivers for the deviation of the control group from the frass treatment groups, since they were both significantly higher in control soil.

In our study, the frass treatments were compared with a control that received an equivalent of 80 kg ha^{-1} nitrogen in the form of NH_4NO_3. In a similar experiment, Ros et al. [61] found that such an amount of mineral N increased the maize yield by 33% compared with an unfertilized control, while N-equivalent additions of compost yielded only 15% increase. Recent observations at field-scale by Beesigamukama et al. showed that even at lower application rates of 30 kg N ha^{-1}, BSFF exceeded the performance of mineral N fertilizer in terms of grain yield and nitrogen fertilizer replacement values when applied at the same rates [16]. Compared with commercial fertilizers, nitrogen recovery rates and nitrogen use efficiency of plants have been shown to be improved when amended with BSFF [11]. Additionally, the higher P concentrations in the frass could facilitate N accumulation in plants by improving N uptake, as P plays an important role in energy transfer [62,63].

Using BSFL instead of aerobic windrow composting has additionally been shown to reduce the global warming potential of treating organic wastes by 50% [64]. The addition of frass did not lead to significant differences in plant growth compared to the mineral fertilizer (Figure 3). In fact, the similar growth progress indicates that the nutrients from frass are readily available for uptake and have no detrimental impact on plant growth. These results, however, do not support the findings of Alattar et al. [13], who reported that the development of plant height and leaves in corn (*Zea mays*) was inhibited by the addition of BSFL frass. In their study, they attributed the negative effects to the low porosity of larval residues that may have created anaerobic conditions. The moisture content of the frass harvested from our preliminary feeding experiment was only 10% (Table 3), thereby facilitating aeration and miscibility in soil. Insufficient oxygen supply can occur when frass has a high moisture content and is not subjected to adequate post-processing. In an environment specialized on insect rearing, a multi-step treatment of frass could increase the efficiency of degradation. With additional downstream composting or anaerobic digestion [65,66], the recovery as soil amendment represents the economically most promising option.

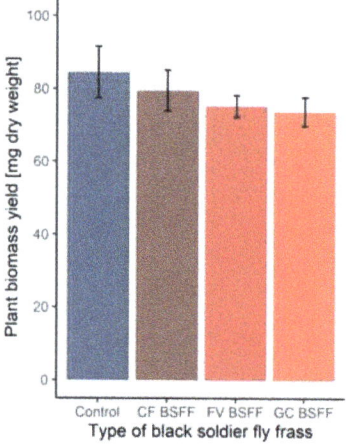

Figure 3. Plant biomass yield of *Lolium perenne* after application of black soldier fly frass (BSFF) obtained from the degradation of various organic substrates. CF BSFF = Chicken feed frass, FV BSFF = Fruit/vegetables frass, GC BSFF = Grass-cuttings frass ($n = 4$).

4. Conclusions

The valorization of organic wastes by insect larvae generates frass as a side-product. From our study we conclude that frass may serve as a soil nutrient source and does not impair soil hygiene. In some cases, however, frass post-processing through anaerobic digestion or composting may be advised to avoid soil nitrogen deficiencies or impairing soil gas permeability. In the light of the increasing importance of insect rearing, the agricultural utilization of frass is demanding further research, in particular, long-term studies.

Supplementary Materials: The following are available online at http://www.mdpi.com/2073-4395/10/10/1578/s1, Figure S1: Influence of three different diets on larval biomass increase, Figure S2: Microbial colonization of larval surfaces.

Author Contributions: Conceptualization, T.K. and M.F.-D.J.; formal analysis, V.T., T.K., and S.O.; funding acquisition, H.I., V.T., and T.K.; investigation, S.O. and V.T.; methodology, V.T. and M.F.-D.J.; resources, H.I.; supervision, T.K. and M.F.-D.J.; visualization, T.K.; writing—original draft, T.K. and M.F.-D.J. All authors have read and agreed to the published version of the manuscript.

Funding: This research was funded by the Austrian Science Fund (FWF; project number: P26444). Thomas Klammsteiner was supported by a PhD grant from the Vizerektorat für Forschung of the Universität Innsbruck (Doktoratsstipendium aus der Nachwuchsförderung). Veysel Turan was supported by a post-doctoral fellowship from the Scientific and Technological Research Council of Turkey (TÜBITAK, grant number, 1059B191601133).

Acknowledgments: The authors show their gratitude to Carina D. Heussler for providing the black soldier fly larvae for this study. Open Access Funding by the Austrian Science Fund (FWF).

Conflicts of Interest: The authors declare no conflict of interest.

References

1. FAO. *Global Food Losses and Food Waste: Extent, Causes and Prevention*; Food and Agriculture Organization of the United Nations: Rome, Italy, 2011; ISBN 978-92-5-107205-9.
2. United Nations. *World Population Prospects. The 2017 Revision*; Department of Economic and Social Affairs—Population Division: New York, NY, USA, 2017; p. 53.
3. European Commission. *811: Green Paper on the Management of Bio-Waste in the European Union*; Commission of the European Communities: Brussels, Belgium, 2008.
4. Pastor, B.; Velasquez, Y.; Gobbi, P.; Rojo, S. Conversion of organic wastes into fly larval biomass: Bottlenecks and challenges. *J. Insects Food Feed* **2015**, *1*, 179–193. [CrossRef]
5. Rumpold, B.A.; Klocke, M.; Schluter, O. Insect biodiversity: Underutilized bioresource for sustainable applications in life sciences. *Reg. Environ. Chang.* **2017**, *17*, 1445–1454. [CrossRef]
6. Sogari, G.; Amato, M.; Biasato, I.; Chiesa, S.; Gasco, L. The potential role of insects as feed: A multi-perspective review. *Animals* **2019**, *9*, 119. [CrossRef] [PubMed]
7. Choudhury, A.R.; Ashok, K.N.; Srinivas, K.; Arutchelvan, V.; Thota, K.R.; Ravi, S.N.; Sandeep, K.D.; Goutham, R.M. Black soldier fly larvae, a viable opportunity for entrepreneurship. *Acta Sci. Agric.* **2018**, *2*, 11–20.
8. Klammsteiner, T.; Walter, A.; Pan, H.; Gassner, M.; Heussler, C.D.; Schermer, M.; Insam, H. On everyone's lips: Insects for food and feed. In Proceedings of the 5th Austrian Citizen Science Conference, Obergurgl, Austria, 26—28 June 2019; Volume 366, p. 6.
9. Quilliam, R.S.; Nuku-Adeku, C.; Maquart, P.; Little, D.; Newton, R.; Murray, F. Integrating insect frass biofertilisers into sustainable peri-urban agro-food systems. *J. Insects Food Feed* **2020**, 1–8. [CrossRef]
10. Beesigamukama, D.; Mochoge, B.; Korir, N.K.; Fiaboe, K.K.M.; Nakimbugwe, D.; Khamis, F.M.; Dubois, T.; Subramanian, S.; Wangu, M.M.; Ekesi, S.; et al. Biochar and gypsum amendment of agro-industrial waste for enhanced black soldier fly larval biomass and quality frass fertilizer. *PLoS ONE* **2020**, *15*, e238154. [CrossRef]
11. Beesigamukama, D.; Mochoge, B.; Korir, N.K.; Fiaboe, K.K.M.; Nakimbugwe, D.; Khamis, F.M.; Subramanian, S.; Dubois, T.; Musyoka, M.W.; Ekesi, S.; et al. Exploring Black Soldier Fly Frass as Novel Fertilizer for Improved Growth, Yield, and Nitrogen Use Efficiency of Maize Under Field Conditions. *Front. Plant Sci.* **2020**, *11*. [CrossRef]
12. Diener, S.; Zurbrügg, C.; Tockner, K. Conversion of organic material by black soldier fly larvae: Establishing optimal feeding rates. *Waste Manag. Res.* **2009**, *27*, 603–610. [CrossRef]
13. Alattar, M.; Alattar, F.; Popa, R. Effects of microaerobic fermentation and black soldier fly larvae food scrap processing residues on the growth of corn plants (*Zea mays*). *Plant Sci. Today* **2016**, *3*, 57–62. [CrossRef]
14. Choi, Y.-C.; Choi, J.-Y.; Kim, J.-G.; Kim, M.-S.; Kim, W.-T.; Park, K.-H.; Bae, S.-W.; Jeong, G.-S. Potential usage of food waste as a natural fertilizer after digestion by *Hermetia illucens* (Diptera: Stratiomyidae). *Int. J. Ind. Entomol.* **2009**, *19*, 171–174.
15. Sarpong, D.; Oduro-Kwarteng, S.; Gyasi, S.F.; Buamah, R.; Donkor, E.; Awuah, E.; Baah, M.K. Biodegradation by composting of municipal organic solid waste into organic fertilizer using the black soldier fly (*Hermetia illucens*) (Diptera: Stratiomyidae) larvae. *Int. J. Recycl. Org. Waste Agric.* **2019**, *8*, 45–54. [CrossRef]
16. Beesigamukama, D.; Mochoge, B.; Korir, N.; Musyoka, M.W.; Fiaboe, K.K.M.; Nakimbugwe, D.; Khamis, F.M.; Subramanian, S.; Dubois, T.; Ekesi, S.; et al. Nitrogen Fertilizer Equivalence of Black Soldier Fly Frass Fertilizer and Synchrony of Nitrogen Mineralization for Maize Production. *Agronomy* **2020**, *10*, 1395. [CrossRef]
17. Klammsteiner, T.; Walter, A.; Bogataj, T.; Heussler, C.D.; Stres, B.; Steiner, F.M.; Schlick-Steiner, B.C.; Arthofer, W.; Insam, H. The core gut microbiome of black soldier fly (*Hermetia illucens*) larvae raised on low-bioburden diets. *Front. Microbiol.* **2020**, *11*. [CrossRef] [PubMed]
18. Osimani, A.; Milanović, V.; Cardinali, F.; Garofalo, C.; Clementi, F.; Pasquini, M.; Riolo, P.; Ruschioni, S.; Isidoro, N.; Loreto, N.; et al. The bacterial biota of laboratory-reared edible mealworms (*Tenebrio molitor* L.): From feed to frass. *Int. J. Food Microbiol.* **2018**, *272*, 49–60. [CrossRef]

19. Wang, H.; Rehman, K.; Liu, X.; Yang, Q.; Zheng, L.; Li, W.; Cai, M.; Li, Q.; Zhang, J.; Yu, Z. Insect biorefinery: A green approach for conversion of crop residues into biodiesel and protein. *Biotechnol. Biofuels* **2017**, *10*, 304. [CrossRef]
20. Erickson, M.C.; Islam, M.; Sheppard, C.; Liao, J.; Doyle, M.P. Reduction of *Escherichia coli* o157:h7 and *Salmonella enterica* serovar enteritidis in chicken manure by larvae of the black soldier fly. *J. Food Prot.* **2004**, *67*, 685–690. [CrossRef] [PubMed]
21. Lalander, C.; Diener, S.; Magri, M.E.; Zurbrugg, C.; Lindstrom, A.; Vinneras, B. Faecal sludge management with the larvae of the black soldier fly (*Hermetia illucens*)—From a hygiene aspect. *Sci. Total Environ.* **2013**, *458–460*, 312–318. [CrossRef] [PubMed]
22. Liu, Q.; Tomberlin, J.K.; Brady, J.A.; Sanford, M.R.; Yu, Z. Black soldier fly (Diptera: Stratiomyidae) larvae reduce *Escherichia coli* in dairy manure. *Environ. Entomol.* **2008**, *37*, 1525–1530. [CrossRef] [PubMed]
23. Vogel, H.; Müller, A.; Heckel, D.G.; Gutzeit, H.; Vilcinskas, A. Nutritional immunology: Diversification and diet-dependent expression of antimicrobial peptides in the black soldier fly *Hermetia illucens*. *Dev. Comp. Immunol.* **2018**, *78*, 141–148. [CrossRef]
24. Zhang, J.; Bisch-Knaden, S.; Fandino, R.A.; Yan, S.; Obiero, G.F.; Grosse-Wilde, E.; Hansson, B.S.; Knaden, M. The olfactory co-receptor IR8a governs larval-frass mediated competition avoidance in a hawkmoth. *Proc. Natl. Acad. Sci. USA* **2019**, *116*, 21828–21833. [CrossRef]
25. Zhang, X.G.; Li, X.; Gao, Y.L.; Liu, Y.; Dong, W.X.; Xiao, C. Oviposition deterrents in larval frass of potato tuberworm moth, *Phthorimaea operculella* (Lepidoptera: Gelechiidae). *Neotrop. Entomol.* **2019**, *48*, 496–502. [CrossRef] [PubMed]
26. Blomquist, G.J.; Figueroa-Teran, R.; Aw, M.; Song, M.; Gorzalski, A.; Abbott, N.L.; Chang, E.; Tittiger, C. Pheromone production in bark beetles. *Insect Biochem. Mol. Biol.* **2010**, *40*, 699–712. [CrossRef] [PubMed]
27. Lorenzana, L.R.J. Frass volatiles as attractant to the mango pulp weevil (*Sternochetus frigidus* (Fabr.) (Coleoptera: Curculionidae)). *Philipp. Agric. Sci.* **2014**, *97*, 385–390.
28. Mitchell, R.F.; Hanks, L.M. Insect frass as a pathway for transmission of bacterial wilt of cucurbits. *Environ. Entomol.* **2009**, *38*, 395–403. [CrossRef]
29. Roy, K.; Ewing, C.P.; Hughes, M.A.; Keith, L.; Bennett, G.M. Presence and viability of *Ceratocystis lukuohia* in ambrosia beetle frass from Rapid 'Ōhi'a Death-affected *Metrosideros polymorpha* trees on Hawai'i Island. *For. Pathol.* **2019**, *49*, e12476. [CrossRef]
30. Khisti, U.V.; Kathade, S.A.; Aswani, M.A.; Anand, P.K.; Bipinraj, N.K. Isolation and identification of saccharomyces cerevisiae from caterpillar frass and their probiotic characterization. *Biosci. Biotechnol. Res. Asia* **2019**, *16*, 179–186. [CrossRef]
31. Frost, C.J.; Hunter, M.D. Recycling of nitrogen in herbivore feces: Plant recovery, herbivore assimilation, soil retention, and leaching losses. *Oecologia* **2007**, *151*, 42–53. [CrossRef]
32. Frost, C.J.; Hunter, M.D. Insect canopy herbivory and frass deposition affect soil nutrient dynamics and export in oak mesocosms. *Ecology* **2004**, *85*, 3335–3347. [CrossRef]
33. Yang, S.-S.; Chen, Y.; Kang, J.-H.; Xie, T.-R.; He, L.; Xing, D.-F.; Ren, N.-Q.; Ho, S.-H.; Wu, W.-M. Generation of high-efficient biochar for dye adsorption using frass of yellow mealworms (larvae of *Tenebrio molitor* Linnaeus) fed with wheat straw for insect biomass production. *J. Clean. Prod.* **2019**, *227*, 33–47. [CrossRef]
34. Schmitt, E.; de Vries, W. Potential benefits of using *Hermetia illucens* frass as a soil amendment on food production and for environmental impact reduction. *Curr. Opin. Green Sustain. Chem.* **2020**. [CrossRef]
35. Goberna, M.; Podmirseg, S.M.; Waldhuber, S.; Knapp, B.A.; García, C.; Insam, H. Pathogenic bacteria and mineral N in soils following the land spreading of biogas digestates and fresh manure. *Appl. Soil Ecol.* **2011**, *49*, 18–25. [CrossRef]
36. Kandeler, E. Nitrate. In *Methods in Soil Biology*; Schinner, F., Öhlinger, R., Kandeler, E., Margesin, R., Eds.; Springer: Berlin/Heidelberg, Germany, 1996; pp. 408–410, ISBN 978-3-642-60966-4.
37. Kandeler, E. Ammonium. In *Methods in Soil Biology*; Schinner, F., Öhlinger, R., Kandeler, E., Margesin, R., Eds.; Springer: Berlin/Heidelberg, Germany, 1996; pp. 406–408, ISBN 978-3-642-60966-4.
38. Illmer, P. Total, organic, inorganic and plant available phosphorus. In *Methods in Soil Biology*; Schinner, F., Öhlinger, R., Kandeler, E., Margesin, R., Eds.; Springer: Berlin/Heidelberg, Germany, 1996; pp. 412–416, ISBN 978-3-642-60966-4.
39. Heinemeyer, O.; Insam, H.; Kaiser, E.A.; Walenzik, G. Soil microbial biomass and respiration measurements: An automated technique based on infra-red gas analysis. *Plant Soil* **1989**, *116*, 191–195. [CrossRef]

40. Anderson, T.-H.; Domsch, K.H. The metabolic quotient for CO_2 (qCO_2) as a specific activity parameter to assess the effects of environmental conditions, such as ph, on the microbial biomass of forest soils. *Soil Biol. Biochem.* **1993**, *25*, 393–395. [CrossRef]
41. *R Core Team R: A Language and Environment for Statistical Computing*; R Foundation for Statistical Computing: Vienna, Austria, 2018; ISBN 3-900051-07-0.
42. Oksanen, J.; Blanchet, F.G.; Friendly, M.; Kindt, R.; Legendre, P.; McGlinn, D.; Minchin, P.R.; O'Hara, R.B.; Simpson, G.L.; Solymos, P.; et al. *Vegan: Community Ecology Package*; R Foundation for Statistical Computing: Vienna, Austria, 2018.
43. Wickham, H. *ggplot2: Elegant Graphics for Data Analysis*; Springer: Berlin/Heidelberg, Germany, 2016; ISBN 978-3-319-24277-4.
44. De Smet, J.; Wynants, E.; Cos, P.; Campenhout, L.V. Microbial community dynamics during rearing of black soldier fly larvae (*Hermetia illucens*) and its impact on exploitation potential. *Appl. Environ. Microbiol.* **2018**, *84*, e2722-17. [CrossRef]
45. Huang, K.; Xia, H.; Cui, G.; Li, F. Effects of earthworms on nitrification and ammonia oxidizers in vermicomposting systems for recycling of fruit and vegetable wastes. *Sci. Total Environ.* **2017**, *578*, 337–345. [CrossRef]
46. Fielding, D.J.; Trainor, E.; Zhang, M. Diet influences rates of carbon and nitrogen mineralization from decomposing grasshopper frass and cadavers. *Biol. Fertil. Soils* **2013**, *49*, 537–544. [CrossRef]
47. McTavish, M.J.; Smenderovac, E.; Gunn, J.; Murphy, S.D. Insect defoliators in recovering industrial landscapes: Effects of landscape degradation and remediation near an abandoned metal smelter on gypsy moth (Lepidoptera: Lymantriidae) feeding, frass production, and frass properties. *Environ. Entomol.* **2019**, *48*, 1187–1196. [CrossRef] [PubMed]
48. Poveda, J.; Jiménez-Gómez, A.; Saati-Santamaría, Z.; Usategui-Martín, R.; Rivas, R.; García-Fraile, P. Mealworm frass as a potential biofertilizer and abiotic stress tolerance-inductor in plants. *Appl. Soil Ecol.* **2019**, *142*, 110–122. [CrossRef]
49. Gómez-Brandón, M.; Juárez, M.F.-D.; Zangerle, M.; Insam, H. Effects of digestate on soil chemical and microbiological properties: A comparative study with compost and vermicompost. *J. Hazard. Mater.* **2016**, *302*, 267–274. [CrossRef]
50. Podmirseg, S.M.; Waldhuber, S.; Knapp, B.A.; Insam, H.; Goberna, M. Robustness of the autochthonous microbial soil community after amendment of cattle manure or its digestate. *Biol. Fertil. Soils* **2019**, *55*, 565–576. [CrossRef]
51. Raaijmakers, J.M.; Mazzola, M. Soil immune responses. *Science* **2016**, *352*, 1392–1393. [CrossRef]
52. Zhu, B.; Gutknecht, J.L.M.; Herman, D.J.; Keck, D.C.; Firestone, M.K.; Cheng, W. Rhizosphere priming effects on soil carbon and nitrogen mineralization. *Soil Biol. Biochem.* **2014**, *76*, 183–192. [CrossRef]
53. Sharp, R.G. A review of the applications of chitin and its derivatives in agriculture to modify plant-microbial interactions and improve crop yields. *Agronomy* **2013**, *3*, 757–793. [CrossRef]
54. Tharanathan, R.N.; Kittur, F.S. Chitin—The undisputed biomolecule of great potential. *Crit. Rev. Food Sci. Nutr.* **2003**, *43*, 61–87. [CrossRef] [PubMed]
55. Dioha, I.; Ikeme, C.H.; Nafiu, T. Effect of carbon to nitrogen ratio on biogas production. *Int. Res. J. Nat. Sci.* **2013**, *1*, 1–10.
56. Wang, L.; Li, Y.; Prasher, S.O.; Yan, B.; Ou, Y.; Cui, H.; Cui, Y. Organic matter, a critical factor to immobilize phosphorus, copper, and zinc during composting under various initial C/N ratios. *Bioresour. Technol.* **2019**, *289*, 121745. [CrossRef] [PubMed]
57. Borkott, H.; Insam, H. Symbiosis with bacteria enhances the use of chitin by the springtail, *Folsomia candida* (Collembola). *Biol. Fertil. Soils* **1990**, *9*, 126–129. [CrossRef]
58. Insam, H.; Merschak, P. Nitrogen leaching from forest soil cores after amending organic recycling products and fertilizers. *Waste Manag. Res.* **1997**, *15*, 277–292. [CrossRef]
59. Spohn, M. Microbial respiration per unit microbial biomass depends on litter layer carbon-to-nitrogen ratio. *Biogeosciences* **2015**, *12*, 817–823. [CrossRef]
60. Leita, L.; De Nobili, M.; Mondini, C.; Muhlbachova, G.; Marchiol, L.; Bragato, G.; Contin, M. Influence of inorganic and organic fertilization on soil microbial biomass, metabolic quotient and heavy metal bioavailability. *Biol. Fertil. Soils* **1999**, *28*, 371–376. [CrossRef]
61. Ros, M.; Klammer, S.; Knapp, B.; Aichberger, K.; Insam, H. Long-term effects of compost amendment of soil on functional and structural diversity and microbial activity. *Soil Use Manag.* **2006**, *22*, 209–218. [CrossRef]

62. Tittonell, P.; Corbeels, M.; van Wijk, M.T.; Vanlauwe, B.; Giller, K.E. Combining Organic and Mineral Fertilizers for Integrated Soil Fertility Management in Smallholder Farming Systems of Kenya: Explorations Using the Crop-Soil Model FIELD. *Agron. J.* **2008**, *100*, 1511–1526. [CrossRef]
63. Fageria, V.D. Nutrient Interactions in Crop Plants. *J. Plant Nutr.* **2001**, *24*, 1269–1290. [CrossRef]
64. Mertenat, A.; Diener, S.; Zurbrügg, C. Black soldier fly biowaste treatment—Assessment of global warming potential. *Waste Manag.* **2019**, *84*, 173–181. [CrossRef] [PubMed]
65. Bulak, P.; Proc, K.; Pawłowska, M.; Kasprzycka, A.; Berus, W.; Bieganowski, A. Biogas generation from insects breeding post production wastes. *J. Clean. Prod.* **2020**, *244*, 118777. [CrossRef]
66. Lalander, C.; Nordberg, A.; Vinneras, B. A comparison in product-value potential in four treatment strategies for food waste and faeces—Assessing composting, fly larvae composting and anaerobic digestion. *Glob. Chang. Biol. Bioenergy* **2018**, *10*, 84–91. [CrossRef]

Publisher's Note: MDPI stays neutral with regard to jurisdictional claims in published maps and institutional affiliations.

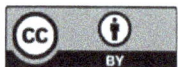

© 2020 by the authors. Licensee MDPI, Basel, Switzerland. This article is an open access article distributed under the terms and conditions of the Creative Commons Attribution (CC BY) license (http://creativecommons.org/licenses/by/4.0/).

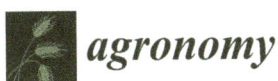

Communication

Earthworms (*Lumbricus terrestris* L.) Mediate the Fertilizing Effect of Frass

Anne-Maïmiti Dulaurent [1],*, Guillaume Daoulas [2], Michel-Pierre Faucon [1] and David Houben [1],*

1. UniLaSalle, AGHYLE, 19 rue Pierre Waguet, 60026 Beauvais, France; michel-pierre.faucon@unilasalle.fr
2. Ÿnsect, 1 rue Pierre Fontaine, 91000 Evry, France; guillaume.daoulas@ynsect.com
* Correspondence: anne-maimiti.dulaurent@unilasalle.fr (A.-M.D.); david.houben@unilasalle.fr (D.H.)

Received: 29 April 2020; Accepted: 29 May 2020; Published: 31 May 2020

Abstract: With the forecasted dramatic growth of insect rearing in the near future, frass (insect excreta) has been increasingly considered a sustainable resource for managing plant nutrition in cropping systems and a promising alternative to conventional fertilizer. However, the impact of soil fauna on its fertilizing effect has not been investigated so far. In this study, we investigated the effect of earthworms (*Lumbricus terrestris* L.) on nitrogen (N), phosphorus (P), potassium (K) and calcium (Ca) uptake and crop growth in the presence of frass from mealworm (*Tenebrio molitor* L.). Using a pot experiment, we found that earthworms increased N, P, K and Ca concentration in barley (*Hordeum vulgare* L.) in the presence of frass, suggesting that earthworm activity enhances the short-term recycling of nutrients from frass. Compared to treatments with and without frass and earthworms, the specific leaf area of barley was the highest in the presence of both earthworms and frass. This confirms that earthworms and frass have a synergistic effect on soil fertility. Overall, our study shows that earthworms may improve the efficiency of organic fertilizers and argues therefore for the importance of developing sustainable agricultural practices that promote earthworm populations.

Keywords: earthworms; frass; insect excreta; insect farming; nitrogen; phosphorus; soil fauna; soil fertility; waste management

1. Introduction

In the context of the massive increase in the human population at an unprecedented level, insect rearing represents an opportunity to answer the growing demand for proteins with a low ecological footprint [1]. Although insect production is highly efficient in converting by-products into biomass, it also yields a waste stream consisting especially of insect feces ("frass"). Given the "zero waste" context and the need to contribute to the circular economy, the possibility of recovering frass as a fertilizer has recently been considered by researchers [2–4]. For instance, Houben et al. [3] have found that frass from mealworm (*Tenebrio molitor* L.) might be as efficient as conventional mineral fertilizer to sustain crop growth due to its rapid mineralization after its incorporation into the soil and the presence of nutrients in a readily-available form. A couple of studies have suggested that microbial activity might partially control the effect of frass on soil fertility, either in natural conditions [5–7] or in cropping systems [2,3]. However, the impact of soil fauna has not been considered so far. It is known that soil fauna, especially earthworms, may positively affect plant growth [8,9] due to, among others, changes in soil structure and water regime [10], improvement of soil organic matter and nutrient cycling [11,12], and stimulation and dispersal of beneficial microorganisms [13]. Moreover, adding exogenous organic amendments generally stimulates earthworm activity which reciprocally improves the fertilizing effect of these amendments [13–15], even though some contradictory results have also been found [12,16].

Since frass is an organic amendment, it is therefore likely that its effect on soil fertility might also be mediated by earthworm activity. Therefore, the aim of this study was to investigate the impact of the earthworm presence on the fertilizer potential of frass. For this purpose, we carried out a pot experiment to determine the effect of earthworms on the frass fertilizing effect. Barley (*Hordeum vulgare* L.) was grown in greenhouse conditions with or without frass from mealworm (*Tenebrio molitor* L.) in the presence or absence of earthworms (*Lumbricus terrestris* L.).

2. Materials and Methods

A pot experiment was conducted to determine the effect of earthworms on the fertilizer potential of frass. Frass (ŸnFrass) from mealworm (*Tenebrio molitor* L.) was provided in the form of powder by Ÿnsect (Paris, France), an industrial company farming this insect at a large-scale. Chemical characteristics of frass are presented in Table 1.

Table 1. Chemical characteristics of frass (data from Houben et al. [3]).

Organic C g kg^{-1}	Total N g kg^{-1}	Total K g kg^{-1}	Total P g kg^{-1}	pH	Soluble Fraction %Corg	Hemicellulose-Like Fraction %Corg	Cellulose-Like Fraction %Corg	Lignin-Like Fraction %Corg
393	50	17	20	5.8	49.3	31	15.2	4.4

The studied soil was sampled in Beauvais (Northern France) and was classified as a Haplic Luvisol (IUSS Working Group WRB, 2015), a soil with properties suitable for soil fauna activity [17]. Soil characterization was carried out by Houben et al. [3] following the procedures described elsewhere [18] and revealed that organic C was 1.54%, total N was 0.18%, the cation exchange capacity (CEC) was 12.5 cmol$_c$ kg^{-1}, and pH was 7.8.

The experimental device was based on our previous study which aimed at estimating the fertilizer potential of frass [3]. Briefly, plastic plant pots were filled with 3500 g of either soil or a mixture of soil and frass at a rate of 10 Mg dry matter ha^{-1} (hereafter called "Frass" treatment), or untreated soil (hereafter called "Control"). Three earthworms (*Lumbricus terrestris* L.) were added in half of the pots (hereafter called "Frass + earthworms" or "Control + Earthworms" treatments) representing biomass of 12.05 ± 0.24 g and 12.25 ± 0.17 g in Frass + Earthworms and Control + Earthworms treatments respectively, according to the recommendations by Vos et al. [19]. Each of the four treatments was replicated four times.

Eight seeds of barley (*Hordeum vulgare* L.) were sown in each pot. After 10 days, excess germinated seedlings were removed (first harvest) so that only four uniform plants per pot were allowed to grow for the following eight weeks (ca. 120 plants m^{-2}). The trials were conducted under controlled greenhouse conditions (temperature 18–25 °C, 16 h photoperiod) with daily sprinkler watering to maintain the soil moisture at field capacity. After 9 weeks, the shoots were harvested with ceramic scissors. Three fully-grown young leaves per replicate were scanned at 600 dpi and then dried at 60 °C for 72 h to determine specific leaf area (SLA). All aboveground biomass was dried at 60 °C for 48 h in a similar manner and weighed. The concentrations of P, K, and Ca in aerial parts were analyzed by inductively coupled plasma-atomic emission spectroscopy (ICP-AES; Jarrell Ash) after *aqua regia* digestion. The concentration of N in aerial parts was analyzed using the Dumas combustion method. Earthworms were extracted from pots, counted, and weighed. As suggested by Coulis et al. [20], available P concentration in soil was assessed using water extraction (soil:water 1:60; w-v) following the procedure described by Sissingh [21]. Available K and Ca concentrations were determined using the acetate ammonium-ethylenediamine tetraacetic acid (AAEDTA) [18,22]. Soil pH was measured in water (soil:water 1:5; w-v).

All recorded data were analyzed using descriptive statistics (mean ± standard error) and normality was determined using the Shapiro-Wilk test. One-way ANOVAs and Tukey's multiple comparison tests or Kruskal-Wallis and Mann-Whitney tests were used to compare biomass, SLA, and nutrient concentrations in the shoot and soil according to whether the distribution was normal or not, respectively. Pearson's correlation coefficient was used to analyze the relationship between SLA and N concentration. All statistical analyses were performed using R software version 3.5.0 [23] and the package Rcmdr [24].

3. Results and Discussion

3.1. Earthworm Survival

At harvest, earthworm survival was 100% for all the treatments and their burrowing activity was clearly visible (Figure 1). In addition, their number and biomass per pot at the end of the experiment were not significantly ($p > 0.05$) different from that before their incorporation into the soil. This indicates that frass had no toxic effect on earthworms and allows us to ascribe the following results to the actual presence of earthworms. The similar earthworm biomass between the beginning and the end of the experiment contrasts with Sizmur et al. [25] who found in a 12-week microcosm experiment a continuous decrease of earthworm (*L. terrestris*) biomass in soil with no amendment or with organic amendments including farmyard manure, anaerobic digestate, and compost. However, Sizmur et al. [25] carried out their experiment without plants, which could possibly explain the discrepancy with our study. Since *L. terrestris* may feed on plant roots [26,27], it is likely that, by providing an additional source of food, the presence of plants contributed to maintaining earthworm biomass all over the experiment.

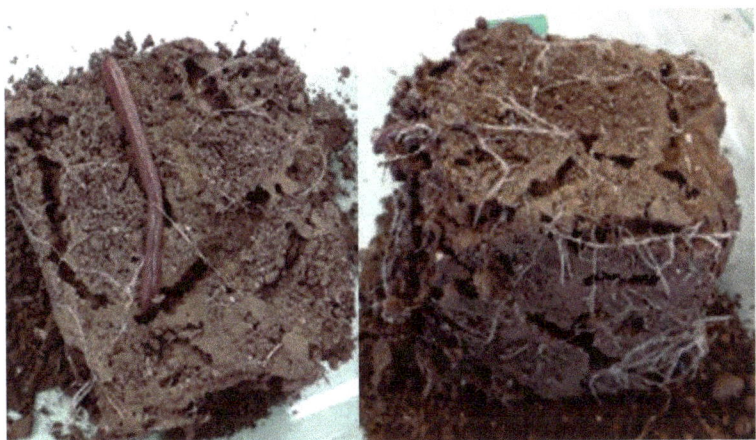

Figure 1. Representative pictures of soil collected in pots at the plant harvest illustrating the intense burrowing activity of earthworms.

3.2. Impact of Earthworms on Nutrient Uptake and Crop Growth

Many studies have reported that earthworm activities significantly increase N concentration in plant tissues [13,28], predominantly due to an earthworm-induced stimulation of N mineralization, which in turn, enhances N availability for plants [29,30]. For instance, Amador et al. [31,32] showed higher N mineralization in the drilosphere of *L. terrestris*, leading to an accumulation of nitrate in earthworm burrow soil. This increase of nitrate can result in higher N uptake, as observed for oilseed rape grown in an earthworm-inoculated (*Metaphire guillemi*) soil [33]. In agreement with these researchers, our results showed that irrespective of the treatment, N concentration in barley shoot was higher with than without earthworms (Figure 2).

More importantly, our results suggest a synergistic effect between frass and earthworms since the Frass + Earthworms treatment displayed the highest N concentration in barley shoot (Figure 2). The positive effect of frass on N uptake by plants has been previously discussed and was attributed to its very rapid mineralization after its incorporation into the soil [3]. Here, our results indicate that earthworms induced a higher uptake of N in the presence of frass. Although the present study did not allow us to identify the pools from which N was taken up by plants, it is likely that the presence of earthworms stimulated the release of N from frass since earthworms generally promote N mineralization from organic fertilizer [8]. For instance, Postma-Blaauw [12] showed that *L. terrestris* enhanced the release of N from crop residue by increasing its mineralization while it had no effect on the mineralization of soil organic matter-derived N. Using ^{15}N, Amador and Görres [34] found that *L. terrestris* could double the amount of litter-derived N taken up by maize grown in mesocosms. In another study, N uptake by maize was 26 and 74% higher from manure and compost treatments, respectively in the presence of earthworms (*Pheretima hawayana*) compared to control without earthworms [14]. This was attributed to an increase of the decomposition of organic N by earthworms which enhanced the N mineralization from the manure and compost treatments, as also observed by Rashid et al. [35]. Besides increasing microbial metabolic activity [3], frass, like other organic amendments, might also have promoted earthworm activity [36], which could further increase N mineralization.

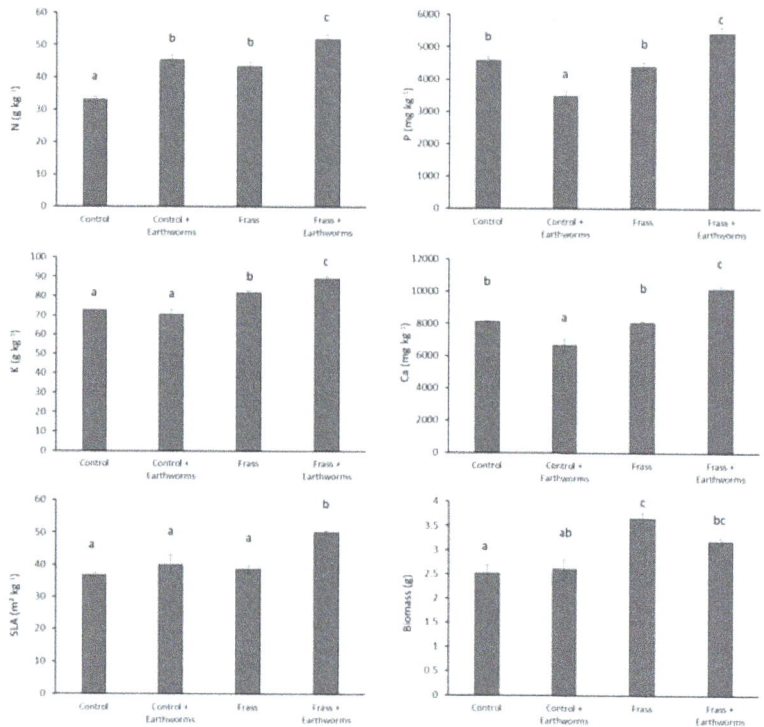

Figure 2. Concentrations of N, P, K, and Ca, specific leaf area (SLA), and biomass of barley. Values are average (n = 4) ± standard error. Columns with the same letter do not differ significantly at the 5% level.

Unlike N, the presence of earthworms decreased P concentration in the shoot of the control (Figure 2), which can be related to the decrease of available P concentration in soil (Figure 3). Earthworms have been reported to enhance P availability in the short run due to changes in complexes induced by competition for sorbing sites between orthophosphates and carboxyl groups of the mucus produced in the gut [37]. However, after three weeks of incubation, Le Bayon and Binet [38] found a dramatic decrease of P availability in the presence of *L. terrestris*, which was ascribed to the immobilization of P by microorganisms. Phosphorus availability may also be reduced due to soil pH increase brought about by earthworm activities [39]. Our results indicate, however, that soil pH was unaffected by the presence of earthworms (Figure 3), which therefore suggests that the lower P availability in the Control + Earthworm treatment would predominantly result from P immobilization by microorganisms.

As reported by Houben et al. [3], application of frass to soil improved P nutrition (Figure 2), which is due to the presence of P in a readily available form as well as to the slightly acidifying effect of frass which can, in turn, increase P solubility (Figure 3). By contrast to the control, the presence of earthworms in the frass treatment increased P concentrations in shoots, suggesting that earthworms promoted the recycling of P from frass. Interestingly, available P concentration was not increased in the Frass + Earthworm treatment and pH was unaffected by earthworms (Figure 3), which indicates that the higher P concentration in barley shoot in this treatment would not result only from a change in the biogeochemical status of P. Improvement of P concentration in barley shoot might be explained by a better distribution of P within the soil due to earthworm activities. Earthworms facilitate P transfer of organic fertilizer within the soil [15,38,40], which can in turn increase the root accessibility to P, especially for plants such as barley, whose spatial soil exploration by roots plays an important role in the acquisition of P from organic fertilizer [41]. Similar to P, available Ca and K concentrations in soil in the presence of frass were not increased by earthworms (Figure 3) while, as for P, the Frass + Earthworm treatment showed the highest Ca and K concentrations in the shoot (Figure 3). This, therefore, suggests that mechanisms responsible for the earthworms-induced recycling of Ca and K from frass are similar to that for P.

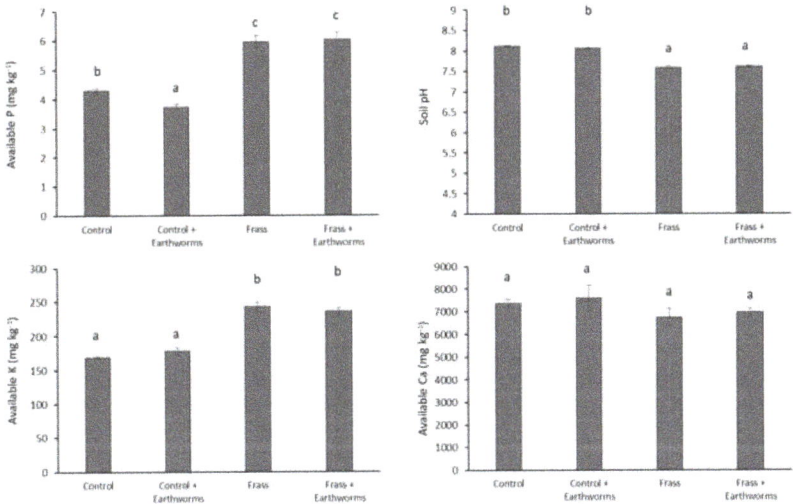

Figure 3. Available P concentration (water extraction), available K and Ca concentrations (AA-EDTA extraction), and pH in the soil. Values are average (n = 4) ± standard error. Columns with the same letter do not differ significantly at the 5% level.

The synergistic effect between earthworms and frass on plant nutrition was reflected by an increase of SLA of barley shoot (Figure 2). Being related to the relative growth rate of plant species [42], SLA is widely used as a target trait to unravel plant responses to soil properties, especially those linked to soil fertility [43], and can explain plant productivity [44]. As a leaf functional trait, its characterization allows us to elucidate the plant response to changes in soil properties at an individual scale. SLA is usually well correlated to N availability and N concentration in plants [45,46], which was also found in our study (r = 0.82; $p < 0.001$). Therefore, its improvement in the Frass + Earthworms treatment corroborates our findings that earthworms improve the fertilizer potential of frass. It is noteworthy that, unexpectedly, shoot biomass was not improved by the presence of earthworms in the frass treatment. Shoot biomass is known to be less sensitive than SLA to a change of soil fertility as many factors can drive it [47]. In the present study, the lack of biomass improvement in the Frass + Earthwoms treatment, in spite of a higher soil fertility status, could be explained by competition for light induced by the higher SLA [48,49]. The perspective is, therefore, to elucidate the plant density which optimizes canopy light interception, crop yield, and nutrient use efficiency from frass. The lack of biomass improvement could also have been due to herbivory by earthworms. Some studies reported *L. terrestris* to commonly consume roots [27], especially in situations of low litter availability [26], which might, in turn, reduce the aboveground biomass production, as shown for other organisms [50]. Therefore, another perspective will be to investigate how the root consumption by earthworms may be affected by organic amendments such as frass.

4. Conclusions

With the forecasted growth of insect farming in the near future, frass is increasingly considered a promising resource for the sustainable management of plant nutrition in cropping systems and an enticing alternative to conventional fertilizer. In this study, we evidenced that earthworms enhance the fertilizer potential of frass. Indeed, their activity increases soil fertility and nutrient (N, P, K and Ca) concentrations in barley in the presence of frass, likely by improving the short-term recycling of nutrients from frass. More generally, our study highlights that, as key biological agents in the transformation of organic matter and waste, earthworms may improve the efficiency of organic fertilizers. Coupled with the other well-documented ecosystem services delivered by earthworms, our findings further argue for the importance of developing sustainable agricultural practices that promote earthworm populations.

Author Contributions: Conceptualization, A.-M.D., G.D., M.-P.F. and D.H.; methodology, A.-M.D. and D.H.; investigation, A.-M.D. and D.H.; writing—original draft preparation, A.-M.D. and D.H.; writing—review and editing, G.D. and M.-P.F. All authors have read and agreed to the published version of the manuscript.

Funding: This research was funded by a private corporation, Ÿnsect.

Acknowledgments: We thank the "ASET 158" students, Céline Roisin, Aurore Coutelier and Vincent Hervé for technical assistance. L. Dulaurent is heartily acknowledged for his contribution to the weightless cloud.

Conflicts of Interest: Although the research was funded by a private corporation, Ÿnsect, we ensure the research is free of bias.

References

1. Dicke, M. Insects as feed and the Sustainable Development Goals. *J. Insects Food Feed* **2018**, *4*, 147–156. [CrossRef]
2. Poveda, J.; Jimenez-Gomez, A.; Saati-Santamaría, Z.; Usategui-Martín, R.; Rivas, R.; García-Fraile, P. Mealworm frass as a potential biofertilizer and abiotic stress tolerance-inductor in plants. *Appl. Soil Ecol.* **2019**, *142*, 110–122. [CrossRef]
3. Houben, D.; Daoulas, G.; Faucon, M.-P.; Dulaurent, A.-M. Potential use of mealworm frass as a fertilizer: Impact on crop growth and soil properties. *Sci. Rep.* **2020**, *10*, 4659. [CrossRef]
4. Schmitt, E.; de Vries, W. Potential benefits of using Hermetia illucens frass as a soil amendment on food production and for environmental impact reduction. *Curr. Opin. Green Sustain. Chem.* **2020**. [CrossRef]
5. Frost, C.J.; Hunter, M.D. Insect Canopy herbivory and frass deposition affect soil nutrient dynamics and export in oak mesocosms. *Ecology* **2004**, *85*, 3335–3347. [CrossRef]
6. Kagata, H.; Ohgushi, T. Positive and negative impacts of insect frass quality on soil nitrogen availability and plant growth. *Popul. Ecol.* **2012**, *54*, 75–82. [CrossRef]
7. Lovett, G.M.; Ruesink, A.E. Carbon and nitrogen mineralization from decomposing gypsy moth frass. *Oecologia* **1995**, *104*, 133–138. [CrossRef]
8. van Groenigen, J.W.; Lubbers, I.M.; Vos, H.M.J.; Brown, G.G.; De Deyn, G.B.; van Groenigen, K.J. Earthworms increase plant production: A meta-analysis. *Sci. Rep.* **2014**, *4*, 6365. [CrossRef]
9. Blouin, M.; Hodson, M.E.; Delgado, E.A.; Baker, G.; Brussaard, L.; Butt, K.R.; Dai, J.; Dendooven, L.; Peres, G.; Tondoh, J.E.; et al. A review of earthworm impact on soil function and ecosystem services. *Eur. J. Soil Sci.* **2013**, *64*, 161–182. [CrossRef]

10. Blanchart, E.; Albrecht, A.; Alegre, J.; Duboisset, A.; Gilot, C.; Pashanasi, B.; Lavelle, P.; Brussaard, L. Effects of earthworms on soil structure and physical properties. In *Earthworm Management in Tropical Agroecosystems*; Lavelle, P., Brussaard, L., Hendrix, P., Eds.; CABI: New York, NY, USA, 1999; pp. 149–171.
11. Chapuis-Lardy, L.; Le Bayon, R.-C.; Brossard, M.; Lopez-Hernandez, D.; Blanchart, E. Role of Soil Macrofauna in Phosphorus Cycling. In *Phosphorus in Action: Biological Processes in Soil Phosphorus Cycling*; Bünemann, E., Oberson, A., Frossard, E., Eds.; Soil Biology; Springer: Berlin/Heidelberg, Germany, 2011; pp. 199–213, ISBN 978-3-642-15271-9.
12. Postma-Blaauw, M.B.; Bloem, J.; Faber, J.H.; van Groenigen, J.W.; de Goede, R.G.M.; Brussaard, L. Earthworm species composition affects the soil bacterial community and net nitrogen mineralization. *Pedobiologia* **2006**, *50*, 243–256. [CrossRef]
13. Medina-Sauza, R.M.; Alvarez-Jimenez, M.; Delhal, A.; Reverchon, F.; Blouin, M.; Guerrero-Analco, J.A.; Cerdan, C.R.; Guevara, R.; Villain, L.; Barois, I. Earthworms Building Up Soil Microbiota, a Review. *Front. Environ. Sci.* **2019**, *7*, 81. [CrossRef]
14. Waqar, A.; Shah, G.M.; Bakhat, H.F.; Shahid, M.; Aslam, M.; Ashraf, M.R.; Hafeez, R.; Murtaza, B.; Rashid, M.I. The earthworm species Pheretima hawayana influences organic wastes decomposition, nitrogen mineralization and maize N recovery. *Eur. J. Soil Biol.* **2019**, *90*, 1–8. [CrossRef]
15. Sharpley, A.; McDowell, R.; Moyer, B.; Littlejohn, R. Land application of manure can influence earthworm activity and soil phosphorus distribution. *Commun. Soil Sci. Plant Anal.* **2011**, *42*, 194–207. [CrossRef]
16. Jouquet, P.; Plumere, T.; Thu, T.D.; Rumpel, C.; Duc, T.T.; Orange, D. The rehabilitation of tropical soils using compost and vermicompost is affected by the presence of endogeic earthworms. *Appl. Soil Ecol.* **2010**, *46*, 125–133. [CrossRef]
17. Clause, J.; Barot, S.; Richard, B.; Decaëns, T.; Forey, E. The interactions between soil type and earthworm species determine the properties of earthworm casts. *Appl. Soil Ecol.* **2014**, *83*, 149–158. [CrossRef]
18. Houben, D.; Meunier, C.; Pereira, B.; Sonnet, P. Predicting the degree of phosphorus saturation using the ammonium acetate–EDTA soil test. *Soil Use Manag.* **2011**, *27*, 283–293. [CrossRef]
19. Vos, H.M.J.; Ros, M.B.H.; Koopmans, G.F.; van Groenigen, J.W. Do earthworms affect phosphorus availability to grass? A pot experiment. *Soil Biol. Biochem.* **2014**, *79*, 34–42. [CrossRef]
20. Coulis, M.; Bernard, L.; Gerard, F.; Hinsinger, P.; Plassard, C.; Villeneuve, M.; Blanchart, E. Endogeic earthworms modify soil phosphorus, plant growth and interactions in a legume–cereal intercrop. *Plant Soil* **2014**, *379*, 149–160. [CrossRef]
21. Sissingh, H.A. Analytical technique of the Pw method, used for the assessment of the phosphate status of arable soils in the Netherlands. *Plant Soil* **1971**, *34*, 483–486. [CrossRef]
22. Gomez-Suarez, A.D.; Nobile, C.; Faucon, M.-P.; Pourret, O.; Houben, D. Fertilizer potential of struvite as affected by nitrogen form in the rhizosphere. *Sustainability* **2020**, *12*, 2212. [CrossRef]
23. R Core Team. *R: A language and Environment for Statistical Computing*; R Foundation for Statistical Computing: Vienna, Austria, 2017; ISBN 3-900051-07-0. Available online: https://www.R-project.org (accessed on 22 December 2019).
24. Fox, J. The R Commander: A Basic-Statistics Graphical User Interface to R. *J. Stat. Softw.* **2005**, *14*, 1–42. [CrossRef]
25. Sizmur, T.; Martin, E.; Wagner, K.; Parmentier, E.; Watts, C.; Whitmore, A.P. Milled cereal straw accelerates earthworm (Lumbricus terrestris) growth more than selected organic amendments. *Appl. Soil Ecol.* **2017**, *113*, 166–177. [CrossRef] [PubMed]
26. Griffith, B.; Türke, M.; Weisser, W.W.; Eisenhauer, N. Herbivore behavior in the anecic earthworm species Lumbricus terrestris L.? *Eur. J. Soil Biol.* **2013**, *55*, 62–65. [CrossRef]
27. Cortez, J.; Bouche, M.B. Do earthworms eat living roots? *Soil Biol. Biochem.* **1992**, *24*, 913–915. [CrossRef]
28. Scheu, S. Effects of earthworms on plant growth: Patterns and perspectives. *Pedobiologia* **2003**, *47*, 846–856. [CrossRef]
29. Baker, G. Differences in nitrogen release from surface and incorporated plant residues by two endogeic species of earthworms (Lumbricidae) in a red–brown earth soil in southern Australia. *Eur. J. Soil Biol.* **2007**, *43*, S165–S170. [CrossRef]
30. Lubbers, I.M.; Brussaard, L.; Otten, W.; Groenigen, J.W.V. Earthworm-induced N mineralization in fertilized grassland increases both N2O emission and crop-N uptake. *Eur. J. Soil Sci.* **2011**, *62*, 152–161. [CrossRef]

31. Amador, J.A.; Gorres, J.H.; Savin, M.C. Effects of Lumbricus terrestris L. on nitrogen dynamics beyond the burrow. *Appl. Soil Ecol.* **2006**, *33*, 61–66. [CrossRef]
32. Amador, J.A.; Gorres, J.H.; Savin, M.C. Carbon and nitrogen dynamics in Lumbricus terrestris (L.) burrow Soil. *Soil Sci. Soc. Am. J.* **2003**, *67*, 1755–1762. [CrossRef]
33. Zhang, S.; Chao, Y.; Zhang, C.; Cheng, J.; Li, J.; Ma, N. Earthworms enhanced winter oilseed rape (Brassica napus L.) growth and nitrogen uptake. *Agric. Ecosyst. Environ.* **2010**, *139*, 463–468. [CrossRef]
34. Amador, J.A.; Gorres, J.H. Role of the anecic earthworm Lumbricus terrestris L. in the distribution of plant residue nitrogen in a corn (Zea mays)–soil system. *Appl. Soil Ecol.* **2005**, *30*, 203–214. [CrossRef]
35. Rashid, M.I.; de Goede, R.G.M.; Corral Nunez, G.A.; Brussaard, L.; Lantinga, E.A. Soil pH and earthworms affect herbage nitrogen recovery from solid cattle manure in production grassland. *Soil Biol. Biochem.* **2014**, *68*, 1–8. [CrossRef]
36. Edwards, C.A. *Earthworm Ecology*, 2nd ed.; CRC Press: Boca Raton, FL, USA, 2004; ISBN 978-0-429-12904-9.
37. Lopez-Hernandez, D.; Lavelle, P.; Fardeau, J.C.; Nino, M. Phosphorus transformations in two P-sorption contrasting tropical soils during transit through Pontoscolex corethrurus (Glossoscolecidae: Oligochaeta). *Soil Biol. Biochem.* **1993**, *25*, 789–792. [CrossRef]
38. Le Bayon, R.C.; Binet, F. Earthworms change the distribution and availability of phosphorous in organic substrates. *Soil Biol. Biochem.* **2006**, *38*, 235–246. [CrossRef]
39. Vos, H.M.J.; Koopmans, G.F.; Beezemer, L.; de Goede, R.G.M.; Hiemstra, T.; van Groenigen, J.W. Large variations in readily-available phosphorus in casts of eight earthworm species are linked to cast properties. *Soil Biol. Biochem.* **2019**, *138*, 107583. [CrossRef]
40. Li, H.; Xiang, D.; Wang, C.; Li, X.; Lou, Y. Effects of epigeic earthworm (Eisenia fetida) and arbuscular mycorrhizal fungus (Glomus intraradices) on enzyme activities of a sterilized soil–sand mixture and nutrient uptake by maize. *Biol. Fertil. Soil* **2012**, *48*, 879–887. [CrossRef]
41. Nobile, C.; Houben, D.; Michel, E.; Firmin, S.; Lambers, H.; Kandeler, E.; Faucon, M.-P. Phosphorus-acquisition strategies of canola, wheat and barley in soil amended with sewage sludges. *Sci. Rep.* **2019**, *9*, 1–11. [CrossRef]
42. Osone, Y.; Ishida, A.; Tateno, M. Correlation between relative growth rate and specific leaf area requires associations of specific leaf area with nitrogen absorption rate of roots. *New Phytol.* **2008**, *179*, 417–427. [CrossRef]
43. Hodgson, J.G.; Montserrat-Martí, G.; Charles, M.; Jones, G.; Wilson, P.; Shipley, B.; Sharafi, M.; Cerabolini, B.E.L.; Cornelissen, J.H.C.; Band, S.R.; et al. Is leaf dry matter content a better predictor of soil fertility than specific leaf area? *Ann. Bot.* **2011**, *108*, 1337–1345. [CrossRef]
44. Madani, N.; Kimball, J.S.; Running, S.W. Improving global gross primary productivity estimates by computing optimum light use efficiencies using flux tower data. *J. Geophys. Res. Biogeosci.* **2017**, *122*, 2939–2951. [CrossRef]
45. Ordoñez, J.C.; Bodegom, P.M.V.; Witte, J.-P.M.; Wright, I.J.; Reich, P.B.; Aerts, R. A global study of relationships between leaf traits, climate and soil measures of nutrient fertility. *Glob. Ecol. Biogeogr.* **2009**, *18*, 137–149. [CrossRef]
46. Lambers, H.; Poorter, H. Inherent variation in growth rate between pigher Plants: A search for physiological causes and ecological consequences. In *Advances in Ecological Research*; Begon, M., Fitter, A.H., Eds.; Academic Press: Amsterdam, The Netherlands, 1992; Volume 23, pp. 187–261.
47. Gong, H.; Gao, J. Soil and climatic drivers of plant SLA (specific leaf area). *Glob. Ecol. Conserv.* **2019**, *20*, e00696. [CrossRef]
48. Yao, H.; Zhang, Y.; Yi, X.; Zhang, X.; Zhang, W. Cotton responds to different plant population densities by adjusting specific leaf area to optimize canopy photosynthetic use efficiency of light and nitrogen. *Field Crops Res.* **2016**, *188*, 10–16. [CrossRef]
49. Knops, J.M.; Reinhart, K. Specific leaf area along a nitrogen fertilization gradient. *Am. Midl. Nat.* **2000**, *144*, 265–272. [CrossRef]
50. Ingham, R.E.; Detling, J.K. Effects of root-feeding nematodes on aboveground net primary production in a North American grassland. *Plant Soil* **1990**, *121*, 279–281. [CrossRef]

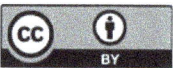

© 2020 by the authors. Licensee MDPI, Basel, Switzerland. This article is an open access article distributed under the terms and conditions of the Creative Commons Attribution (CC BY) license (http://creativecommons.org/licenses/by/4.0/).

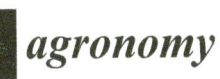

Biochar-Compost Interactions as Affected by Weathering: Effects on Biological Stability and Plant Growth

Marie-Liesse Aubertin [1,2,*], Cyril Girardin [2], Sabine Houot [2], Cécile Nobile [3], David Houben [3], Sarah Bena [4], Yann Le Brech [4] and Cornelia Rumpel [1,*]

1. Institute of Ecology and Environmental Sciences, UMR 7618, CNRS-UPMC-UPEC-INRA-IRD, Sorbonne University, 75005 Paris, France
2. National Institute for Agricultural Research, Ecosys Soil, UMR INRA-AgroParisTech, 78820 Thiverval-Grignon, France; cyril.girardin@inrae.fr (C.G.); sabine.houot@inrae.fr (S.H.)
3. UniLaSalle, AGHYLE, 60026 Beauvais, France; cecile.nobile@cirad.fr (C.N.); david.houben@unilasalle.fr (D.H.)
4. LRGP–CNRS, Lorraine University, 54000 Nancy, France; sarah.bena@univ-lorraine.fr (S.B.); yann.le-brech@univ-lorraine.fr (Y.L.B.)
* Correspondence: marie-liesse.aubertin@inrae.fr (M.-L.A.); cornelia.rumpel@inrae.fr (C.R.)

Abstract: Biochar addition to compost is of growing interest as soil amendment. However, little is known about the evolution of material properties of biochar-compost mixtures and their effect on plants after exposure to physical weathering. This study aimed to investigate the physico-chemical characteristics of fresh and weathered biochar-compost mixtures, their biological stability and their effect on ryegrass growth. To this end, we used the contrasting stable isotope signatures of biochar and compost to follow their behavior in biochar-compost mixtures subjected to artificial weathering during 1-year of incubation. We assessed their impact on ryegrass growth during a 4-week greenhouse pot experiment. Weathering treatment resulted in strong leaching of labile compounds. However, biochar-compost interactions led to reduced mass loss and fixed carbon retention during weathering of mixtures. Moreover, weathering increased carbon mineralization of biochar-compost mixtures, probably due to the protection of labile compounds from compost within biochar structure, as well as leaching of labile biochar compounds inhibiting microbial activity. After soil application, weathered mixtures could have positive effects on biomass production. We conclude that biochar-compost interactions on soil microbial activity and plant growth are evolving after physical weathering depending on biochar production conditions.

Keywords: biochar; compost; isotopic signature; carbon mineralization; plant growth

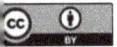

1. Introduction

According to the last report of the Intergovernmental Panel of Climate Change (IPCC), global temperatures have increased by 1 °C above pre-industrial levels due to human activity [1]. Further increase should be limited to 1.5 °C in order to prevent dangerous climate change. To achieve this goal, active carbon dioxide removal from the atmosphere and its storage is needed [1]. Soil carbon sequestration and biochar application to soils may be used for this purpose. As negative emission technologies (NETs), their implementation may be able to achieve long-term carbon sequestration and may have advantages over the other NETs related to their effect on land use, water use and energy requirement [2].

Soil carbon (C) sequestration may be enhanced by the addition of organic amendments. While organic residues such as plant material or manure are usually transformed into amendments through composting, they may also be the feedstock for biochar production [3]. Biochar is a solid pyrolysis product intended to be used as soil amendment [4]. It is mainly composed of aromatic C and has favourable properties such as large porosity and surface area in addition to high cation exchange capacity, depending on feedstock, pyrolysis conditions and particle size [5–7]. Biochar is known to improve soil properties such as water retention under drought conditions [8], and soil aggregate stability and porosity [9,10]. Due to its low nutrient content, biochar should be combined with nutrient additions through mineral fertilizers, compost and/or growth promoting micro-organisms to further increase its beneficial effects on plant growth when applied to soil [3]. On the other hand, compost is rapidly mineralized after soil application and its carbon sequestration potential may be enhanced by combination with organic and inorganic additives [11]. Mixtures of both materials may therefore be an innovative practice, leading to more efficient soil amendment as compared to their single use.

Biochar combination with other organic amendments may have synergistic effects on organic C retention, which were attributed to physical protection of compost by its occlusion into aggregates or adsorption on biochar surface [12–14]. Other studies found that biochar and mature compost mixtures induced a negative priming effect [15] or a neutral effect [16] on C mineralization when compared to application of compost. Soil addition of biochar-compost mixtures was shown to promote plant growth, biomass accumulation, yield and to improve soil properties such as water holding capacity [17–22]. Yet the synergistic effects of freshly applied biochar-compost mixtures on plant growth and performance are still under debate [23]. Indeed, application of fresh biochar-compost mixture has been found to have neutral [18] or even antagonisms effects [23]. This may be due to release of toxic compounds contained in the biochars' labile fraction [24–27] or to low availability of nutrients due to the biochars' high sorption capacity [23].

When applied to the field and exposed to weathering, the mixture effects may prevent carbon and nitrogen losses as compared to the single use of compost and biochar [28]. Physical weathering may increase the biological stability of biochars and reduce their priming effect on native SOM mineralization [29]. Moreover, weathering may change the biochar structure [30] and its effects on soil properties [8]. These effects may also change the compost-biochar interactions in mixtures and their amendment effects. Indeed several studies observed an alleviation of beneficial effects of biochar-compost addition on biomass production over time [31–33]. However, to the best of our knowledge, no studies have focused on the effect of weathering on biochar-compost mixture properties and their biological stability.

Therefore, the aim of the present study was to investigate the effect of artificial weathering on chemical characteristics and biological stability of biochar-compost mixtures and the consequences for plant biomass production after soil amendment. We used two industrially produced biochars from maize and *Miscanthus*, a green-waste compost and the corresponding biochar-compost mixtures. The mixtures and pure media were subjected to a physical weathering to mimic natural aging mechanisms. Thanks to contrasting stable carbon isotope ratios of biochars derived from C4 plants and compost derived from C3 plants, we were able to monitor the mineralization of the two components of the mixtures during a 1-year of laboratory incubation with a soil inoculum. In addition, we investigated in a 4-weeks pot experiment the effect of fresh and weathered biochar-compost mixtures on ryegrass growth growing on two different soils. We hypothesized that (i) biochar addition to compost would induce synergetic effects on biological stability and plant growth and that (ii) physical weathering would weaken these interactions.

2. Materials and Methods

2.1. Biochar and Compost

Biochars were produced from maize cobs (*Zea mays* L.) and elephant grass (*Miscanthus × giganteus*, Greef and Deuter), through pyrolysis without oxygen during 10 min at respectively 450 and 550 °C. Pyrolysis was performed by VTGreen (Allier, France), using an industrial pyrolysis reactor (Biogreen®Pyrolysis Technology, ETIA, Oise, France). The compost was made from green wastes at the platform of Fertivert (Normandy, France). The composting process consisted of 4 months fermentation and 2 months maturation. Three compost turnings were applied. The biochar from maize cobs and the compost are the same than the ones used in Nobile et al. [34]. General parameters of the biochars and the compost are listed in Tables 2 and 3. Biochar-compost mixtures were prepared by mixing 20 % (w/w) of each biochar with 80% (w/w) of the compost. The biochars and mixtures were air-dried at ambient temperature and the compost was stored at 4 °C.

2.2. Physical Weathering

The mixtures and pure media were subjected to a physical weathering through wet-drying and freeze-thawing cycles to mimic natural aging mechanisms. The weathering procedure was inspired by Naisse et al. [29]. Briefly, we placed 100 g (d.w.) of compost or biochar-compost mixtures in PVC cylinders (ø 9.5 cm). Two PVC cylinder (ø 5 cm) were used for the weathering of 30 g of maize and *Miscanthus* biochars. We covered the bottom of all tubes with a polyamide canvas with 20 µm mesh size (SEFAR-Nitex, Sefar AG, Haiden, Switzerland) and placed them on smaller tubes of 10 cm height to elevate the device. All was then put in a 10 cm ø beaker, in order to recover the lixiviates (Supplementary Material, Figure S1). We mimicked weathering processes through three successive cycles including three cycles of wetting/drying and three cycles of freezing/thawing. Wetting/drying steps consisted of saturating the samples with distilled water, leaving them at room temperature during 3 h followed by drying of the sample at 60 °C overnight. Freezing/thawing steps consisted of saturating samples with distilled water with the same amount as for the previous cycles, freezing at −20 °C overnight and thawing during 6–7 h at 28 °C. We replicated these experiments 2 times. At the end of the weathering procedure, we dried the solid samples at 60 °C during 2 days and lixiviates until complete evaporation. Mass and carbon loss after artificial weathering were assessed by mass balance.

2.3. Material Properties: Physico-Chemical, Elemental and Thermogravimetric Analysis

To measure pH and electrical conductivity (EC), 2 g of sample were mixed with 40 mL of distilled water and centrifugated for 1 h. The pH (780 pH meter, Metrohm, Herisau, Switzerland) was measured in the supernatant and the mixtures were filtered (glass microfibres paper, Fisherbrand) before EC (InLab® 738-ISM, Mettler Toledo, Columbus, Ohio, USA) measurement. We evaluated the effect of weathering on dissolved organic carbon content (DOC) and elemental content. For DOC determination, 2 g of dried samples were sieved at 2 mm and mixed with 40 mL of distilled water, (1:20 w/v) ratio. The samples were shaken during 1 h, centrifugated at 4750 t/min during 20 min and the supernatant recovered by filtration (glass microfibres paper, Fisherbrand). DOC was analysed using a Total organic carbon analyzer (TOC-5050A, Shimadzu, Marne-la-Vallée, France). The determination of C, H, N and O of solid samples was performed using a CHN-O analyzer (FlashEA 1112 Series, Thermo-Fisher Scientific, Illkirch, France).

Ash content, volatile matter and fixed carbon of dry matter were determined by thermogravimetric analyses (TGA/DSC1 STAR System, Mettler-Toledo, Viroflay, France). The samples (in 70 µL crucibles, approx. 6–7 mg) were first heated at 105 °C during 30 min to determine the moisture content. Thereafter, the temperature was increased by 15 °C min^{-1} to 900 °C during 40 min under N_2 atmosphere to determine volatile content. Temperature was then kept at 900 °C under air flux (50 mL min^{-1}) for 6 min to determine ash content.

2.4. Biological Stability: Incubation

Laboratory incubation was carried out under optimum conditions after the addition of a microbial inoculum (4 mL soil inoculum per 100 g of sample). The inoculum was prepared with 50 g of soil from a cropland field (Haplic Luvisol [35], Beauvais, Northern France), by preparing a water extract with 200 mL of distilled water. The soil was not carbonated, contained 154 mg g^{-1} organic C, 18 mg g^{-1} total N and had a pH (water) of 7.7 (Table 1). After inoculum addition, 20 g of sample were placed in 100 mL glass vials and covered with rubber septa. We carried out the incubation in triplicate for 8 treatments (2 biochar/compost mixtures, a compost and one biochar (all fresh and weathered) at 20 °C during 12 months. As we hypothesized that pure biochars will behave similarly, we used only *Miscanthus* biochar as control sample. We adjusted the water content to 60 % at the beginning of the incubation, when the flask's atmosphere was free of CO_2. We monitored the decomposition of the materials by measuring release of CO_2-C using a micro-GC (490 Micro-GC, Agilent Technologies, Les Ulis, France) and the stable carbon isotope ratio of CO_2-C with an isotopic ratio mass spectrometer (Vario isotope select, Elementar, UK-Ltd Cheadle, UK) at day 1, 3, 7, 16, 24, and then once a month until the end of the incubation. At each CO_2-C measurement date, we also determined the isotopic signature of the CO_2 emitted by compost, biochar and compost-biochar mixtures. Thanks to the isotopic ^{13}C signature of the C4-biochar, which is distinctly different from C3 compost, we were able to determine the contribution of carbon mineralized from biochar or compost in CO_2 emitted from the biochar-compost mixtures. After each measurement, we flushed the bottles with synthetic CO_2 free-air. The results are expressed as cumulated CO_2-C emitted form fresh and aged samples in terms of initial total C content of the compost or biochar within the fresh samples.

Table 1. Characteristics of the Calcaric Cambisol and Haplic Luvisol used for the pot experiment.

	Unit (Dry Matter)	Calcaric Cambisol	Haplic Luvisol
Clay	%	33.3	17.6
Silt	%	46.1	66.9
Sand	%	20.6	15.6
CaCO3	g kg^{-1}	563.3	0.0
organic C	g kg^{-1}	9.5	15.4
total N	g kg^{-1}	2.6	1.8
C/N		3.6	8.6
pH KCl		7.8	7.4
pH water		8.0	7.8
CEC	cmolc kg^{-1}	14.0	12.5
P water	mg kg^{-1}	1.2	3.9
Available P	mg kg^{-1}	19.7	71.2
Available K	mg kg^{-1}	326.8	291.9
Available Mg	mg kg^{-1}	271.1	100.7
Available Ca	mg kg^{-1}	46727.4	3868.6

2.5. Effect on Biomass Production: Pot Experiment

A pot experiment was carried out with fresh and weathered compost and mixtures added to two different agricultural soils sampled in Beauvais (Northern France) and classified as a silt loam Haplic Luvisol and a clay loam Calcaric Cambisol [35]. Soil characteristics are shown in Table 1.

After sieving the soil (4 mm), the composts and mixtures were applied at respectively 16t ha^{-1} and 20 t ha^{-1} to 0.4 kg of soil. Both fresh and weathered amendments were applied to soil at a similar rate, considering the mass loss during the weathering treatment. The pots were sown with 0.15 g pot^{-1} of Italian ryegrass (*Festuca perennis* Lam. ex *Lolium multiflorum*) seeds. Thereafter, they were kept in a growth chamber under controlled conditions: 16 h day^{-1} of light, a temperature of 24 °C (day) and 20 °C (night) and addition of distilled water every two days (Supplementary Material, Figure S2). We harvested the plants 4 weeks after sowing by cutting at 2 cm from soil surface. Biomass production was determined gravimetrically after 72 h drying at 60 °C.

2.6. Calculations and Statistics

The stable C isotope signatures were used to estimate the contribution of biochar and compost to the mixtures and the CO_2 emissions from the mixtures. The partitioning was done with Equation (1):

$$C_{biochar,mix} = (\delta^{13}C_{mixture} - \delta^{13}C_{compost})/(\delta^{13}C_{biochar} - \delta^{13}C_{compost}) \qquad (1)$$

where $C_{biochar,mix}$ is biochar carbon in the mixture or in CO_2-C emitted from the mixture (%); $\delta^{13}C_{mixture}$ is the stable C isotope signature of the mixture, $\delta^{13}C_{biochar}$ is the stable C isotope signature of biochar and $\delta^{13}C_{compost}$ is the stable isotope signature of compost.

To evaluate interactions between biochar and compost in mixtures, we calculated expected values for the mixtures according to Equation (2). The comparison between the expected and the measured values of the mixtures were used to assess interactions between biochar and compost.

$$m_{biochar,mix}/m_{mixture} = C_{mixture} \times C_{biochar,mix}/C_{biochar} \qquad (2)$$

where $m_{biochar,mix}$ is the mass of biochar within the mixture (g); $m_{mixture}$ is the mass of the mixture (g); $C_{mixture}$ is the C content of the mixture; and $C_{biochar}$ is the C content of biochar.

To calculate differences between fresh and weathered materials, we tested for normality using the Shapiro-Wilk test. For the normally distributed data, we performed analysis of variances (ANOVA) and Tukey multiple comparison. When data did not follow a normal distribution, we used Kruskal-Wallis tests with Bonferroni corrections. The level of significance was set at $p = 0.05$. We performed all statistical analyses using the R software (version 3.5.2).

3. Results

3.1. Leaching Due to Physical Weathering

Material losses ranged from about 20 mg g^{-1} for maize biochar to about 150 mg g^{-1} for compost (Figure 1). Artificial physical weathering thus resulted in twice as much material loss from compost as compared to biochars. Mass losses for both mixtures were around 75 mg g^{-1}. They were about two times lower than expected from the losses of individual materials (Figure 1).

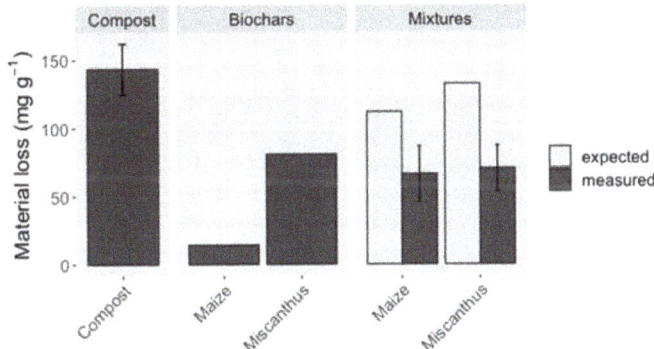

Figure 1. Total mass loss during physical weathering of compost, biochars and their mixtures. Data are presented as mean ± sd ($n = 2$ for the compost and the mixture and $n = 1$ for the biochars). Expected values for mixtures were calculated based on mass losses measured for individual components.

3.2. Properties of the Fresh and Weathered Materials

3.2.1. Elemental Composition

Fresh compost was composed of 226 mg g^{-1} C, 20 mg g^{-1} H, 112 mg g^{-1} O and 23 mg g^{-1} N (Table 2). Fresh biochars contained at least twice more C than the fresh compost, with biochar from maize and *Miscanthus* containing respectively 591 and 778 mg g^{-1} C (Table 2). Hydrogen content of biochars were similar to compost, whereas O and N content of biochars were at least twice lower than for compost. Following the mixing ratio, carbon content of the mixtures ranged between 298 mg g^{-1} and 332 mg g^{-1} and all other elemental components had similar values for both mixtures. The mixtures showed similar C/N ratios independently from biochar feedstocks.

Table 2. Elemental composition of fresh (F) and weathered (W) compost, biochars and biochar compost mixtures. Expected (exp) values were calculated for the weathered mixtures. Data are presented as means ± sd (n = 3). The letters represent differences among treatments.

			C (mg g^{-1})	H (mg g^{-1})	O (mg g^{-1})	N (mg g^{-1})	C/N
Compost							
Compost	F		226 ± 1 [i]	20 ± 1 [ab]	112 ± 4 [a]	23 ± 0 [a]	10 ± 0 [g]
	W		209 ± 5 [j]	17 ± 5 [abc]	99 ± 4 [b]	21 ± 1 [ab]	10 ± 0 [g]
Biochars							
Maize	F		591 ± 1 [d]	21 ± 1 [ab]	48 ± 3 [d]	8 ± 0 [gh]	72 ± 0 [c]
	W		618 ± 0 [c]	21 ± 0 [ab]	76 ± 5 [c]	9 ± 0 [fg]	65 ± 0 [d]
Miscanthus	F		778 ± 1 [a]	13 ± 1 [c]	18 ± 3 [e]	4 ± 0 [hi]	186 ± 0 [b]
	W		742 ± 1 [b]	16 ± 2 [bc]	58 ± 6 [d]	4 ± 0 [i]	189 ± 0.3 [a]
Mixtures							
Maize	F		298 ± 3 [h]	19 ± 1 [ab]	103 ± 0 [ab]	17 ± 0 [ef]	17 ± 0 [f]
	W		350 ± 3 [f]	22 ± 1 [a]	78 ± 1 [c]	18 ± 0 [cd]	20 ± 0 [ef]
		exp	321	18	92	18	18
Miscanthus	F		332 ± 1 [g]	19 ± 2 [ab]	107 ± 3 [ab]	19 ± 0 [bc]	17 ± 0 [f]
	W		374 ± 3 [e]	20 ± 1 [ab]	83 ± 1 [c]	17 ± 0 [de]	22 ± 0 [e]
		exp	355	16	87	16	22

Compost weathering induced decreasing contents of all elements, while mostly C and O were affected for biochars. As a result of weathering, C content respectively increased and decreased for the maize and *Miscanthus* biochars, while O content more than doubled for both biochars. The expected C content of the weathered mixtures were slightly lower than the measured ones ranging between 321 and 355. As for biochars, weathering affected mainly the C and O contents of the mixtures; O contents of the weathered mixtures were slightly lower than the expected values. For both mixtures, weathering increased the C/N ratio (Table 2).

3.2.2. Physico-Chemical Properties, Dissolved Organic Carbon and Stable δ^{13}C Ratio

Table 3 shows physico-chemical properties and the dissolved organic carbon content (DOC) of the materials. pH and electrical conductivity (EC) ranged from 8.1 to 10.5 and from 109 to 1598 µS cm^{-1}, respectively. Compost had lower pH (8.4), and EC (944 µS cm^{-1}) than both biochars. Both biochars showed similar pH (around 10.5), but maize biochar had higher EC than *Miscanthus* biochar. The pH and EC of fresh mixtures were in between the values from compost and biochars.

Fixed C content ranged between 0.6 and 67.8 %, DOC varied between 2.2 and 277.2 mg g^{-1} C, whereas ash content ranged between 13.6 and 59.3 % and volatile matter content between 17.8 and 38.8 %. Compost showed lower fixed C and higher DOC, ash content and volatile matter than biochars. Both biochars had similar volatile C but varied in ash content and fixed C; maize biochar presented a twice-higher ash content and a lower fixed C content (45.6 vs. 63.6%) than *Miscanthus* biochar. We assumed that differences between the two biochars were mainly driven by production temperature rather than initial feedstock, as it has been found to be the main driver of biochar chemical composition [36–38]. Maize mixtures showed higher pH (9.1 vs. 8.9) and ash contents (54.0 vs. 51.2%) and lower volatile matter contents (35.1 vs. 38.2%) compared to *Miscanthus* mixture.

Weathering induced an increase of fixed C from around 10% to 17.1% and 16.6% for maize and *Miscanthus* mixtures. In contrast, EC and DOC showed 4 times lower values after weathering. When compared to the expected values, slightly higher EC values than expected were recorded for both mixtures after weathering. In addition, the weathered mixture with maize biochar showed lower DOC (50.1 vs. 57.6 mg g C^{-1}) and higher fixed C (17.1 vs. 11.6%) than expected. The weathered *Miscanthus* mixture showed higher volatile matter than expected (37.1 vs. 31.3%) (Table 3). During weathering, the isotopic signatures remained unchanged for compost, biochars and the mixture containing maize biochar, but decreased for the mixture containing *Miscanthus* biochar. The $\delta^{13}C$ ratios of the weathered mixtures (21.9‰) were lower than expected (25.4 and 25.2‰).

Table 3. Chemical characteristics of fresh (F) and weathered (W) compost, biochars and biochar-compost mixtures. Expected (exp.) values were calculated for the weathered mixtures. EC: electric conductivity; DOC: dissolved organic carbon. Data are presented as means ± sd (n = 3) for pH, EC, DOC and $\delta^{13}C$. Proximate analysis was carried out for 1 sample. The letters represent differences among treatments.

			pH *	EC (µS cm^{-1})	DOC (mg g^{-1} C)	$\delta^{13}C$ (‰)	Ash (%)	Volatile (%)	Fixed C (%)
Compost									
Compost	F		8.4 g	944 ± 18 cd	277.2 ± 49.0 a	−28.9 ± 0.1 gh	59.3	38.8	1.9
	W		7.9 h	215 ± 4 fg	73.5 ± 2.4 cd	−29.2 ± 0.0 h	63.0	36.4	0.6
Biochars									
Maize	F		10.5 a	1640 ± 62 a	36.7 ± 1.6 f	−15.3 ± 0.1 bc	28.5	25.9	45.6
	W		8.7 e	109 ± 3 g	15.5 ± 0.1 fg	−15.3 ± 0.0 c	23.5	35.7	40.8
Miscanthus	F		10.4 a	1516 ± 14 bc	3.6 ± 0.7 g	−14.9 ± 0.1 ab	13.6	22.8	63.6
	W		9.4 b	129 ± 3 g	2.2 ± 0.1 g	−14.5 ± 0.1 a	14.4	17.8	67.8
Mixtures									
Maize	F		9.1 c	1588 ± 12 ab	203.2 ± 7.9 bc	−22.3 ± 0.3 ef	54.0	35.1	10.9
	W	real	8.6 e	224 ± 3 ef	50.1 ± 1.1 ef	−21.9 ± 0.0 de	48.9	34.0	17.1
		exp	8.1	186	57.6	−25.4	52.2	36.2	11.6
Miscanthus	F		8.9 d	1598 ± 20 a	210.3 ± 9.3 ab	−23.2 ± 0.1 fg	51.2	38.2	10.6
	W	real	8.5 f	238 ± 15 de	54.3 ± 1.5 de	−21.9 ± 0.1 d	46.3	37.1	16.6
		exp	8.3	192	54.0	−25.2	49.7	31.3	19.0

* standard deviations of pH were <0.05.

3.3. Biological Stability

Cumulative CO_2-C released during 1-year of incubation from fresh and weathered compost, *Miscanthus* biochar and both mixtures are presented in Figure 2. After 1 year of incubation, the fresh compost showed the highest cumulative C mineralization with values up to 30 mg g^{-1} of initial carbon. In contrast, very few C was mineralized from *Miscanthus* biochar. The isotopic signatures of carbon were used to assess the origin of C mineralized from biochar-compost mixtures. The data indicated that compost released between 15 and 20 mg g^{-1} C when incubated in mixtures, while biochar released between 10 and 15 mg g^{-1} C when incubated in mixtures. Compost showed lower C-mineralization in mixture compared to individual incubation. Conversely, biochar showed higher C-mineralization when combined with compost compared to individual incubation.

After weathering, cumulative compost C mineralization amounted to 10 mg g^{-1} C, which was significantly lower than C mineralization of fresh compost (Figure 2). Biochar C-mineralization was not significantly affected by weathering when individually incubated. When combined with compost it mineralized significantly less than in fresh mixtures. In contrast, compost mineralized significantly more in weathered mixtures as compared to fresh mixtures and reached values between 20 and 25 mg g^{-1} C after 1-year incubation.

3.4. Ryegrass Growth

Biomass of Italian ryegrass was higher when grown on Haplic Luvisol as compared to Calcaric Cambisol, as shown for the unamended controls (Figure 3). All organic amendments stimulated ryegrass growth, when applied to Calcaric Cambisol. However, when applied to Haplic Luvisol, organic amendments induced neutral or negative effects on biomass. For both soils, application of fresh biochar-compost mixtures did not lead to significant differences in ryegrass biomass as compared to fresh compost alone. Physical weathering decreased the effect of compost addition to Calcaric Cambisol on biomass, but the effect was still positive as compared to the control. Concerning the Haplic Luvisol compost addition tended to decrease biomass. For both soils and after weathering, the mixture containing *Miscanthus* biochar induced significantly higher biomass than the compost alone, while the mixture containing maize biochar showed similar effects as compost alone.

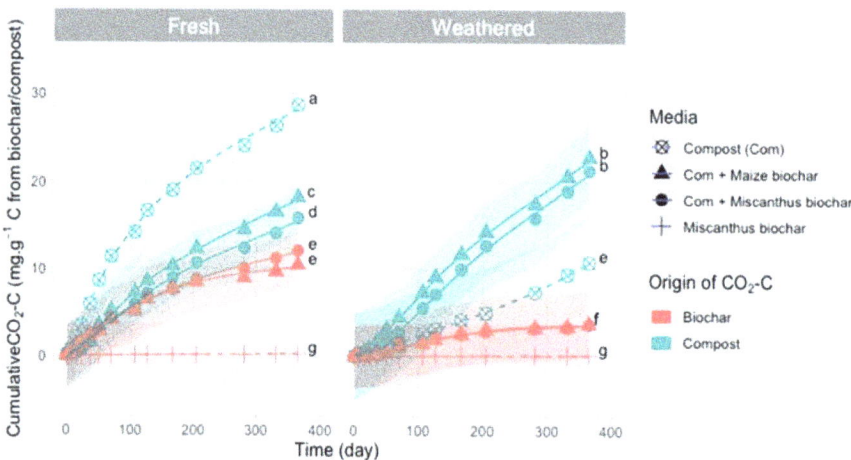

Figure 2. Cumulative CO_2-C mineralized from biochar and compost when incubated alone or in mixture. Turquoise and red colors represent C mineralized from compost and biochar respectively. Data represent means from 3 replicated samples. The colored ribbon represents the standard deviations. The letters represent the significant differences from a two-ways ANOVA analysis ($n = 3$).

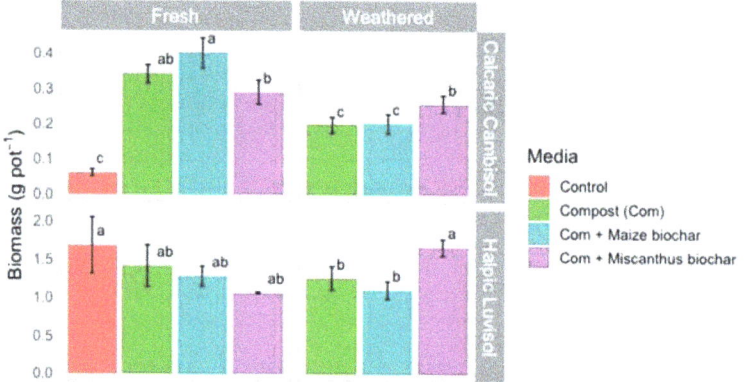

Figure 3. Biomass of ryegrass after addition of compost or its mixture with maize and *Miscanthus* biochars, grown on two soil types. Data are presented as means ± sd ($n = 3$). The letters represent the significant differences from a one-way ANOVA analysis ($n = 4$) within each treatment and soil type.

4. Discussion

4.1. Weathering Effects on Material Properties

Physical weathering induced much higher mass loss from compost as compared to biochar and mixtures. This may probably be explained by the high leaching losses. Biochar mass loss amounted to 75 mg g^{-1}, which is much lower than observed for gasification biochar [29]. This may be due to the lower friability of biochar produced by pyrolysis making it less prone to particle losses [30]. Lower mass loss for the mixtures than expected (Figure 1), may be explained by protection of compost from leaching losses by its association with the biochar structure [12,39]. Both weathering cycles may affect release of dissolved organic matter and cause cracking on biochar-surfaces, thus leading to changes in pore structure [40]. While DOC was lower than expected in weathered mixtures, EC values were higher than expected (see below). We therefore suggest that there may be interactions between biochar and compost leading to solid particles retention during weathering treatment.

Compost weathering induced a decrease of the content of all main elements, following strong leaching due to weathering treatment (Table 2). However, weathering of biochars affected only C and O contents and led to decreasing C content and increasing O content. Our results are consistent with data of Naisse et al. [29], who suggested that these observations may indicate oxidation processes induced by weathering [41]. In contrast, weathering of the mixtures increased their C contents, while it decreased their O contents. This might be related to a preferential elimination of O relative to C in the labile fraction of the mixtures. This hypothesis may be supported by the visual observation of high loss of soluble compounds during weathering. Indeed, strong decreases of DOC and EC of the remaining substrates indicated that soluble compounds were removed by leaching during artificial weathering (Table 3). In contrast to the mixture containing *Miscanthus* biochar, the DOC content of the mixture containing maize biochar decreased slightly stronger than expected. The strong decrease of EC as a result of weathering is consistent with the results of Yao et al. [42], who evidenced a rapid decline of EC from 0.7 to 0.2 mS cm^{-1} following leaching losses from biochar. EC reduction after weathering may be due to the leaching of mineral biochar compounds. This is supported by the lower ash content of the material remaining after weathering. Ashes and volatile compounds were both partly removed during weathering, except for volatile compounds of maize biochar. Both ashes and volatile compounds compose the labile fraction of all materials and are more likely to be leached than the more stable compounds. In particular, ash represents the mineral material contribution, which may be an indicator of nutrient content [43].

Fixed C slightly decreased for compost and biochars following weathering treatment, while it increased for the mixtures (Table 3). Fixed C is mainly composed by fused aromatic C structures and may be used as an indicator of the C sequestration potential of biochars [44]. Higher fixed C of the mixtures than the expected values after weathering might result from the increasing chemical recalcitrance of the materials due to labile compounds leaching. These observations are in agreement with the lower than expected $\delta^{13}C$ ratios of the mixtures, might indicate preferential leaching of ^{12}C enriched compounds, e.g., C3-compost or labile polysaccharides, which are ^{13}C enriched compared to recalcitrant compounds [45].

4.2. Biological Stability

4.2.1. Biological Stability of the Fresh Materials

During the incubation, compost showed the highest cumulative C-mineralization, while biochar C hardly mineralized. C-mineralization of the mixtures ranged between those of its individual components. These results are in agreement with other studies [13,14,16] and may be explained by a higher content of labile C in compost than in biochar [5]. It was interesting to note that compost showed a lower C-mineralization when combined with biochar than when incubated individually. Two mechanisms could explain observation: the adsorption of labile fraction on the biochar surface [13], and the presence of phenolic compounds or salts originating from biochar [24,25,27], which might inhibit microbial activity in compost-biochar mixtures. The opposite effect was observed for biochar, since biochar C mineralized more when combined with compost than when individually applied. Indeed, several studies showed positive priming effect when labile substrates were added to biochar [46–48].

4.2.2. Effect of Weathering on the Biological Stability

The cumulative C-mineralization from compost after 1 year of incubation was significantly lower for weathered compost compared to fresh compost when individually incubated (10 vs. 30 mg g^{-1}). This negative effect of weathering on C-mineralization from compost was attributed to the strong leaching of easily mineralizable labile components. On the other hand, the absence of weathering effects on biochar C mineralisation may be explained by the high stability of biochar with only few labile compounds [48].

C-mineralization from compost in the mixture increased significantly after weathering when compared to the fresh mixtures (Figure 2). This may be due to the protection of labile compounds by biochar and/or the removal of biochar compounds, which inhibited microbial activity and thus C-mineralization from compost (see above). Indeed, fresh biochar may contain large amounts of salts, which may inhibit microbial activity when applied to soil [49–51]. This could lead to the negative priming effect of biochar on native C often observed immediately after soil addition [52].

Weathering also reduced biochar C-mineralization, within the mixtures (Figure 2) most probably due to the leaching of easily mineralizable C and nutrients from compost which stimulated biochar C-mineralization before weathering (see above). Our results thus indicate that weathering affects biochar-compost interaction in mixtures, which might also impact their effects on plant growth.

4.3. Ryegrass Growth

4.3.1. Effect of the Fresh Media on Ryegrass Growth

Higher ryegrass biomass was recorded when grown on Haplic Luvisol as compared to Calcaric Cambisol, regardless the organic amendment (Figure 3). Moreover, the addition of organic amendments containing compost had positive effects on biomass when applied on Calcaric Cambisol, but the effects were neutral or negative when applied to Haplic Luvisol (Figure 3). Our results were consistent with the results of Von Glisczynski et al. [53] who also did not find any plant growth promoting effect of biochar-compost mixtures application on Haplic Luvisol. As reviewed by Faucon et al. [54], organic amendments such as compost may promote plant growth by providing readily available nutrients or releasing them through mineralization. The available P concentration of the Calcaric Cambisol was much lower than that of the Haplic Luvisol (19.66 vs. 71.18 mg kg^{-1}) (Table 1), suggesting a possible P-limitation for plant growth in this soil, which might have been alleviated by compost application.

Addition of biochar compost mixtures led to similar ryegrass biomass than compost along (Figure 3). As reported in the literature, the combination of biochar with compost can have synergic [32,55], antagonistic [23,56] or neutral effects [16,18,23,57,58] on plant growth. Several factors may impact plant growth after biochar-compost mixtures addition and the mechanisms are still poorly understood [17]. It was suggested that pre-treatment of biochar may be beneficial for plant growth before its soil application [59]. Moreover, it was shown that weathering may alter biochar properties [29]. Therefore, we tested in the following, if weathering of biochar/compost mixtures influenced plant growth.

4.3.2. Effect of Weathered Amendments on Ryegrass Growth

Irrespective of the soil type, weathered compost had negative or neutral effects on biomass when individually applied (Figure 3). This is most likely due to the weathering-induced loss of readily-available nutrients and easily-mineralizable C compounds (Table 3 and Figure 2).

The addition of weathered biochar-compost mixtures to both soils had neutral or positive effects on biomass compared to the effect of compost applied individually depending on the biochar feedstock (Figure 3). The positive effect of the weathered *Miscanthus* mixture on biomass may result from better compost mineralisation through the removal of compounds, which inhibit microbial activity as discussed above (Section 4.3.1). However, the weathered maize mixture showed neutral effect on biomass when compared to the effects of weathered compost alone. Our results showed that weathering of biochar-compost mixtures could lead to positive growth effect. These results are in agreement with a recent field study, showing positive growth effects on the second crop after soil application [60]. In addition, our results also showed that neutral effects of weathering depending on biochar feedstocks and/or soil type may occur [60,61]. Further studies would be needed to investigate the mechanisms controlling the variation of biochar-compost interactions on plant growth over time.

5. Conclusions

We investigated the effect of two biochar-compost mixtures and weathering on their material properties, biological stability and on plant growth after addition to two contrasting soils. Our results showed that the physical weathering led to the alteration of material properties of the mixtures, in particular through leaching of labile compounds. These effects could impact the mineralisation of the mixture and also plant growth after soil addition. We suggest that the mixtures contained inhibitive compounds for microbial activity in their labile fraction, as shown by the negative effect on compost mineralisation when combined with biochar. The increase of compost mineralisation within the mixtures after weathering may have provided more plant available nutrients, which could promote plant biomass production when compared to individual compost application. On the other hand, biochar mineralisation was also affected by weathering, indicating that weathering may influence its C sequestration potential.

We conclude that biochar-compost interactions are evolving after physical weathering most probably due to its effect on leaching of soluble compounds. The effect of fresh and weathered biochar-compost mixtures on plant growth depend on biochar production conditions. Further studies should focus on mechanisms influencing the nutrient supply of biochar-compost mixtures.

Supplementary Materials: The following are available online at https://www.mdpi.com/2073-4395/11/2/336/s1, Figure S1: Experimental set up used for physical weathering of organic amendments, Figure S2: Pot experiment with ryegrass.

Author Contributions: M.-L.A., C.G., S.H., C.N., D.H. and C.R. designed the study. M.-L.A. and C.N. carried out the laboratory work, and exploited the results. Y.L.B. and S.B. contributed data. M.-L.A. wrote the first draft of the manuscript. All authors discussed the results and commented on the manuscript. All authors have read and agreed to the published version of the manuscript.

Funding: The study was funded by FUI (project BIOCHAR21). ADEME provided a PhD grant.

Data Availability Statement: Data will be made available upon request.

Acknowledgments: We thank FUI for funding under the framework of the project BIOCHAR21. MLA acknowledges ADEME for providing her PhD grant. We thank Valérie Pouteau for help with the laboratory work.

Conflicts of Interest: The authors declare no conflict of interest.

References

1. Field, C.B.; Barros, V.R.; Mastrandrea, M.D.; Mach, K.J.; Abdrabo, M.A.-K.; Adger, N.; Anokhin, Y.A.; Anisimov, O.A.; Arent, D.J.; Barnett, J.; et al. Summary for Policymakers. Available online: https://epic.awi.de/id/eprint/37531/ (accessed on 4 February 2021).
2. Smith, P. Soil carbon sequestration and biochar as negative emission technologies. *Glob. Chang. Biol.* **2016**, *22*, 1315–1324. [CrossRef] [PubMed]
3. Abbott, L.; Macdonald, L.; Wong, M.; Webb, M.; Jenkins, S.; Farrell, M. Potential roles of biological amendments for profitable grain production—A review. *Agric. Ecosyst. Environ.* **2018**, *256*, 34–50. [CrossRef]
4. Lehmann, J.; Joseph, S. (Eds.) *Biochar for Environmental Management. Science, Technology and Implementation*; Routledge: London, UK, 2015.
5. Liu, W.-J.; Jiang, H.; Yu, H.-Q. Development of Biochar-Based Functional Materials: Toward a Sustainable Platform Carbon Material. *Chem. Rev.* **2015**, *115*, 12251–12285. [CrossRef] [PubMed]
6. Glaser, B.; Lehmann, J.; Zech, W. Ameliorating physical and chemical properties of highly weathered soils in the tropics with charcoal—A review. *Biol. Fertil. Soils* **2002**, *35*, 219–230. [CrossRef]

7. Alghamdi, A.G. Biochar as a potential soil additive for improving soil physical properties—A review. *Arab. J. Geosci.* **2018**, *11*, 766. [CrossRef]
8. Paetsch, L.; Mueller, C.W.; Kögel-Knabner, I.; Von Lützow, M.; Girardin, C.; Rumpel, C. Effect of in-situ aged and fresh biochar on soil hydraulic conditions and microbial C use under drought conditions. *Sci. Rep.* **2018**, *8*, 1–11. [CrossRef]
9. Obia, A.; Mulder, J.; Martinsen, V.; Cornelissen, G.; Børresen, T. In situ effects of biochar on aggregation, water retention and porosity in light-textured tropical soils. *Soil Tillage Res.* **2016**, *155*, 35–44. [CrossRef]
10. Sun, F.; Lu, S. Biochars improve aggregate stability, water retention, and pore-space properties of clayey soil. *J. Plant. Nutr. Soil Sci.* **2013**, *177*, 26–33. [CrossRef]
11. Barthod, J.; Rumpel, C.; Dignac, M.-F. Composting with additives to improve organic amendments. A review. *Agron. Sustain. Dev.* **2018**, *38*, 17. [CrossRef]
12. Jien, S.-H.; Wang, C.-C.; Lee, C.-H.; Lee, T.-Y. Stabilization of Organic Matter by Biochar Application in Compost-amended Soils with Contrasting pH Values and Textures. *Sustainability* **2015**, *7*, 13317–13333. [CrossRef]
13. Ngo, P.-T.; Rumpel, C.; Ngo, Q.-A.; Alexis, M.; Vargas, G.V.; Gil, M.D.L.L.M.; Dang, D.-K.; Jouquet, P.; Ngô, Q.-A. Biological and chemical reactivity and phosphorus forms of buffalo manure compost, vermicompost and their mixture with biochar. *Bioresour. Technol.* **2013**, *148*, 401–407. [CrossRef]
14. Jien, S.H.; Chen, W.C.; Ok, Y.S.; Awad, Y.M.; Liao, C.S. Short-term biochar application induced variations in C and N mineralization in a compost-amended tropical soil. *Environ. Sci. Pollut. Res.* **2018**, *25*, 25715–25725. [CrossRef]
15. Qayyum, M.F.; Liaquat, F.; Rehman, R.A.; Gul, M.; ul Hye, M.Z.; Rizwan, M.; ur Rehaman, M.Z. Effects of co-composting of farm manure and biochar on plant growth and carbon mineralization in an alkaline soil. *Environ. Sci. Pollut. Res.* **2017**, *24*, 26060–26068 [CrossRef] [PubMed]
16. Teutscherova, N.; Vazquez, E.; Santana, D.; Navas, M.; Masaguer, A.; Benito, M. Influence of pruning waste compost maturity and biochar on carbon dynamics in acid soil: Incubation study. *Eur. J. Soil Biol.* **2017**, *78*, 66–74. [CrossRef]
17. Agegnehu, G.; Srivastava, A.; Bird, M.I. The role of biochar and biochar-compost in improving soil quality and crop performance: A review. *Appl. Soil Ecol.* **2017**, *119*, 156–170. [CrossRef]
18. Trupiano, D.; Cocozza, C.; Baronti, S.; Amendola, C.; Vaccari, F.P.; Lustrato, G.; Di Lonardo, S.; Fantasma, F.; Tognetti, R.; Scippa, G.S. The Effects of Biochar and Its Combination with Compost on Lettuce (Lactuca Sativa L.) Growth, Soil Properties, and Soil Microbial Activity and Abundance. Available online: https://www.hindawi.com/journals/ija/2017/3158207/ (accessed on 25 May 2020).
19. Naeem, M.A.; Khalid, M.; Aon, M.; Abbas, G.; Amjad, M.; Murtaza, B.; Khan, W.; Ahmad, N. Combined application of biochar with compost and fertilizer improves soil properties and grain yield of maize. *J. Plant. Nutr.* **2018**, *41*, 112–122. [CrossRef]
20. Manolikaki, I.; Diamadopoulos, E. Positive Effects of Biochar and Biochar-Compost on Maize Growth and Nutrient Availability in Two Agricultural Soils. *Commun. Soil Sci. Plant. Anal.* **2019**, *50*, 512–526. [CrossRef]
21. Zulfiqar, F.; Younis, A.; Chen, J. Biochar or Biochar-Compost Amendment to a Peat-Based Substrate Improves Growth of Syngonium podophyllum. *Agronomy* **2019**, *9*, 460. [CrossRef]
22. Tsai, C.-C.; Chang, Y.-F. Carbon Dynamics and Fertility in Biochar-Amended Soils with Excessive Compost Application. *Agronomy* **2019**, *9*, 511. [CrossRef]
23. Seehausen, M.L.; Gale, N.V.; Dranga, S.; Hudson, V.; Liu, N.; Michener, J.; Thurston, E.; Williams, C.; Smith, S.M.; Thomas, S.C. Is There a Positive Synergistic Effect of Biochar and Compost Soil Amendments on Plant Growth and Physiological Performance? *Agronomy* **2017**, *7*, 13. [CrossRef]
24. Gale, N.V.; Sackett, T.E.; Thomas, S.C. Thermal treatment and leaching of biochar alleviates plant growth inhibition from mobile organic compounds. *PeerJ* **2016**, *4*, e2385. [CrossRef] [PubMed]
25. Kołtowski, M.; Oleszczuk, P. Toxicity of biochars after polycyclic aromatic hydrocarbons removal by thermal treatment. *Ecol. Eng.* **2015**, *75*, 79–85. [CrossRef]
26. Buss, W.; Mašek, O. Mobile organic compounds in biochar—A potential source of contamination—Phytotoxic effects on cress seed (Lepidium sativum) germination. *J. Environ. Manag.* **2014**, *137*, 111–119. [CrossRef]
27. Deenik, J.L.; McClellan, T.; Uehara, G.; Antal, M.J.; Campbell, S. Charcoal Volatile Matter Content Influences Plant Growth and Soil Nitrogen Transformations. *Soil Sci. Soc. Am. J.* **2010**, *74*, 1259–1270. [CrossRef]
28. Ngo, P.T.; Rumpel, C.; Janeau, J.-L.; Dang, D.-K.; Doan, T.T.; Jouquet, P. Mixing of biochar with organic amendments reduces carbon removal after field exposure under tropical conditions. *Ecol. Eng.* **2016**, *91*, 378–380. [CrossRef]
29. Naisse, C.; Girardin, C.; Lefevre, R.; Pozzi, A.; Maas, R.; Stark, A.; Rumpel, C. Effect of physical weathering on the carbon sequestration potential of biochars and hydrochars in soil. *GCB Bioenergy* **2015**, *7*, 488–496. [CrossRef]
30. Spokas, K.A.; Novak, J.M.; Masiello, C.A.; Johnson, M.G.; Colosky, E.C.; Ippolito, J.A.; Trigo, C. Physical Disintegration of Biochar: An Overlooked Process. *Environ. Sci. Technol. Lett.* **2014**, *1*, 326–332. [CrossRef]
31. Prodana, M.; Bastos, A.; Amaro, A.; Cardoso, D.; Morgado, R.; Machado, A.; Verheijen, F.; Keizer, J.; Loureiro, S. Biomonitoring tools for biochar and biochar-compost amended soil under viticulture: Looking at exposure and effects. *Appl. Soil Ecol.* **2019**, *137*, 120–128. [CrossRef]
32. Doan, T.T.; Henry-Des-Tureaux, T.; Rumpel, C.; Janeau, J.-L.; Jouquet, P. Impact of compost, vermicompost and biochar on soil fertility, maize yield and soil erosion in Northern Vietnam: A three year mesocosm experiment. *Sci. Total. Environ.* **2015**, *514*, 147–154. [CrossRef]

3. Schmidt, H.-P.; Kammann, C.; Niggli, C.; Evangelou, M.W.; Mackie, K.A.; Abiven, S. Biochar and biochar-compost as soil amendments to a vineyard soil: Influences on plant growth, nutrient uptake, plant health and grape quality. *Agric. Ecosyst. Environ.* **2014**, *191*, 117–123. [CrossRef]
4. Nobile, C.; Denier, J.; Houben, D. Linking biochar properties to biomass of basil, lettuce and pansy cultivated in growing media. *Sci. Hortic.* **2020**, *261*, 109001. [CrossRef]
5. IUSS Working Group WRB. World Reference Base for Soil Resources 2014. In *International Soil Classification System for Naming Soils and Creating Legends for Soil Maps*; FAO: Rome, Italy, 2014; ISBN 9789251083697.
6. Uchimiya, M.; Wartelle, L.H.; Klasson, K.T.; Fortier, C.A.; Lima, I.M. Influence of Pyrolysis Temperature on Biochar Property and Function as a Heavy Metal Sorbent in Soil. *J. Agric. Food Chem.* **2011**, *59*, 2501–2510. [CrossRef]
7. Enders, A.; Hanley, K.; Whitman, T.; Joseph, S.; Lehmann, J. Characterization of biochars to evaluate recalcitrance and agronomic performance. *Bioresour. Technol.* **2012**, *114*, 644–653. [CrossRef]
8. Wiedner, K.; Naisse, C.; Rumpel, C.; Pozzi, A.; Wieczorek, P.; Glaser, B. Chemical modification of biomass residues during hydrothermal carbonization—What makes the difference, temperature or feedstock? *Org. Geochem.* **2013**, *54*, 91–100. [CrossRef]
9. Cooper, J.; Greenberg, I.; Ludwig, B.; Hippich, L.; Fischer, D.; Glaser, B.; Kaiser, M. Effect of biochar and compost on soil properties and organic matter in aggregate size fractions under field conditions. *Agric. Ecosyst. Environ.* **2020**, *295*, 106882. [CrossRef]
10. Wang, L.; O'Connor, D.; Rinklebe, J.; Ok, Y.S.; Tsang, D.C.; Shen, Z.; Hou, D. Biochar Aging: Mechanisms, Physicochemical Changes, Assessment, And Implications for Field Applications. *Environ. Sci. Technol.* **2020**, *54*, 14797–14814. [CrossRef]
11. Baldock, J.A.; Smernik, R.J. Chemical composition and bioavailability of thermally altered Pinus resinosa (Red pine) wood. *Org. Geochem.* **2002**, *33*, 1093–1109. [CrossRef]
12. Yao, F.; Arbestain, M.C.; Virgel, S.; Blanco, F.; Arostegui, J.; Maciá-Agulló, J.; Macías, F. Simulated geochemical weathering of a mineral ash-rich biochar in a modified Soxhlet reactor. *Chemosphere* **2010**, *80*, 724–732. [CrossRef]
13. Aller, M.F. Biochar properties: Transport, fate, and impact. *Crit. Rev. Environ. Sci. Technol.* **2016**, *46*, 1183–1296. [CrossRef]
14. Enders, A.; Lehmann, J. *Proximate Analyses for Characterising Biochars*; Singh, B., CampsArbestain, M., Lehmann, J., Eds.; Csiro Publishing: Melbourne, Australia, 2017; ISBN 978-1-4863-0509-4.
15. Amelung, W.; Brodowski, S.; Sandhage-Hofmann, A.; Bol, R. Combining Biomarker with Stable Isotope Analyses for Asses-sing the Transformation and Turnover of Soil Organic Matter. In *Advances in Agronomy*; Sparks, D.L., Ed.; Academic Press Inc: Cambridge, MA, USA, 2008; Volume 100, pp. 155–250. ISBN 978-0-12-374361-9.
16. Yousaf, B.; Liu, G.; Wang, R.; Abbas, Q.; Imtiaz, M.; Liu, R. Investigating the biochar effects on C-mineralization and sequestration of carbon in soil compared with conventional amendments using the stable isotope (δ13C) approach. *GCB Bioenergy* **2017**, *9*, 1085–1099. [CrossRef]
17. Zimmerman, A.R.; Gao, B.; Ahn, M.-Y. Positive and negative carbon mineralization priming effects among a variety of biochar-amended soils. *Soil Biol. Biochem.* **2011**, *43*, 1169–1179. [CrossRef]
18. Wang, J.; Xiong, Z.; Kuzyakov, Y. Biochar stability in soil: Meta-analysis of decomposition and priming effects. *GCB Bioenergy* **2016**, *8*, 512–523. [CrossRef]
19. Setia, R.; Marschner, P.; Baldock, J.; Chittleborough, D.; Smith, P.; Smith, J. Salinity effects on carbon mineralization in soils of varying texture. *Soil Biol. Biochem.* **2011**, *43*, 1908–1916. [CrossRef]
20. Wen, Y.; Bernhardt, E.S.; Deng, W.; Liu, W.; Yan, J.; Baruch, E.M.; Bergemann, C.M. Salt effects on carbon mineralization in southeastern coastal wetland soils of the United States. *Geoderma* **2019**, *339*, 31–39. [CrossRef]
21. Luo, M.; Huang, J.-F.; Zhu, W.-F.; Tong, C. Impacts of increasing salinity and inundation on rates and pathways of organic carbon mineralization in tidal wetlands: A review. *Hydrobiologia* **2019**, *827*, 31–49. [CrossRef]
22. Ventura, M.; Alberti, G.; Viger, M.; Jenkins, J.R.; Girardin, C.; Baronti, S.; Zaldei, A.; Taylor, G.; Rumpel, C.; Miglietta, F.; et al. Biochar mineralization and priming effect on SOM decomposition in two European short rotation coppices. *GCB Bioenergy* **2015**, *7*, 1150–1160. [CrossRef]
23. Von Glisczynski, F.; Sandhage-Hofmann, A.; Amelung, W.; Pude, R. Biochar-compost substrates do not promote growth and fruit quality of a replanted German apple orchard with fertile Haplic Luvisol soils. *Sci. Hortic.* **2016**, *213*, 110–114. [CrossRef]
24. Faucon, M.-P.; Houben, D.; Reynoird, J.-P.; Mercadal-Dulaurent, A.-M.; Armand, R.; Lambers, H. Chapter Two—Advances and Perspectives to Improve the Phosphorus Availability in Cropping Systems for Agroecological Phosphorus Management. In *Advances in Agronomy*; Sparks, D.L., Ed.; Academic Press: Cambridge, MA, USA, 2015; Volume 134, pp. 51–79.
25. Kumar, S.; Bharti, A. *Management of Organic Waste*; BoD—Books on Demand: Norderstedt, Germany, 2012; ISBN 978-953-307-925-7.
26. Schulz, H.; Glaser, B. Effects of biochar compared to organic and inorganic fertilizers on soil quality and plant growth in a greenhouse experiment. *J. Plant. Nutr. Soil Sci.* **2012**, *175*, 410–422. [CrossRef]
27. Sanchez-Monedero, M.; Cayuela, M.; Roig, A.; Jindo, K.; Mondini, C.; Bolan, N. Role of biochar as an additive in organic waste composting. *Bioresour. Technol.* **2018**, *247*, 1155–1164. [CrossRef]
28. Libutti, A.; Rivelli, A.R. Quanti-Qualitative Response of Swiss Chard (Beta Vulgaris L. Var. Cycla) to Soil Amendment with Biochar-Compost Mixtures. *Agronomy* **2021**, *11*, 307. [CrossRef]
29. Kammann, C.I.; Schmidt, H.-P.; Messerschmidt, N.; Linsel, S.; Steffens, D.; Müller, C.; Koyro, H.-W.; Conte, P.; Joseph, S. Plant growth improvement mediated by nitrate capture in co-composted biochar. *Sci. Rep.* **2015**, *5*, 11080. [CrossRef] [PubMed]

60. Doan, T.T.; Sisouvanh, P.; Sengkhrua, T.; Sritumboon, S.; Rumpel, C.; Jouquet, P.; Bottinelli, N. Site-specific effects of organic amendments on parameters of tropical agricultural soil and yield: A field experiment in three countries in Southeast Asia. *Agronomy* **2021**, *10*. in press.
61. Von Glisczynski, F.; Pude, R.; Amelung, W.; Sandhage-Hofmann, A. Biochar-compost substrates in short-rotation coppice: Effects on soil and trees in a three-year field experiment. *J. Plant. Nutr. Soil Sci.* **2016**, *179*, 574–583. [CrossRef]

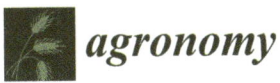

Article

Cover Crop Selection by Jointly Optimizing Biomass Productivity, Biological Nitrogen Fixation, and Transpiration Efficiency: Application to Two *Crotalaria* Species

Verónica Berriel [1,*], Jorge Monza [2] and Carlos H. Perdomo [3]

1. Centre for Applications of Nuclear Technology in Sustainable Agriculture (CATNAS), Soil and Water, Department, Agronomy College, University of the Republic, Av. Garzón 809, Montevideo CP 12.900, Uruguay
2. Plant Biology Department, Agronomy College, University of the Republic, Av. Garzón 780, Montevideo CP 12.900, Uruguay; jmonza@fagro.edu.uy
3. Soil and Water Department, Agronomy College, University of the Republic, Av. Garzón 780, Montevideo CP 12.900, Uruguay; chperdom@fagro.edu.uy
* Correspondence: vberriel@gmail.com or vberriel@fagro.edu.uy

Received: 24 May 2020; Accepted: 24 July 2020; Published: 1 August 2020

Abstract: *Crotalaria spectabilis* and *Crotalaria juncea* are cover crops (CC) that are used in many different regions. Among the main attributes of these species are their high potential for biomass production and biological fixation of nitrogen (BNF). Attempting to maximize these attributes, while minimizing water consumption through high transpiration efficiency (TE), is a challenge in the design of sustainable agricultural rotations. In this study, the relationship between biomass productivity, BNF, and TE in *C. spectabilis* and *C. juncea* was evaluated. For this purpose, an experiment was carried out under controlled conditions without water limitations and using non-inoculated soil. BNF was determined by the natural abundance of ^{15}N, while TE was estimated by several different methods, such as gravimetric or isotopic method (^{13}C). *C. juncea* produced 42% less dry matter, fixed 28% less nitrogen from the air, and had 20% less TE than *C. spectabilis*. TE results in both species were consistent across methodologies. Under simulated environmental conditions of high temperature and non-limiting soil water content, *C. spectabilis* was a relatively more promising species than *C. juncea* to be used as CC.

Keywords: *Crotalaria spectabilis*; *C. juncea*; ^{15}N natural abundance; ^{13}C isotopic composition; transpiration efficiency

---

1. Introduction

The use of legumes as cover crops (CC) in agricultural rotations makes it possible to reduce the production costs associated with a lower use of nitrogenous fertilizers, which also results in environmental benefits [1,2]. CCs are also used to reduce soil erosion caused by high precipitation, minimize surface runoff, and provide channels to the subsurface layers of the soil, allowing an increased infiltration rate [3,4].

The use of the genus *Crotalaria*, in particular *C. juncea* and *C. spectabilis*, as CCs has been recommended for warm and temperate regions [5]. Some of the main attributes of these species are their rapid and high productivity of biomass (8 Mg ha^{-1}) [6–8] and their high content of foliar nitrogen, obtained by biological nitrogen fixation (BNF) at an average of 150 kg N ha^{-1} [9–11]. In addition, a characteristic of these species is that they have the ability to establish a promiscuous and functional symbiosis with the native rhizobia of the soil [12]. The biomass production of CCs, including *C. juncea* and *C. spectabilis*, is positively correlated with the recycling of nutrients, the entry of carbon (C) into the soil [13–15], and a decrease in the rate of erosion [3]. Furthermore, high concentrations of foliar N derived from BNF determine a low C/N ratio, which favors the rapid decomposition of plant remains [16,17]. The ease of degradation of this material also facilitates net N mineralization, which can be used by subsequent crops [18].

For these reasons, in a sustainable production system, it is necessary that plant species used as CCs, if they are legumes, have a high BNF and also high biophysical gain rates (biomass productivity) in relation to the consumed or transpired water [19,20]; in other words, a high water use efficiency (WUE) or transpiration efficiency (TE). A low TE and excessive water consumption can not only waste soil water reserves, but can also induce a water deficit in the subsequent cash crop and reduce its yield [21]. For the genus of *Crotalaria*, there is little information about TE, so it was interesting to evaluate this attribute and its relationship with others that have been more studied, such as biomass production and BNF [6–8,10].

However, as there are different methodological approaches to assess TE, we needed to find a simple but robust indicator for these species. The reference technique consists of computing the ratio between total biomass productivity and transpired water during the whole crop cycle [20,22], providing an integrated value of TE for the entire plant growing period. Two other methods provide only a one-time "snapshot" of TE. The instantaneous foliar WUE is the ratio of the photosynthetic rate (A) to the transpiration rate (E), while the intrinsic foliar WUE is the proportion of A to stomatal conductance (g) [23,24]. In contrast, the ^{13}C isotopic composition (δ^{13}C) of plants with C3 photosynthetic metabolism has also been used to estimate the TE of plants in a time-integrated manner [25,26]. Through models, it is possible estimate from δ^{13}C the intrinsic WUE (iWUE) [25,27,28].

In a previous work, we compared the biomass productivity and the WUE of these two *Crotalaria* species, but under conditions of a moderate deficit of water in the soil. We found *C. spectabilis* showed superior behavior [29]. In this work, under controlled conditions and non-limited water, our objective was to relate the productivity of the biomass, BNF, and TE in these species. In addition, another secondary objective was to study the consistency between the methodologies that estimate TE, to understand its robustness and precision.

2. Materials and Methods

2.1. Plant Materials and Growing Conditions

Crotalaria juncea, *Crotalaria spectabilis* (obtained from Brseeds Sementes Co., Araçatuba, Brazil), and corns the seeds were planted in plastic pots containing 4 kg Argiudol soil from the south of Uruguay (latitude—34.6 S and longitude—55.6 W). Soil characteristics: soil organic carbon = 11.6 g kg^{-1} soil; organic matter = 20.0 g kg^{-1} soil; sand = 245 g kg^{-1} soil; silt = 487 g kg^{-1} soil; clay = 268 g kg^{-1} soil). The plants were not inoculated and noduled with the rhizobia in the soil. Ten days after the initial emergence of seedlings, the plants were thinned to one per pot, and perlite was placed on the soil surface to minimize water evaporation. The pots were kept in a growth chamber at 30 ± 3 °C, with variable relative humidity between 30% and 50%, and a light intensity of 1200 µmol m^{-2} s^{-1} with a 16/8 h cycle (light/dark). The growth chamber was continuously monitored by a computer system.

Soil moisture was kept constant at 100% (*w/w*) at container capacity for 75 days. The amount of water needed to achieve soil water capacity was estimated daily as the difference between the target gravimetric content and the actual water content in the soil. The sum of these daily differences was the evapotranspiration (ET) accumulated during the plant growing cycle. Transpiration (T) was determined as the accumulated loss of water from pots with plants, minus the average value determined in pots without plants and with perlite on the surface.

2.2. Biomass Productivity and Characteristics of Nodules

Seventy five days after starting the experiment (before flowering), the aerial parts of the plants (leaves, stems, and leaves + stems = shoots) were harvested and dried at 60 °C until they reached a constant weight, and then the dry mass of each plant was weighed. The roots were washed and the nodules were considered, according to their size, as larger or smaller nodules, the latter being about half the size of the large ones.

2.3. Determination of Transpiration Efficiency

Gravimetric method

The TE was calculated based on Equation (1) as the quotient between the biomass produced by the aerial part (shoot) and the accumulated plant transpiration throughout the experiment:

$$TE = \frac{shoot\ dry\ mass}{T}. \tag{1}$$

2.4. Gas Exchange Measurements

Intercellular CO_2 concentration, A, g, and E were determined using the youngest fully expanded leaf of all plants 70 days after sowing. These determinations were made using a portable photosynthesis system (LI-6400, LI-COR Inc., Lincoln, NE, USA); the photosynthetically active radiation was set to 1200 µmol m^{-2} s^{-2}, and the leaf temperature at 25 °C. The CO_2 concentration of the chamber was adjusted to 400 µL L^{-1}.

2.5. Determination of Nitrogen Concentration and Stable Isotopic Composition of Plant Parts

Samples from different plant parts (leaves, stems, and leaves + stems = shoots) were first ground with a fixed and mobile knife mill (Marconi MA-580) until a particle size of less than 2 mm was achieved, and then with a rotary mill (SampleTek 200 vial Rotator). Determination of N-total concentration and natural abundance of ^{13}C and ^{15}N was determined on a Flash EA 1112 elemental analyzer coupled to a Thermo Finnigan DELTAplus mass spectrometer (Bremen, Germany). Isotopic relationships were expressed in delta notation (δ) in parts per thousand (‰), using the following equation [30]:

$$\delta^{13}C\ or\ \delta^{15}N = \left(\frac{R_{sample}}{R_{standard}} - 1\right) \times 1000. \tag{2}$$

Carbon ^{13}C isotope discrimination ($\Delta^{13}C$) was calculated according to Farquhar et al. [25], where $\delta^{13}C_{atmosphere}$ is the $\delta^{13}C$ value of air (−8‰) and $\delta^{13}C_{plant}$ is the $\delta^{13}C$ value of the plant sample:

$$\Delta^{13}C = \left(\frac{\delta^{13}C_{atmosphere} - \delta^{13}C_{plant}}{1 + \frac{\delta^{13}C_{atmosphere}}{1000}} - 1\right) \times 1000. \tag{3}$$

The ratios between the intercellular (in the plant) and air CO_2 concentration and the intrinsic WUE (iWUE) were determined from the following equations [25]:

$$iWUE = \frac{Ci}{Ca} = \frac{\Delta^{13}C_{plant} - 4.4}{22.6} [4]. \tag{4}$$

Biological nitrogen fixation was estimated with Equation [6], according to Unkovich et al. [25]:

$$BNF = \left(\frac{\delta^{15}N_{ref} - \delta^{15}N_{fix}}{\delta^{15}N_{ref} - B}\right) \times 100, \tag{5}$$

where:

BNF is the percentage of N in the plant, derived from BNF.
δ^{15}Nref is the δ^{15}N value of the non-fixing reference plant.
δ^{15}Nfix is the δ^{15}N value of the fixing plant.
B is the δ^{15}N value of a fixing plant growing in N-free growth medium.

Corn was the non-fixing reference plant used, with an δ^{15}N isotopic composition of −8‰ (average value of 12 plants), while in *C. juncea* and *C. spectabilis*, the reported B values of −2.25‰ [31] and −1.0‰ [32] were respectively assumed.

2.6. Experimental Setup

A completely randomized design was used; the pot was the experimental unit and the species was considered the treatment. The experiment was repeated in the same plant growth chamber in two time periods (with the same set of environmental parameters and the same duration in time), that were named batch 1 and batch 2. Nine pots of each *Crotalaria* species were used in each batch. Close to the *C. spectabilis* and *C. juncea* pots, six pots with corn plants and eight with soil but without plants were randomly placed. Between the two batches, 17 plants of *C. spectabilis* and 14 of *C. juncea* plants culminated the experiment. The scheme of the experiment is shown in Figure 1.

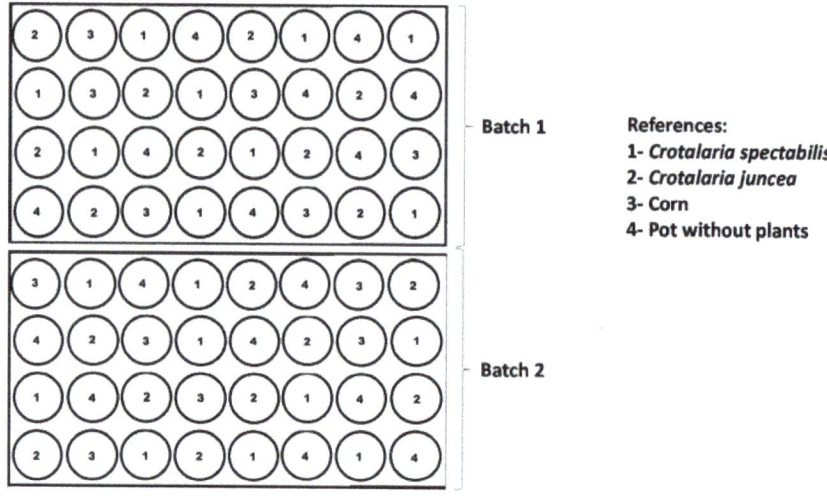

Figure 1. Design of the experiment. Circles represent the pots in the plant growth chamber.

2.7. Statistical Analysis

In order to test if there was a difference in five variables (foliar concentration of N, T, TE, A, and E) in each *Crotalaria* species between the two batches, we carried out a Shapiro–Wilks test to evaluate normality, an F-test and a Student's t-test. According to the results obtained, the F-test showed that the variances could be considered as equal because the p-value was superior to 0.05. In the Student's t-test, the null hypothesis (the differences between means is equal to 0) could not be rejected in any of the species at a significance level of 0.05. Within a specie, no statistically significant difference at $\alpha = 0.05$ was found between batches for any of the evaluated parameters. For this reason, the data for the two batches were pooled for each species.

In the pooled data, also the normality was evaluated with the Shapiro–Wilks test, while the assumption of equality of variances was evaluated with Levene's test. After, the species effect was analyzed by ANOVA in those variables with a normal distribution (N, T, TE, A, E, and A/E), and by the Kruskal Wallis test for variables without a normal distribution (shoot dry mass, g, A/g, δ^{15}N, BNF, δ^{13}C, and iWUE). Pearson correlation analyses were also performed. The statistical packages InfoStat [33] and XLSTAT [34] were used in the statistical analyses.

3. Results and Discussion

3.1. Biomass and Nitrogen Productivity from Fixation

In simulated environmental conditions, with a high temperature and non-limited soil water availability, the two species differed both in terms of biomass productivity (Tables 1 and 2) and foliar N concentration (Tables 1 and 3). *C. spectabilis* was the species that produced the highest biomass and had the higher leaf N concentration (Table 1). All *C. spectabilis* plants and 57% of *C. juncea* presented large pink nodules. The remaining 43% of the *C. juncea* plants also had pink nodules, but these were small. The same trend with respect to nodulation was observed between the two analyzed batches of *C. juncea* plants, most of them presented larger and a minority smaller nodules.

Due the species of the genus *Crotalaria* sp. showing promiscuous behavior and establishing more or less efficient symbiosis with rhizobia from the soil, the plants were not inoculated. Therefore, in this experiment, the symbiotic efficiency of the rhizobia strains present in the soil was evaluated. The difference in the size of *C. juncea* nodules may be a consequence of its nodulation by less efficient and competitive strains, as has been observed in white clover [35].

When were compared the biomass productivity and leaf N concentration in the two *C. juncea* groups (with larger and smaller nodules), a statistically significant difference in favor of the group with larger nodules was found (Tables 1 and 3). Furthermore, shoot dry matter and foliar N concentration were correlated positively with each other (shoot dry mass = 2.4415 × [N] + 0.0286, R^2 = 0.3783, p = 0.0004). This finding is in agreement with the findings of Adams et al. [36], which stated that an increase in foliar N concentration favors photosynthetic capacity [37].

The ^{15}N isotopic composition of the leaves (δ^{15}N) significantly varied between the two species; while the δ^{15}N mean in *C. spectabilis* was negative, in *C. juncea* it was positive (Table 1). Contrarily, when only the *C. juncea* group with large nodules was included in this comparison, no significant difference was found (Table 2). In turn, the mean values of δ^{15}N in the *C. juncea* groups with larger and smaller nodules were different, being negative in the first group and positive in the second (Table 1), although they were always less than the δ^{15}N values of the reference plant. Negative values of δ^{15}N would indicate that the main N source was atmospheric N_2 acquired by BNF, while positive values seem to point to the soil as the main N source.

The BNF proportion, estimated form the average δ^{15}N values of whole plants, was higher in *C. spectabilis* than in *C. juncea* (Table 1). On the contrary, there was no difference in BNF between these two species when only the *C. juncea* plants with large nodules were compared with *C. spectabilis* plants (Table 2). Within the *C. juncea* plants, the BNF values were close to 85% in the group with larger nodules, but decreased to 45% in the group with smaller nodules (Table 1). In *C. spectabilis*, on the other hand, all individuals had BNF values equal to or greater than 90% (Table 1). In any case, the BNF proportion was high for both species, which is in agreement with reports from Brazilian authors [11,38]. Overall, this result suggests that *C. spectabilis* maintained high BNF values in the simulated environment, while *C. juncea* showed high variability among plants. This result contrasts, however, with that of another Uruguayan field study, in which these species, despite having been inoculated, failed to nodulate [17].

Table 1. Mean values of total dry matter (Total DM), transpired water mass (T), foliar N concentration (N_{leaf}), net photosynthesis (A), leaf stomatal conductance (g), instantaneous transpiration rate (E), ^{13}C isotopic composition ($\delta^{13}C$), ^{15}N isotopic composition ($\delta^{15}N$), transpiration efficiency (TE), foliar intrinsic water efficiency (A/g), foliar instantaneous water efficiency (A/E), intrinsic water efficiency of the whole plant (iWUE), and proportion of biological N fixation (BNF) in *Crotalaria spectabilis* and *C. juncea*, evaluated according to a visual criterion in plants with large (+) and small (−) nodules.

Species	Nodules	Shoot DM g	T kg	N_{leaf} gN/100gDM	A μmol/m² s	g mol/m² s	E mmol/m² s	$\delta^{13}C$ ‰	$\delta^{15}N$ ‰
C. spectabilis	+	6.29 ± 1.16	2.11 ± 0.56	2.26 ± 0.43	6.78 ± 2.15	0.11 ± 0.06	1.70 ± 0.80	−27.75 ± 0.56	−0.45 ± 0.72
C. juncea	+/−	3.60 ± 2.61	1.48 ± 0.76	1.85 ± 0.70	5.09 ± 3.72	0.15 ± 0.09	2.21 ± 1.14	−29.46 ± 0.78	1.13 ± 2.27
	+	5.05 ± 2.72	1.87 ± 0.81	2.23 ± 0.70	7.06 ± 3.96	0.19 ± 0.10	2.72 ± 1.15	−29.23 ± 0.90	−0.74 ± 0.95
	−	1.91 ± 1.05	1.03 ± 0.39	1.40 ± 0.37	2.80 ± 1.63	0.10 ± 0.07	1.61 ± 0.87	−29.74 ± 0.55	3.30 ± 0.87

Species	Nodules	Water-Use Efficiency				N fixation
		TE g/kg	A/g μmol/mol	A/E mmol/mol	iWUE μmol/mol	BNF %
C. spectabilis	+	3.10 ± 0.58	68.95 ± 17.86	4.25 ± 0.93	74.06 ± 6.57	92.65 ± 7.50
C. juncea	+/−	2.21 ± 0.68	33.44 ± 13.01	2.17 ± 0.89	54.15 ± 8.91	67.08 ± 22.90
	+	2.54 ± 0.74	35.22 ± 7.59	2.43 ± 0.70	57.00 ± 10.30	85.30 ± 9.27
	−	1.81 ± 0.34	31.37 ± 18.09	1.87 ± 1.06	50.83 ± 6.24	45.82 ± 8.50

Table 2. Statistical results of the Kruskal–Wallis analysis for total dry matter (Total DM), isotopic composition of ^{15}N (δ^{15}N), proportion BNF (BNF), leaf stomatal conductance (g), intrinsic leaf water-use efficiency (A/g), isotopic composition of ^{13}C (δ^{13}C), and intrinsic plant water-use efficiency (iWUE) in *Crotalaria spectabilis* and *C. juncea*, evaluated in plants with large (+) and small nodules (−).

	Nodules	Shoot DM	δ^{15}N	BNF	g	A/g	δ^{13}C	iWUE
					p			
Model		0.0026	<0.0001	<0.0001	NS	0.0003	0.0001	0.0001
Species		Ranks mean and Groups						
C. juncea	−	4.8A	26.50A	3.50A	-	6.67A	5.83A	5.83A
C. juncea	+	14.9B	10.14B	17.4B	-	9.00A	9.29A	9.29A
C. spectabilis	+	18.9B	12.81B	19.2B	-	20.75B	20.94B	20.94B

Means with a common letter are not significantly different (*p* > 0.05), NS: not significant.

Table 3. Statistical results of an ANOVA for foliar N concentration (N$_{leaf}$), transpired water (T), transpiration efficiency (TE), net photosynthesis rate (A), instantaneous transpiration rate (E), and instantaneous water-use efficiency (A/E) in *Crotalaria spectabilis* and *C. juncea*, evaluated in plants with large (+) and small nodules (−).

	N$_{leaf}$	T	TE	A	E	A/E
Model			*p*			
Species	0.0352	0.0099	0.0004	NS	NS	<0.0001
Species > Fix	0.0061	0.0173	0.0339	0.0067	0.0363	NS
Contrasts			*p*			
C. juncea vs. C. spectabilis	0.0245	0.0071	0.0003	0.0687	NS	<0.0001
C. juncea (+) vs. C. juncea (−)	0.0061	0.0173	0.0339	0.0067	0.0363	NS
C juncea (+) vs. C. spectabilis	NS	0.4011	0.0467	NS	0.0421	0.0002

Means with a common letter are not significantly different (*p* > 0.05), NS: not significant.

On the other hand, the two *Crotalaria* species did not differ in terms of photosynthetic rate (Table 3), stomatal conductance (Table 2), and transpiration rate (Table 3). However, the transpiration and photosynthetic rate were significantly higher in *C. juncea* plants with large nodules and a higher BNF (Table 3). Moreover, the transpiration rate (E) in the *C. juncea* group with higher nodulation was significantly higher than in *C. spectabilis* (Table 3).

The mass of transpired water (T) during the plant growing cycle was higher in *C. spectabilis* than in *C. juncea* (Tables 1 and 3), and besides, T was positively correlated with the aerial biomass (Figure 2). This result was consistent with what was reported for these two same species when they grew under controlled conditions but went through a period of moderate water deficit [29]. Contrarily, no significant T difference was found when *C. spectabilis* plants were compared with *C. juncea* with larger nodules (Table 3). The T mean, however, was significantly higher in the *C. juncea* group with larger nodules and a higher BNF.

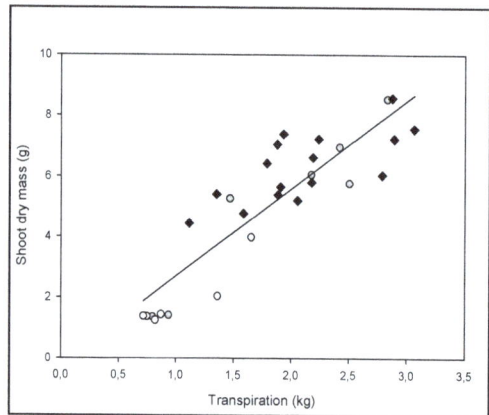

Figure 2. Relationship between shoot dry mass and water transpiration expressed for *Crotalaria spectabilis* (rhombuses) and *Crotalaria juncea* (circles). *C. juncea* was evaluated at two nodulation levels. Plants with large nodules are identified with gray circles, and those with small nodules with white circles. Regression lines: $y = 2.893x - 0.2$. $R^2 = 0.7896$ ($p < 0.0001$).

The water footprint, which corresponds to the amount of water used to generate 1 kg of dry matter, was on average 515 and 342 L water/Kg dry matter for *C. juncea* and *C. spectabilis*, respectively. Therefore, *C. juncea* was less efficient in the use of water resources than *C. spectabilis*. If the water supply of these crops in the field were only rainwater, the water footprint of both species could be classified as green [39].

The isotopic composition of ^{13}C, evaluated as $\delta^{13}C$, was different between species and lower in *C. juncea* (Tables 1 and 2), which was due to the greater isotopic fractionation of $^{13}CO_2$ in this species [40]. As comparisons between species were made in the same environment and developmental circumstances, the $\delta^{13}C$ values are related to genetic differences [41]. In addition, the ^{13}C isotopic composition within *C. juncea* plants was not related to BNF, because there were no differences between the groups with the largest and smallest nodules; that is, plants that fixed more and less N (Table 2).

3.2. Transpiration Efficiency and Water Use Efficiency

In both species, the mean values of the different WUE indicators evaluated in this work (TE, A/E, A/g, iWUE) were consistent, and showed that *C. spectabilis* was more efficient than *C. juncea* in the use of water resources (Table 1). Interestingly, the mean TE of *C. spectabilis* was higher than that of *C. juncea*, (Table 1), regardless of the size of the nodules and the BNF values of the latter species (Table 3). Regarding A/E, A/g, and iWUE, significant differences were observed between the species, but not between *C. juncea* plants with different nodule sizes (Table 2).

When both species were grouped, positive correlations between iWUE and the other instantaneous WUE indicators, such as A/g, were found (Figure 3; Table 4). This outcome agrees which the findings of Johnson et al. [42] and Read et al. [43]; they found negative correlations between A/g and $\Delta^{13}C$ in different *Agropyron desertorum* clones, observed both under conditions without hydric limitation and under drought conditions. Overall, these results highlight the robustness of the isotopic methodology for the study of these parameters.

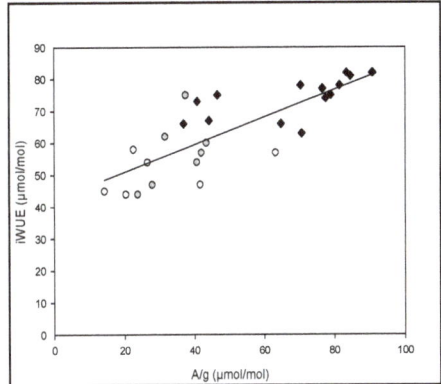

Figure 3. Relationship between the integrated intrinsic water use efficiency (iWUE) and foliar water use efficiency [quotient: photosynthesis (A) and stomatal conductance (g)] for *Crotalaria spectabilis* (rhombuses) and *Crotalaria juncea* (circles). *C. juncea* was evaluated at two nodulation levels. Plants with large nodules are identified with gray circles, and those with small nodules with white circles. Regression lines in a): $y = 0.43x + 42.2$. $R^2 = 0.66$ ($p < 0.0001$).

Table 4. Pearson's correlation matrix of transpiration efficiency (TE) in *C. spectabilis* and *C. juncea*, efficiency in the use of leaf intrinsic water (A/g), isotope composition of ^{15}N (δ^{15}N), proportion of biological fixation of N (BNF), foliar N concentration (N), and efficiency in the use of intrinsic water from the entire plant (iWUE).

Variable	TE	A/g	δ^{15}N	BNF	N	iWUE
TE	1					
A/g	0.49 **	1				
δ^{15}N	−0.56 **	−0.36 NS	1			
BNF	0.62 ***	0.34 NS	−0.99 ***	1		
N	0.44 *	0.37 *	−0.52 **	0.54 ***	1	
iWUE	0.54 **	0.81 ***	−0.58 **	0.58 ***	0.40 *	1

*** Significant at the 0.001 level (2-tailed), ** Significant at the 0.01 level (2-tailed), * Significant at the 0.05 level (2-tailed), NS: non-significant.

A positive correlation was also established between BNF and iWUE (Table 4), as also reported by Kumarasinghe et al. [44]. These authors found a negative correlation between BNF and ^{13}C isotopic discrimination in different *Glycine max* cultivars subjected to saline stress conditions. However, Knight et al. [45], working in greenhouse conditions, reported a positive correlation between both variables. They attributed this result to the ^{13}C depletion that occurred at the leaf level, which was caused by isotopic fractionation mechanisms within N-fixing plants.

The foliar N concentration was also positively correlated with TE and iWUE (Table 4). Results obtained by Evans et al. [36] through metadata analysis of multiple plant species suggested that low Δ^{13}C values (or high δ^{13}C values) in fixing plants with high N contents were a consequence of relatively high A/g ratios.

The results indicate that *C. spectabilis* is more promising than *C. juncea* for use as a CC in this evaluation under controlled conditions. Although the results in these conditions may not be fully extrapolated to field conditions, it is important to highlight that the plants were able to nodulate with rhizobia present in soil with no history of these CCs. This is auspicious for regions where there is no commercial availability of specific rhizobia for *Crotalaria*. Similarly, the plants were harvested in the same phenological state as that used in the field to finish the CC, so it is expected that the same trends will be maintained regarding the evaluated attributes. In any case, although this first approach is necessary, field evaluation must also be carried out with the use of the same isotopic technique used in this work to determine TE, given its consistency with other forms of evaluation of this attribute and being that its main advantages are the simplicity of sampling and the precision of the results.

4. Conclusions

This study shows that under simulated conditions of high temperature and non-limiting soil water content C. spectabilis has advantages for use as a CC over C. juncea in terms of biomass production, BNF, and transpiration efficiency. Furthermore, these results suggest that the ^{13}C isotopic technique is a robust indicator to differentiate TE between these species. In C. juncea, the ^{13}C isotope indicator was not useful to distinguish between plants with low and high TE. In contrast, the ^{15}N isotope was useful to detect differences in TE between plants. Finally, although these results are valid only for these two species, this methodology of selecting legumes based on multiple objectives could also be applied to other species or cultivars—not only those destined to be used as CCs, but also cash crops.

Author Contributions: Conceptualization, V.B. and C.H.P.; methodology, V.B.; formal analysis, V.B and C.H.P.; investigation, V.B and C.H.P.; resources, V.B.; data curation, V.B and C.H.P.; writing—original draft preparation, V.B, J.M. and C.H.P.; writing—review and editing, V.B, J.M. and C.H.P.; visualization, V.B. and C.H.P.; supervision, J.M. and C.H.P.; project administration, V.B.; funding acquisition, V.B. All authors have read and agreed to the published version of the manuscript.

Funding: This research was funded by National Research and Innovation Agency of Uruguay, Funds: María Viñas, grant number FMV_125492; University of Republic of Uruguay Funds: Fellowship CAP grants; and Faculty of Science, Funds: Fellowship Biotechnology Postgraduate. The APC was funded by the National Research and Innovation Agency of Uruguay.

Acknowledgments: The authors give thanks to J. Berriel and G. Galindo for the experimental work in growth plant chamber, G. Quero for photosynthesis measurements, and S. Álvarez for the graphical design.

Conflicts of Interest: The authors declare no conflict of interest.

References

1. Cherr, C.M.; Scholberg, J.M.S.; McSorley, R. Green manure approaches to crop production: A synthesis. *Agron. J.* **2006**, *98*, 302–319. [CrossRef]
2. Martins, F.; Hungria, M.; de Carvalho, L.; Bueno, F.; Souza, D. *Fixação biológica de nitrogeno em adubos verdes In Adubação Verde e Plantas de Cobertura no Brasil: Fundamentos e Práticas*; Lima Filho, O.F., Ambrosano, E.J., Rossi, F., Carlos, J.A.D., Eds.; Embrapa. Brasília—DF: Brasilia, Brazil, 2014; pp. 309–334.
3. Folorunso, O.A.; Rolston, D.E.; Lovi, D.T. Soil surface strength and infiltration rate as affected by winter cover crops. *Soil Technol.* **1992**, *5*, 189–197. [CrossRef]
4. Pacheco, J.S.; Silva-López, R.E.S. Genus Crotalaria L. (*Leguminoseae*). *Rev. Fitos* **2010**, *5*, 43–52.
5. Meena, R.S.; Lal, R. Legumes and Sustainable Use of Soils. In *Legumes for Soil Health and Sustainable Management*; Meena, R., Das, A., Yadav, G., Lal, R., Eds.; Springer: Singapore, 2018; pp. 1–31.
6. Soratto, R.P.; Crusciol, C.A.C.; Costa, C.H.M.; Ferrani Neto, J.; Castrp, G.S.A. Produção, decomposição e ciclagem de nutrientes em resíduos de crotalária e milheto, cultivados solteiros e consorciados. *Pesqui. Agropecu. Bras.* **2012**, *47*, 1462–1470. [CrossRef]
7. Menezes, L.A.S.; Leandro, W.M.; de Oliveira Junior, J.P.; Ferreira, A.C.B.; das Santana, J.G.; Barros, R.G. Produção de fitomassa de diferentes espécies, isoladas e consorciadas, com potencial de utilização para cobertura do solo. *Biosci. J.* **2009**, *25*, 7–12.
8. Perin, A.; Santos, R.H.S.; Urquiaga, S.C.; Guerra, J.G.M.; Cecon, P.R. Produção de fitomassa, acúmulo de nutrientes e fixação biológica de nitrogênio por adubos verdes em cultivo isolado e consorciado. *Pesqui. Agropecu. Bras.* **2004**, *39*, 35–40. [CrossRef]
9. Balkcom, K.S.; Reeves, D.W. Sunn-hemp utilized as a legume cover crop for corn production. *Agron. J.* **2005**, *97*, 26–31. [CrossRef]
10. Wutke, E.B.; Calegari, A.; Wildner, L.P. Espécies de adubos verdes e plantas de cobertura e recomendações para seu uso. In *Adubação Verde e Plantas de Cobertura no Brasil: Fundamentos e Práticas*; Lima Filho, O.F., Ambrosano, E.J., Rossi, F., Carlos, J.A.D., Eds.; Embrapa, Brasília—DF: Brasilia, Brazil, 2014; pp. 59–167.

11. Mendonça, E.; Lima, P.C.; Guimarães, G.P.; Moura, W.; Andrade, F.V. Biological Nitrogen Fixation by Legumes and N Uptake by Coffee Plants. *Rev. Bras. Ciênc. Solo Viçosa* **2017**, *41*, e0160178. [CrossRef]
12. Lombardi, M.L.; Moreira, M.; Ambrosio, L.A.; Cardoso, E.J. Occurence and host specificity of indigenous rhizobia from soils of São Paulo State, Brazil. *Sci. Agric.* **2009**, *66*, 543–548. [CrossRef]
13. Crusciol, C.A.C.; Arf, O.; Soratto, R.P.; Andreotti, M.; Rodrigues, R.A.F. Absorção, exportação e eficiência de utilização de nutrientes pela cultura do arroz de terras altas em função de lâminas de agua aplicadas por aspersão. *Acta Sci. Agron.* **2003**, *25*, 97–102. [CrossRef]
14. Li, D.; Niu, S.; Luo, Y. Global patterns of the dynamics of soil carbon and nitrogen stocks following afforestation: A meta-analysis. *New Phytol.* **2012**, *195*, 172–181. [CrossRef] [PubMed]
15. Poeplau, C.; Don, A. Carbon sequestration in agricultural soils via cultivation of cover crops—A meta-analysis. *Agric. Ecosyst. Environ.* **2015**, *200*, 33–41. [CrossRef]
16. de Alves, F.J.S.; Miranda, J.P.H.V.; Moura, D.A.; Reis, B.R.; Soares, J.P.G.; Fernandes, F.D.; Ramos, A.K.B.; Malaquias, J.V. Produção de biomassa e valor nutricional do Cajanus Cajan cv. Mandarin sob manejo orgânico e convencional. In Proceedings of the XXIV Congresso Brasileiro de Zootecnia, Vitória, Brazil, 12–14 May 2014.
17. Macedo, I.; Otaño, C.; Barrios, E.; Beyhaut, E.; Rossi, C.; Sawchick, J.; Terra, J.A. Leguminosas anuales de verano como opciones de cobertura en sistemas agrícolas. *Rev. INIA Urug.* **2015**, *43*, 50–54.
18. Matos, E.S.; Mendoca, E.S.; Lima, P.C.; Coelho, M.S.; Mateus, R.F.; Cardoso, I.M. Green manure in coffee systems in the region of Zona da Mata, Minas Gerais: Characteristics and kinetics of carbon and nitrogen mineralization. *Rev. Bras. Cienc. Solo* **2008**, *32*, 2027–2035. [CrossRef]
19. Fishman, R.; Devineni, N.; Raman, S. Can improved agricultural water use efficiency save India's groundwater? *Environ. Res. Lett.* **2015**, *10*, 084022. [CrossRef]
20. Ren, C.F.; Guo, P.; Yang, G.Q.; Li, R.H.; Liu, L. Spatial and temporal analyses of water resources use efficiency based on data envelope analysis and malmquist index: Case study in Gansu Province, China. *J. Water Resour. Plan. Manag.* **2016**, *142*, 04016066. [CrossRef]
21. Wunsch, E.M.; Bell, L.W.; Bell, M.J. Can legumes provide greater benefits than millet as a spring cover crop in southern Queensland farming systems? *Crop Pasture Sci.* **2017**, *68*, 746. [CrossRef]
22. Gregory, P.J. Concepts of water use efficiency. In *Soil and Crop Management for Improved Water Use Efficiency in Rainfed Areas*; Harris, H.C., Cooper, P.J.M., Pala, M., Eds.; Proceedings of International Workshop; ICARDA: Ankara, Turkey; Aleppo, Syria, 1991; pp. 9–20.
23. Franks, P.J.; Doheny-Adams, T.W.; Britton-Harper, Z.J.; Gray, J.E. Increasing water-use efficiency directly through genetic manipulation of stomatal density. *New Phytol.* **2015**, *207*, 188–195. [CrossRef]
24. Bhattacharya, A. Water-use efficiency under changing climatic conditions. In *Changing Climate and Resource Use Efficiency in Plants*; Bhattacharya, A., Ed.; Academic Press: Cambridge, MA, USA, 2019; pp. 111–180.
25. Farquhar, G.D.; Ehleringer, J.R.; Hubick, K.T. Carbon isotope discrimination and photosynthesis. *Annu. Rev. Plant Physiol. Plant Mol. Biol.* **1989**, *40*, 503–537. [CrossRef]
26. Pronger, J.; Campbell, D.I.; Clearwater, M.J.; Mudge, P.L.; Rutledge, S.; Wall, A.M.; Schipper, L.A. Toward optimisation of water use efficiency in dryland pastures using carbon isotope discrimination as a tool to select plant species mixtures. *Sci. Total Environ.* **2019**, *665*, 698–708. [CrossRef]
27. Farquhar, G.D.; Richards, R.A. Isotopic composition of plant carbon correlates with water-use efficiency of wheat genotypes. *Aust. J. Plant Physiol.* **1984**, *11*, 539–552. [CrossRef]
28. Condon, A.G.; Richards, R.A.; Rebetzke, G.J.; Farquhar, G.D. Improving intrinsic water-use efficiency and crop yield. *Crop Sci.* **2002**, *42*, 122–131. [PubMed]
29. Berriel, V.; Perdomo, C.; Monza, J. Carbon Isotope Discrimination and Water-Use Efficiency in Crotalaria Cover Crops under Moderate Water Deficit. *J. Soil Sci. Plant Nutr.* **2020**, *20*, 537–545. [CrossRef]
30. Sulzman, E.W. Stable isotope chemistry and measurement: A primer. In *Stable Isotopes in Ecology and Environmental Science*, 2nd ed.; Michener, R., Lajtha, K., Eds.; Blackwell Publishing: Boston, NJ, USA, 2007; pp. 1–21.
31. Unkovich, M.; Herridge, D.; Peoples, M.; Boddey, R.; Cadisch, G.; Giller, K.; Alves, B.; Chalk, P. *Measuring Plant-Associated Nitrogen Fixation in Agricultural Systems*; Australian Center of International Agricultural Research (ACIAR): Canberra, Australia, 2008; p. 258.
32. Okito, A.; Alves, B.J.R.; Urquiaga, S.; Boddey, R.M. Isotopic fractionation during N_2 fixation by four tropical legumes. *Soil Biol. Biochem.* **2004**, *36*, 1179–1190. [CrossRef]

33. Di Rienzo, J.A.; Casanoves, F.; Balzarini, M.G.; Gonzalez, L.; Tablada, M.; Robledo, C.W. *InfoStat Version 2011*; Grupo InfoStat, FCA, Universidad Nacional de Córdoba: Córdoba, Argentina, 2018.
34. Addinsoft. *XLSTAT*; Statistical Software: Paris, France, 2020.
35. Irisarri, P.; Cardozo, G.; Tartaglia, C.; Reyno, R.; Gutiérrez, P.; Lattanzi, F.A.; Rebuffo, M.; Monza, J. Selection of Competitive and Efficient Rhizobia Strains for White Clover. *Front. Microbiol.* **2019**, *10*, 768. [CrossRef] [PubMed]
36. Adams, M.A.; Buchmann, N.; Sprent, J.; Buckley, T.N.; Turnbull, T.L. Crops, Nitrogen, Water: Are Legumes Friend, Foe, or Misunderstood Ally? *Trends Plant Sci.* **2018**, *23*, 539–550. [CrossRef]
37. Evans, J.R. Photosynthesis and nitrogen relationships in leaves of C_3 plants. *Oecologia* **1989**, *78*, 9–19. [CrossRef]
38. Sant'Anna, S.A.C.; Martins, M.R.; Goulart, J.M.; Araújo, S.N.; Araújo, E.S.; Zaman, M.; Jantalia, C.P.; Alves, B.J.R.; Boddey, R.M.; Urquiaga, S. Biological nitrogen fixation and soil N_2O emissions from legume residues in an Acrisol in SE Brazil. *Geoderma Reg.* **2018**, *15*, e00196. [CrossRef]
39. Veettil, A.V.; Mishra, A.K. Water security assessment using blue and green water footprint concepts. *J. Hydrol.* **2016**, *542*, 589–602. [CrossRef]
40. Sinclair, T.R. Is transpiration efficiency a viable plant trait in breeding for crop improvement? *Funct. Plant Biol.* **2012**, *39*, 359–365. [CrossRef]
41. Fu, Q.A.; Button, T.W.; Ehleringer, J.R.; Flager, R.B. Environmental and Developmental effects on carbon isotope discrimination by two species of Phaseolus. In *Stable Isotopes and Plant Carbon-Water Relations*; Ehleringer, J.R., Hall, A.E., Farquhar, G.D., Eds.; Academic Press: San Diego, CA, USA, 1993; pp. 297–310.
42. Johnson, R.C.; Basset, L.M. Carbon isotope discrimination and water use efficiency in four cool season grasses. *Crop Sci.* **1991**, *31*, 157–162. [CrossRef]
43. Read, J.J.; Johnson, D.A.; Asay, K.H.; Tieszen, L.T. Carbon isotope discrimination, gas exchange, and water use efficiency in crested wheatgrass clones. *Crop Sci.* **1991**, *31*, 1203–1208. [CrossRef]
44. Kumarasinghe, K.S.; Kirda, C.; Mohamed, A.R.A.G.; Zapata, F.; Danso, S.K.A. ^{13}C isotope discrimination correlates with biological nitrogen fixation in soybean (Glycine max (L.) Merrill). *Plant Soil* **1992**, *139*, 145–147. [CrossRef]
45. Knight, J.D.; Verhees, F.; Van Kessel, C.; Slinkard, A.E. Does carbon isotope discrimination correlate with biological nitrogen fixation? *Plant Soil* **1993**, *153*, 151–153. [CrossRef]

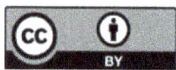

© 2020 by the authors. Licensee MDPI, Basel, Switzerland. This article is an open access article distributed under the terms and conditions of the Creative Commons Attribution (CC BY) license (http://creativecommons.org/licenses/by/4.0/).

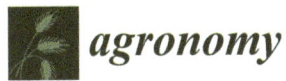

Article

Improving Productivity in Integrated Fish-Vegetable Farming Systems with Recycled Fish Pond Sediments

Chau Thi Da [1,2], Phan Anh Tu [3], John Livsey [4,*], Van Tai Tang [2], Håkan Berg [4] and Stefano Manzoni [4]

1. Environmental Engineering and Management Research Group, Ton Duc Thang University, 19 Nguyen Huu Tho Street, Tan Phong Ward, District 7, Ho Chi Minh 72915, Vietnam; chauthida@tdtu.edu.vn
2. Faculty of Environment and Labor Safety, Ton Duc Thang University, Ho Chi Minh 72915, Vietnam; tangvantai@tdtu.edu.vn
3. Department of Crop Sciences, Loc Troi Groups of Vietnam, 23 Ha Hoang Ho Street, My Xuyen Ward, Long Xuyen 90108, Vietnam; phananhtu170385@gmail.com
4. Department of Physical Geography and Bolin Center for Climate Research, Stockholm University, 10691 Stockholm, Sweden; hakan.berg@natgeo.su.se (H.B.); stefano.manzoni@natgeo.su.se (S.M.)
* Correspondence: john.livsey@natgeo.su.se

Received: 27 May 2020; Accepted: 14 July 2020; Published: 16 July 2020

Abstract: The increasing intensification of aquaculture systems requires the development of strategies to reduce their environmental impacts such as pollution caused by the discharge of nutrient rich sediments into local water bodies. Recycling of fish pond sediments (FPS) as fertilizer has been proposed as a possible solution that may also reduce the reliance on synthetic fertilizers. With a case study in the Mekong Delta, Vietnam, we determined suitable mixtures of striped catfish (*Pangasianodon hypophthalmus*) pond sediment (PPS) and locally sourced organic amendments of rice straw (RS), or common water hyacinth (WH) to fertilize cucumber plants (*Cucumis sativus* L.) in an integrated cucumber–giant gourami fish (*Osphronemus goramy*) farming system. Highest nutrient concentrations were found when mixing 30% PPS with 70% RS or WH. When used in combination with chemical fertilizer, it was found that a 25% to 75% reduction in chemical fertilizer application could be achieved, while also increasing cucumber yields, with the highest yields found when RS was used in organic amendments. In combination with the additional income from fish production, integrated farming systems such as that demonstrated in this study, may increase both farm income and production diversity.

Keywords: pond sediments; organic fertilizer; mineral fertilizer; cucumber; integrated fish-vegetable farming; Mekong Delta

---

1. Introduction

Inland aquaculture is one of the fastest growing animal production sectors in the world, and provides a promising way to improve livelihoods and provide export revenues in Asian countries [1]. Production is predicted to continue increasing, by optimizing resource use and intensifying existing aquaculture practices [2,3]. In Vietnam, more than half of inland aquaculture fish are striped (also referred to as *Pangasius*) catfish (*Pangasianodon hypophthalmus*), which are produced in freshwater earthen ponds and are exported to over 130 countries [3,4]. The total area of ponds used for striped catfish aquaculture has increased approximately 8-fold over the last 20-year period, while total production has increased 64-fold, indicating a rapid and dramatic intensification. This is particularly evident in the Mekong Delta, where striped catfish account for almost 70% of total fish production [5–7]. As an important commodity, this equates to an export value of US $2.26 billion for Vietnam [4].

Whilst this development of industrial aquaculture generates large profit and income, it also creates risks stemming from negative environmental impacts [8,9]. These impacts include landscape modification and biodiversity loss [10,11], and eutrophication [12,13] caused by the discharge of nutrient rich sediments into local water bodies. Sediments and sludge from intensive aquaculture ponds are enriched with organic matter (OM), nitrogen (N), phosphorus (P), and macro and micronutrients that have accumulated in pond sediments [13–17]. The bulk of the dissolved and suspended inorganic and organic matter contained within the aquaculture pond effluents are derived from feed inputs, either directly in the form of the end-products of feed digestion and metabolism or from uneaten/wasted feed, or indirectly through eutrophication in the ponds. Oláh et al. [14] and Boyd [18] also reported that 30%–95% of the N and a high fraction of P compounds applied to fishponds accumulated in pond sediments.

Effluent and sediments from the bed of striped catfish ponds in the Mekong Delta are removed and disposed of approximately every two months during the fish farming cycle. As fish pond sediments (FPS) and sludge are enriched with OM and nutrients, they potentially represent a continuously available fertilizer supplement and soil conditioner, which could enhance the soil environment for crop production [2,13,19]. Nowadays, there are many research examples of integrated aquaculture-agriculture farming systems that are economically and environmentally sustainable as well as practically applicable in a local context [17,20–22]. However, previous studies in Vietnam, Thailand, Bangladesh, and China have focused on reusing wastewater from striped catfish pond farming or fish pond sediments for rice, vegetable (green bean), fodder grass production, or Triticeae crops [12,13,17,23–25], whilst the recycling of sediments has mostly been neglected.

In recent years, the use of inorganic fertilizer in Vietnam has risen steadily and the country faces a large fertilizer deficit [26]. Using the nutrient rich sediments from Pangasius catfish ponds in crop production could reduce the reliance on inorganic fertilizer, and potentially decrease production costs while also reducing the negative impacts on aquaculture on the environment [13].

A lack of cost-effective technologies and inappropriate disposal for organic waste has caused environmental pollution from FPS [15,16,27–29]. Similarly, rice straw as a by-product of rice production is abundant in the Mekong Delta, but is not considered suitable for animal feed due to its low digestibility, low protein, high lignin, and high silica concentration [28,30]. Composting is an effective approach to reuse FPS and agricultural residues, thereby converting them into a relatively valuable agronomic resource for use as organic fertilizers [28,31,32]. Composting of FPS mixed with locally sourced organic residues can offer both a solution to mitigate pollution in the region and an opportunity to improve agricultural soils. To explore this potential, we combined—in different proportions—sediments from striped catfish ponds and agricultural residues such as rice straw and water hyacinth (*Eichhornia crassipes*), and assessed how these amendments affected cucumber (*Cucumis sativus* L.) vegetable growth and yield. Furthermore, we conducted the experiment in an integrated cucumber–fish production system, aiming to optimize the mutual benefits of growing fish and vegetables in such a system (Figure 1). Similar integrated fish–crop production systems have been shown to have both economic and environmental benefits greater than mono-production systems [17]. The hypothesis tested in the present study is that nutrients contained in organic fertilizers produced from Pangasius catfish pond sediment (PPS) and locally sourced organic amendments can replace the inorganic fertilizers for cucumber vegetable production.

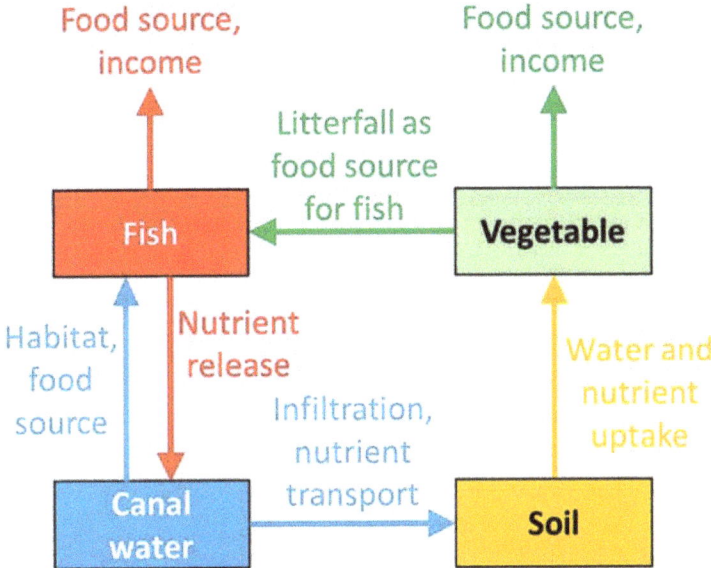

Figure 1. Potential benefits of integrated fish and cucumber production.

2. Materials and Methods

Two linked experiments were conducted. One experiment focused on organic fertilizer production. This experiment was carried out in the laboratory of An Giang University, An Giang Province, Vietnam. The second experiment focused on cucumber growth performance with different organic and chemical fertilizer combinations, using compost from the first experiment as an organic amendment. The second experiment was implemented both in the September–December 2016 wet season, and the February–June 2017 dry season. The timeline and the work flow of experiments one and two are shown in Figure 2 and described in detail in the following sections.

2.1. Site Description

The cucumber experimental plots were established in the Truong Long A commune, Chau Thanh District, Hau Giang Province, Vietnam. This site is characterized by a marked seasonality in precipitation and an average annual temperature of 27 °C. The rainy season is from May to November, accounting for 92%–97% of the annual rainfall. Annual precipitation is between 1800 and 2500 mm. The wet season during 2016 was characterized by temperatures in the range of 26.7–33.2 °C and 2304 mm of rainfall; the dry season of 2017 was slightly warmer (30.2–37.3 °C), and much drier, with 54.3 mm of rainfall [6].

2.2. Experiment One: Organic Fertilizer Production

Experiment one was designed to determine a suitable mixture of Pangasius catfish (*Pangasianodon hypophthalmus*) pond sediment (PPS) and locally sourced organic amendments, from rice straw (RS) (*Oryza sativa* L.) or common water hyacinth (WH) (*Eichhornia crassipes*), to produce organic fertilizers for cucumber cultivation.

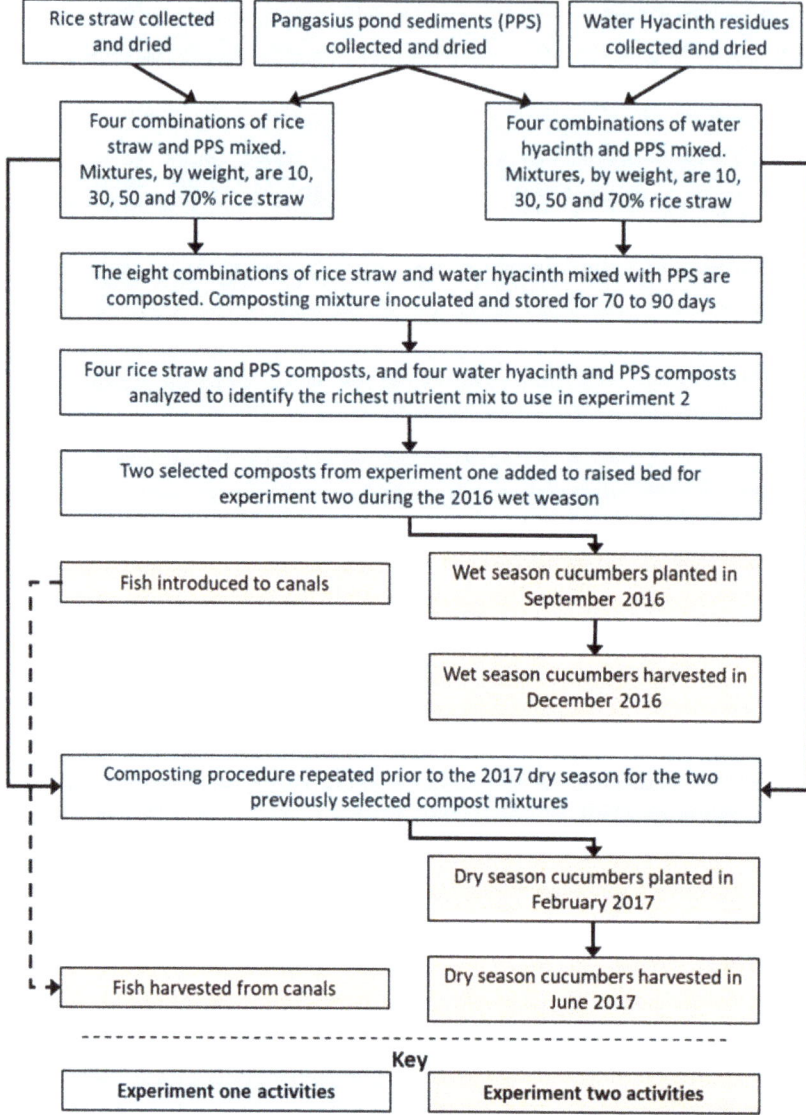

Figure 2. The work flow of experiments one and two. Light blue boxes represent activities included in experiment one; orange boxes are the activities of experiment two.

2.2.1. Collection of Rice Straw and Water Hyacinth Residues for Fertilizer Amendments

The RS and WH were collected to create organic amendments. Both RS and WH are common in the Mekong Delta, making them suitable for the production of organic amendments. RS was collected from rice farms during the harvest period and WH was collected from streams in Thoai Son, An Giang Province. Leaves and stems of water hyacinth were cleaned with freshwater and sun-dried for 2–3 days before use. All RS and WH samples were cut into approximately 5 cm-long segments and weighed before and after sun-drying. Three 1 kg (dry weight) samples of RS and WH were collected, homogenized, and stored in separately labeled plastic bags for chemical analysis. Results of the chemical analysis can be found in Table 1.

Table 1. Chemical composition of Pangasius pond sediments, rice straw, and common water hyacinth used in the first experiment, and soil where cucumber was grown before and after the second experiment.

Parameters	Pond Sediments	Rice Straw	Water Hyacinth	Soil (Initial)	Soil (Final)
pH	6.97	-	-	5.01	5.92
Organic carbon (% C)	4.51	47.31	40.19	5.17	5.24
Total N (% N)	0.35	0.81	2.32	0.28	0.30
Total P (% P_2O_5)	0.82	-	0.05	0.05	0.06
Total K (% K_2O)	1.07	2.24	1.46	1.72	1.10
Phosphate (Bray II) (PO_4^{3-}, ppm)	43.71	-	-	19.97	70.98
Ammonium (NH_4^+, mg kg^{-1})	37.16	-	-	13.76	325.0
Nitrate (NO_3^-, mg kg^{-1})	2.103	-	-	2.64	431.1

Note: All concentrations are expressed on a dry weight basis and all measurements refer to homogenized pooled samples.

2.2.2. Collection of Pond Sediments for Fertilizer Amendments

PPS was obtained from the sludge and sediment of Pangasius catfish ponds. The farm ponds from which this material was collected are located in My Thanh Ward, Long Xuyen City, An Giang Province. The pond sediments were collected during the fourth month of Pangasius catfish growth using a pump. The obtained sediments were then sun-dried for 5–7 days and transported to An Giang University, where they were air-dried for three additional days. Once dry, the samples were thoroughly mixed and three 1 kg samples were collected and stored separately in labeled plastic bags for chemical analysis. The results of the chemical analysis are given in Table 1.

2.2.3. Selection of Optimal Rice Straw-Pond Sediment and Water Hyacinth-Pond Sediment Organic Fertilizer Combinations

Two types of organic fertilizer were produced (Figures 2 and 3). One contained a mixture of PPS and RS (PPS_{RS}), the other a mixture of PPS and WH (PPS_{WH}). Both types of fertilizer were made by mixing sediments and residues in different proportions, so that they contained 10%, 30%, 50%, or 70% of either RS or WH mixed with 90%, 70%, 50%, and 30% PPS, respectively, creating eight organic fertilizer combinations (Figure 3). The PPS_{RS} and PPS_{WH} fertilizers were produced following the methods of Hein [33]. Briefly described, a measured quantity of the dried PPS was mixed with a measured quantity of RH or WH to achieve the mixing percentages noted above. The mixtures were turned regularly and then composted. A microbial fungal inoculum was added to each mixture. The inoculum used (TRICODHCT-LUA VON) contains a combination of *Trichoderma asperellum* spp. (80%, v/v) and *Trichoderma atroviride* Karsten (20%, v/v), with 5 g added, diluted in 3 liters of water, per 10 kg of compost. The inoculum was provided by the Department of Biotechnology at Can Tho University and was used to accelerate the composting process. The composting fertilizers were incubated in plastic incubator bags, which were turned over every 4–5 days during the first month to ensure homogeneity. The incubation temperature was 60 °C during 70 and 90 days for the treatments of rice straw and water hyacinth, respectively. The material was deemed ready for use when the color of the composting fertilizers in the incubation bags changed from brown to green [33]. To identify the PPS_{RS} and PPS_{WH} combination for use in the growth performance experiments, samples from each of the eight fertilizer combinations were collected for chemical analysis. The PPS_{RS} and PPS_{WH} combinations with the greatest nutrient concentrations were selected for the cucumber growing experiment.

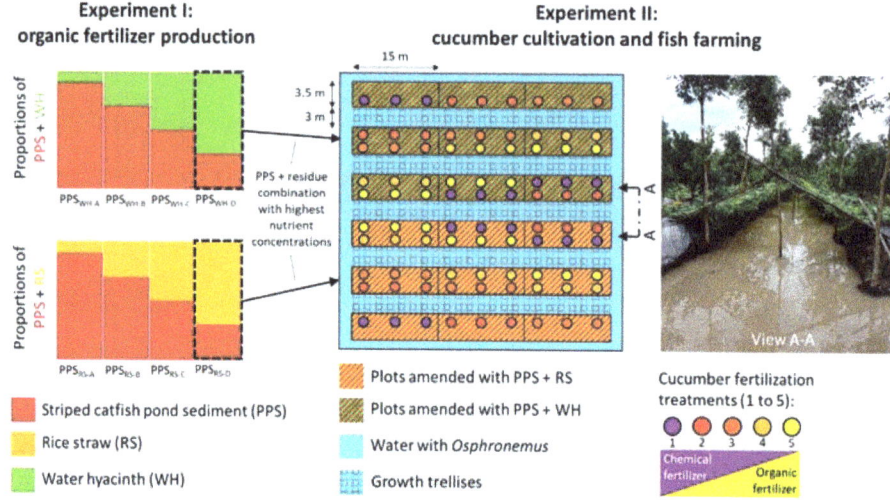

Figure 3. Schematic of the organic fertilizer production in experiment one (left); and layout of the integrated cucumber–fish cultivation with the organic–chemical fertilizer combinations in experiment two (right). In the latter, three replicate plots were amended with different levels of fish pond sediments and water hyacinth (WH, green background) or rice straw (RS, orange background). The organic fertilizer levels are indicated by colored circles (increasing organic fertilizer amount from violet to yellow); note that circles do not indicate individual plants, which were planted at a higher density (40–45 cm apart). View A-A shows a canal with growth trellises.

2.2.4. Preparation of Organic Fertilizer for Wet Season and Dry Season Cucumber Production

The PPS$_{RS}$ and PPS$_{WH}$ combinations prepared and identified in the previous section were used in fertilizer applications for the 2016 wet season (Figure 2). To create organic fertilizer for the 2017 dry season, the methods above were repeated prior to the start of the dry season, but only for the two selected PPS$_{RS}$ and PPS$_{WH}$ combinations.

2.3. Experiment Two: Integrated Cucumber–Fish Cultivation with Organic–Chemical Fertilizer Combinations

2.3.1. Fertilizer Application

Experiment two tested the use of different organic–chemical fertilizer mixes, from entirely organic to entirely chemical nutrient sources, on cucumber production. The PPS$_{RS}$ and PPS$_{WH}$ identified as having the highest nutrient concentrations were used in combination with different quantities of chemical fertilizer to fertilize cucumbers in the wet and dry seasons. The PPS$_{RS}$ and PPS$_{WH}$ amendments used in experiment two were prepared in two batches, before the start of each cucumber growth season, based on the selected combinations from experiment one (Figures 2 and 3). Five different treatment levels, T1–T5, which represent a gradient from 100% chemical fertilizer to 100% organic fertilizer were used:

- T1—control treatment with cucumbers grown using 100% chemical fertilizer at an average rate for Vietnam (220 N-180 P$_2$O$_5$-140 K$_2$O) [34];
- T2—75% of chemical fertilizer input used within T1, and 25% of organic fertilizers (PPS$_{RS}$ or PPS$_{WH}$) used in T5;
- T3—50% of chemical fertilizer input used within T1, and 50% of organic fertilizers (PPS$_{RS}$ or PPS$_{WH}$) used in T5;

- T4—25% of chemical fertilizer input used within T1, and 75% of organic fertilizers (PPS$_{RS}$ or PPS$_{WH}$) used in T5; and
- T5—100% of organic fertilizer input of PPS$_{RS}$ or PPS$_{WH}$ at 100 kg per plot.

2.3.2. Production Area Preparation

A series of raised beds, surrounded by canals, were used for experiment two (Figure 3). Each bed measured 3.5 × 45 × 0.4 m (width × length × height above water surface). The canals in between the raised beds measured 3 × 45 × 1 m (width × length × depth), and were connected by a channel at each end. The total experimental area was 1945 m^2, of which 945 m^2 were raised beds. Each 45 m long raised bed was divided into three 15 m long plots. These plots were then divided along their length to create sub-plots. In total, this resulted in 30 plots, on which the PPS$_{RS}$ and PPS$_{WH}$ fertilizers were added, in triplicate, at the five treatment levels. The layout of the experiment can be seen in Figure 3.

To prepare the plots for planting, they were first ploughed and allowed to dry for four days, and then covered by an agro-polymer plastic to maintain soil moisture and prevent weeds and pathogens before seedling establishment. The plot and agro-plastics were pierced to make a hole with a diameter of 5–6 cm and 7–8 cm depth to raise the cucumbers. The canals were prepared before the experiment by removing wastewater and surface sediments and left empty to dry for about two weeks. The bottom of the pond was treated with 20 kg of lime per 100 m^2 and left to dry for an additional week. Water from the nearby river was then pumped into the canal to a depth of 2 m.

2.3.3. Cucumber and Fish Preparation

A high yielding cucumber (*Cucumis sativus* L.; seed variety: AG208) was obtained from the Loc Troi Group of My Xuyen Ward, Long Xuyen City, An Giang Province. This cucumber variety is recommended to local farmers by the Agricultural Extension Center, Department of Agriculture and Rural Development, An Giang Province. With a cultivation period of around 60 days, it is one of the most popular cucumber varieties in the province.

Fish fingerlings of the herbivore (*Osphronemus goramy*) were obtained from the Research Center for Aquaculture Seed Production of Can Tho City, Can Tho Province. All fish fingerlings were treated with a 3% NaCl solution for 15 min on arrival to eliminate ectoparasite infections. Approximately 1000 fingerlings were nursed together in a big hapa net (5 m × 7 m × 1.5 m) and fed commercial feed that contained 28%–35% crude protein (Proconco Cuu Long Aquafeed Corporation, Long Duc Industry Zone, Tra Vinh City, Tra Vinh Province, Vietnam) for two weeks before the experiment started. The fingerlings were then introduced into canals that lay between the cucumber beds and had a fish density of 2 fish m^{-2}. At the beginning and end of the experiment, all fish were individually weighed using a digital scale. Except for a small amount of supplementary commercial feed, the fish relied only on the natural productivity of the canal ecosystem, fallen leaves, and discarded cucumber fruits as well as water spinach growing in the canal as a food source. The layout of the integrated fish–cucumber cultivation system can be seen in Figure 3.

2.3.4. Cucumber Planting and Growth Conditions

Cucumbers were grown in three replicated plots at each of the five fertilization treatments and during two consecutive cropping cycles (Figure 3). Cucumber vegetable seeds were soaked in warm water for 2-3 h and then incubated in damp paper towels for 3–4 days. The individual sprouted seeds, with white papillary, were sown in soil pots and nursery trays. When the seedlings had two 5 cm-long leaves, they were transplanted in the experiment plots. Plants were spaced about 0.4 m apart, with about 37 plants in each experimental plot, resulting in a planting density of approximately 5700 plants ha^{-1} considering the integrated field setup. Cucumbers were grown on the raised beds between the canals, with pairs of melaleuca poles (2–2.5 m tall) tied diagonally over each canal and covered by ribbed mesh (10 cm of mesh size), providing the climbing-frame for cucumber plants (view A-A in Figure 3).

Where organic fertilizers were used, these were added into each plot just after the soil was plowed, while the chemical fertilizers were added at 5–10 days after sowing (DAS), 15–20 DAS, and 30–35 DAS. Cucumber plants were irrigated by pumping water from the fish canal near each plot.

2.3.5. Plot Soil Sampling

At the beginning and end of the cucumber growth experiment, soil from the top 5 cm in the cucumber plots was collected at five different locations in each plot. A single homogenized soil sample, combining the samples from all plots, was used to analyze pH, NH_4^+ (mg L^{-1}), NO_3^- (mg L^{-1}), TN, TP, soil organic carbon (SOC) and available phosphorus (mg kg^{-1}). Soil pH was measured in a mixture of 20 g soil and 20 mL of distilled water with a glass electrode [35]. Analysis of TN followed the Kjeldahl method for soil analysis [36,37]. TP concentrations were determined by digesting soil with 60% perchloric acid [38] and measuring the available phosphorus in the digested fraction by the vanadomolybdophosphoric acid colorimetric method [39]. SOC was measured by the Walkley–Black dichromate oxidation technique [40]. Average soil properties at the beginning and end of the experiment can be seen in Table 1.

2.3.6. Data Collection and Calculation

During the cucumber growing period, plant length and vine length, width and number of leaves, and root length of six plants in each treatment were measured twice in each crop cycle at approximately 10 and 20 DAS. Cucumber fruits were harvested from all plots daily between 16:00–18:00. Harvested fruits were counted and weighted until the end of the growth season to estimate final yields in each treatment. At the beginning and end of the experiment, giant gourami fish were counted and individually weighed. The following parameters were calculated: survival rate SR% = TF_f/TF_i × 100, where TF_f is the total number of fish at the final harvest and TF_i is the initial number of fish; specific growth rate (SGR) (% day^{-1}) = $[\ln(W_f) - \ln(W_i)]/T \times 100$; daily weight gain (DWG) (g day^{-1}) = $(W_f - W_i)/T$, where W_f and W_i refer to the mean final and initial weights, respectively, and T is the growth period in days; and fish yield (kg) = total W_f − total W_i, where totals are calculated by summing up the final and initial weights of all harvested fish.

2.3.7. Data Analysis

Samplings for growth performance and production of cucumber were conducted at fixed intervals, three times over one month during the experimental period. Differences in plant traits between individual treatments were analyzed using Duncan's multiple range test, and deemed significant when $p < 0.01$. These statistical analyses were carried out using IBM SPSS Statistics (version 25). To present the changing effect of total nitrogen, phosphorous, and potassium inputs on yield between the five fertilizer mixtures, second order polynomial curves were fitted to cucumber yield data. Curves were fitted using the Curve Fitting toolbox within MATLAB, version R2017a (The Mathworks Inc., Natick, Massachusetts, USA).

3. Results

3.1. Experiment One: Organic Fertilizer Production

Chemical analysis of PPS, RS, and WH found that the pH ranged between 5.5–6.9. Concentrations of OM in RS and WH were over ten times higher than in PSS. The TN concentration was highest in WH and lowest in PPS. Moreover, the phosphate (PO_4^{3-}) − Bray II (ppm), NH_4^+ (mg kg^{-1}), and NO_3^- (mg kg^{-1}) concentrations were highest in PPS (Table 1).

Analysis of the different PPS to RS or WH fertilizer combinations found that the highest nutrient concentrations at the end of the composting process were in the PPS_{RS} and PPS_{WH} that contained 30% PPS and 70% RS or WH (Table 2). These mixtures were therefore chosen to create the organic fertilizer used in the cucumber growth experiments.

Table 2. Chemical composition of organic fertilizer produced from Pangasius pond sediments (PPS) mixed with rice straw (RS) or common water hyacinth (WH).

Parameters	PPS + RS (PPS$_{RS}$)				PPS + WH (PPS$_{WH}$)			
	PPS$_{RS-10}$	PPS$_{RS-30}$	PPS$_{RS-50}$	PPS$_{RS-70}$ [1]	PPS$_{WH-10}$	PPS$_{WH-30}$	PPS$_{WH-50}$	PPS$_{WH-70}$ [1]
Plant residues (%)	10	30	50	70	10	30	50	70
Organic carbon (% C)	6.03	11.70	11.39	16.68	6.53	10.11	9.94	16.54
TN (% N)	0.42	0.70	0.70	1.12	0.63	0.70	0.70	0.98
TP (% P_2O_5)	0.88	0.63	0.68	0.65	0.68	0.67	0.63	0.83
TK (% K_2O)	22.75	26.63	25.98	24.90	25.46	26.39	26.53	24.58
C/N	14.36	16.71	16.27	14.89	10.41	14.44	14.20	16.88

Note: All concentrations are expressed as % on a dry weight basis and all measurements refer to homogenized pooled samples. [1] The organic fertilizer mixtures used in experiment two.

3.2. Experiment Two: Integrated Cucumber–Fish Cultivation with Organic–Chemical Fertilizer Combinations

3.2.1. Fertilizer and Soil Properties

The chemical compositions of the experimental organic fertilizers (PPS$_{RS-70}$ and PPS$_{WH-70}$) obtained both before the wet season and before the dry season are reported in Table 3. The nutrient concentrations of organic fertilizers produced before the two growing seasons differed slightly, with concentrations of OM, P, and K in the dry season being higher than in the wet season (Table 3). Moreover, nutrient concentrations were slightly lower than the standard values for organic fertilizers (Table 3). The total nutrient inputs for each treatment in the wet and dry seasons, derived by combining different proportions of chemical fertilizer and PPS$_{RS-70}$ or PPS$_{WH-70}$ inputs can be found in Table 4. The pH, organic matter (OM%), total nitrogen TN (%N), total potassium TK (%K_2O), and total phosphorus TP (%P_2O_5) in the soil of the experimental area did not differ markedly between the beginning and end of experiment two (although we could not test differences statistically as we reported concentrations from pooled samples). However, higher available phosphorus (PO_4^{3-}), NH_4^+, and NO_3^- concentrations in soils were recorded at the end of experiment two (Table 1).

Table 3. Chemical composition of the organic fertilizers obtained from Pangasius pond sediments mixed with rice straw (PPS$_{RS}$) and with water hyacinth (PPS$_{WH}$) that were used in the wet and dry season cucumber cultivation, as well as the national standards for organic fertilizer.

Parameters	Wet Season		Dry Season		Standard for Organic Fertilizer [1]
	PPS$_{RS-70}$	PPS$_{WH-70}$	PPS$_{RS-70}$	PPS$_{WH-70}$	
pH	6.85	7.38	7.35	7.26	6.0–8.0
Organic carbon (% C)	12.67	11.41	18.10	12.91	>13
TN (% N)	1.33	0.77	1.05	0.91	>2.5
TP (% P_2O_5)	0.84	1.14	1.36	1.80	>2.5
TK (% K_2O)	1.35	2.06	1.76	2.14	>1.5
C/N	9.52	14.82	17.24	14.19	-
Phosphate (Bray II) (PO_4^{3-}, ppm)	62.77	65.41	35.36	42.98	-
Ammonium (NH_4^+, mg kg^{-1})	34.49	7.12	50.42	12.10	-

Note: All concentrations are expressed on a dry weight basis and are obtained from pooled samples for each treatment. [1] Standard of organic fertilizer: industrial standard 10TCN 526: 2002 applied for microorganism organic fertilizer processing from domestic solid waste of Ministry of Agriculture and Rural Development, Vietnam (2002).

Table 4. Composition and doses of chemical and organic fertilizers and total amount of nutrients (N–P–K) applied in the cucumber vegetable production during the wet and dry season growing periods.

Treatment	Fertilizer Composition (kg per Plot)		Total N-P-K from Chemical+PPS$_{WH-70}$ Fertilizer Combinations (kg ha^{-1})						Total N-P-K from Chemical+PPS$_{RS-70}$ Fertilizer Combinations (kg ha^{-1})					
			Wet Season			Dry Season			Wet Season			Dry Season		
	Chemical	Organic N	N	P	K	N	P	K	N	P	K	N	P	K
T1	4.5	0	171	147	95	171	147	95	171	147	95	171	147	95
T2	3.4	25	137	116	79	130	112	73	134	118	83	134	121	84
T3	2.3	50	102	85	64	89	77	50	96	88	71	98	95	72
T4	1.2	75	68	53	48	47	42	28	59	58	61	61	69	61
T5	0	100	30	19	30	23	30	39	17	25	46	20	40	48

3.2.2. Growth Performance and Plant Traits

Growth performance and plant indices at 10 days after sowing (DAS) for the wet and dry season crops are given in Table S1. While not always significant, plant traits (plant length, leaf length, leaf width) were generally greater in the 100% chemical treatments (T1) compared to where 100% organic amendments were used (T5) in both the wet and dry seasons. Growth performance and plant indices of cucumber growth experiments recorded at 20 DAS for the crops during the dry season and wet season are given in Table S2. Almost all the plant indices at 20 DAS were smallest in the two treatments with the lowest quantity of chemical fertilizer applied (T4 and T5) in both seasons and with both types of residues used.

The trends in plant indices at 10 and 20 DAS as a function of the total nitrogen inputs including chemical and organic amendments are presented in Figures 4 and 5. During the early plant development stages at 10 DAS, increasing the total additions of nutrient inputs appears to increase the plant length. Leaf length and leaf width indices showed opposing trends between the two types of residue used (Figure 4). Both leaf length and width were smallest when rice straw was used in the organic amendments and total nitrogen inputs were the smallest. Conversely, leaf length and width were greatest at the lowest total nitrogen addition levels when water hyacinth was used as an organic residue. Similarly, at 20 DAS (Figure 5), there was an increasing trend in plant indices as nutrient inputs increased. However, after the nitrogen inputs increased above approximately 100 kg ha^{-1}, there was no additional benefit to increasing the nitrogen inputs on plant indices, and possibly a mild negative effect.

Figure 6 shows how fruit yields in experiment two varied with increasing total amount of added nutrient (N, P, and K) including chemical and organic amendments. Curves represent the fitted second-degree polynomials, all of which had high adjusted-R^2 values (all > 0.88) to present the general trend in treatment effect. Lower plots (d, e, f) presented the fraction of nutrient inputs from chemical fertilizer compared to total inputs (chemical + organic addition nutrients). For all four experiments (two crops, two organic amendment type), the highest yields were produced at the medium chemical fertilizer input rates. At these rates, whilst there was a reduction in chemical fertilizer input, their input rates were still a relatively high fraction of the total nutrient inputs. However, the addition of nutrients as organic matter appears to have had a positive impact on crop yields compared to simply increasing the amount of chemical fertilizer added to the field.

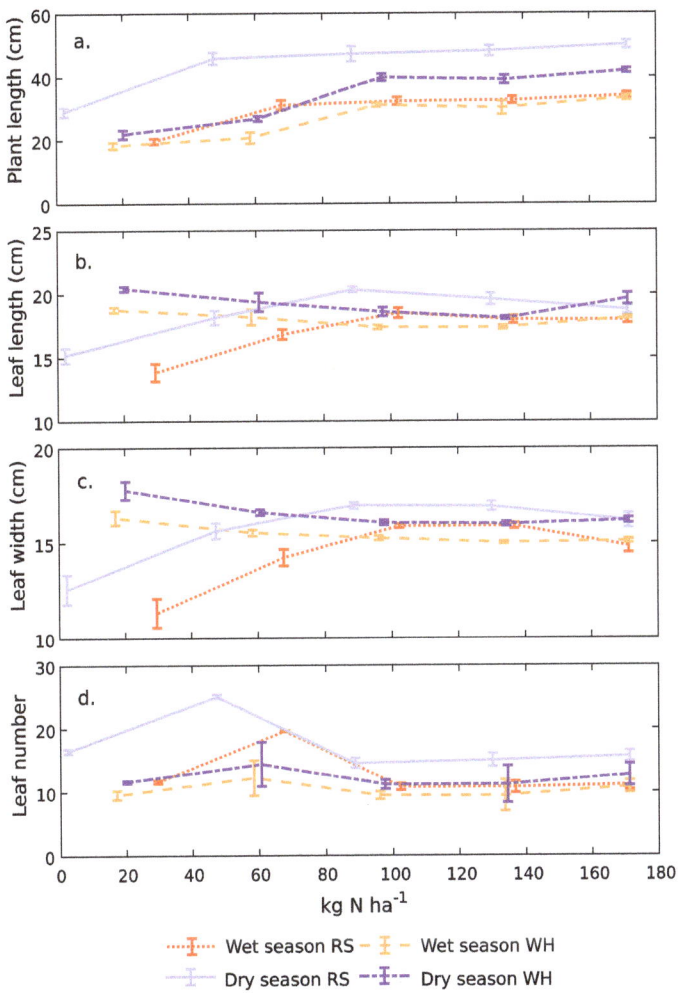

Figure 4. Plant traits as a function of total nitrogen input: (**a**) plant length, (**b**) leaf length, (**c**) leaf width, and (**d**) leaf number. Data were compared between each treatment (organic amendment made with rice straw (RS) or water hyacinth (WH)) and between growing seasons at 10 days after sowing. Vertical bars are standard errors ($n = 3$).

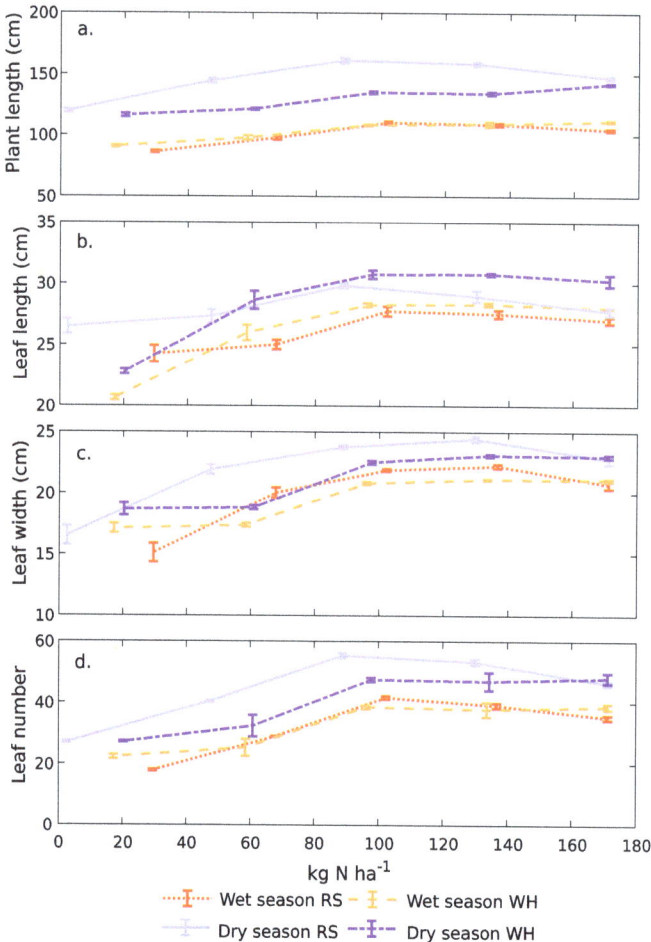

Figure 5. Plant traits as a function of total nitrogen input: (**a**) plant length, (**b**) leaf length, (**c**) leaf width, and (**d**) leaf number. Data are compared between each treatment (organic amendment made with rice straw (RS) or water hyacinth (WH)) and between growing seasons at 20 days after sowing. Vertical bars are standard errors ($n = 3$).

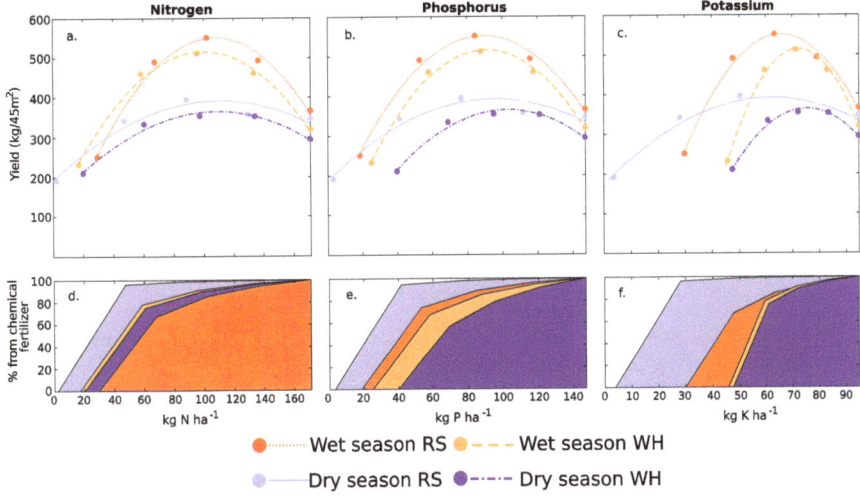

Figure 6. The top panels show the relationship between the total additions of (**a**) nitrogen; (**b**) phosphorus; and (**c**) potassium within the four treatments conducted within the study (organic amendment made with rice straw (RS) or water hyacinth (WH); wet or dry season). Second-degree polynomial curves were fitted to demonstrate the changing yield with increasing nutrient inputs and fractions derived from chemical and organic nutrient additions. Lower panels (**d**,**e**) present the percentage of nutrient inputs from the chemical fertilizer compared to the total nutrient additions for the nutrients in the corresponding upper plots.

3.2.3. Final Yield of Fish and Cucumber

The final body weight of the giant gourami grown for eight months in the canals surrounding the cucumber plots was 459.3 g per fish, with a total fish yield of 0.387 kg m^{-2} of water. There were at least an additional 20 kg of wild fish species in the canals, but this was not included in the final yield of fish in this study. The survival rate (%), specific growth rate (SGR), daily weight gain (DWG) of giant gourami were 70.2%, 0.69% day^{-1}, and 1.3 g day^{-1}, respectively.

For both seasons, considering both RS and WH mixtures, the greatest cucumber yields were found in T3 and the smallest were in T5 (Table 5), and the wet season yields were consistently higher than their comparative dry season yields. However, comparing the T1 in both the wet season and dry season, when plants were fertilized with only chemical fertilizer, yields from plots within the RS growing area were consistently (but marginally) higher than in the respective water hyacinth growing area.

Table 5. Final yield (number of fruits or kg wet weight per treatment) of cucumber vegetable production in the integrated fish–farming system in each treatment and crop cycle.

Crop	Fruit	RS					WH				
		T1	T2	T3	T4	T5	T1	T2	T3	T4	T5
Wet Season	Tot No. of fruit	4380	6001	6596	5826	3323	3517	5536	6091	5981	2992
	Tot fruit weight (kg)	364	491.8	549.9	489.1	249.4	317	459.1	510.6	459.5	230.8
Dry Season	Tot No. of fruit	3288	3425	3903	3248	2114	2935	3608	3359	3389	2311
	Tot fruit weight (kg)	344.4	355.9	393.3	340.5	190.7	292.3	350.9	352.4	332.2	209.4

4. Discussion

The development of integrated fish–vegetable farming systems are often considered as sustainable agricultural models for smallholders and provide opportunities for improved food security, economic liberalization, climate change adaptation, and additional income for the resources-poor in developing countries [23,41,42]. Thus, integrated farming systems have been shown to provide sustainable alternatives to less integrated systems, which are also often practically applicable in a local context [21]. However, there are limited studies on the effects of organic fertilizer produced from PPS and RS or WH on *Brassica juncea* and *Ipomoea aquatica* [31]. In contrast, there are many studies on compost from other agricultural wastes combined with fish pond sediment [28], sewage [43], sludge rock phosphate and ammonium sulfate [44], swine manure [45], rape cake, poultry manure [46], and dairy manure [39]. In this work, we assessed how chemical fertilizers and organic residues can be combined to reduce dependence on chemical additions while also increasing vegetable yields. Specifically, we tested whether this could be achieved in an integrated cucumber–fish production system, where the benefits of FPS and residue recycling were combined with those of fish farming (Figure 1).

4.1. Characteristics of Individual Organic Amendments

As summarized in Table 1, the total nitrogen concentration of RS and WH residues used in this study were higher than the earlier data published for RS, wheat straw (*Triticum aestivum* L.), potato plant residues (*Solanum tuberosum* L.), and mustard stover (*Brassica juncea* L.) [28]. However, carbon, nitrogen, and phosphate concentrations of RS and WH were slightly lower than the values measured in market crop waste [47].

Previous studies indicate that PPS amendments are rich in OM, N, and P, and have high water holding capacity. These properties make it suitable as a bulking agent to speed up the composting of agricultural residues [16,48,49]. As PPS is rich in macro- and micronutrients, it can serve as a potential organic fertilizer and soil conditioner, which could enhance the soil environment for crop production [2,50]. We showed that PPS contained higher levels of the major nutrients required for crop fertilization (N, P, K) than the initial soil in the experimental plots (Table 1). In general, the concentrations of major nutrients in PPS were comparable to values reported for Pangasius and other FPS used as organic fertilizer for rice, morning glory (*Brachiaria mutica*), chinese mustard (*Brassica juncea*), water spinach (*Ipomoea aquatica*), and fodder grass (*Ipomoea reptans*) grown in tropical regions [2,13,16,31,51–53]. Moreover, Boyd et al. [51] reported that the major nutrient concentrations of PPS were similar to or higher than those of manure from chicken, cattle, and horses.

These results suggest that combining RS or WH residues with PPS has the potential to provide a nutrient-rich organic amendment for vegetable cultivation. To use these organic amendments, however, they first need to be composted.

4.2. Characteristics of the Organic Fertilizer after Composting

The physico-chemical properties of the organic fertilizer are summarized in Table 3. The concentrations of some important nutrients (P, K) in the organic fertilizer were slightly higher in the dry season than in the wet season (Table 3). However, Saldarriaga et al. [32] stated that the physical and chemical properties of the composting products for organic fertilizer depend on the type of initial material, duration of the decomposition step, and conditions during the process (e.g., temperature, moisture content, degree of aeration, pH, and C/N ratio, and the physical structure of the raw materials), so it is not surprising to find some variation between our two batches of compost. The physico-chemical properties of our organic fertilizer were within the range reported in previous studies [28,31,49,54]. The pH (6.85–7.38) was in the range measured in the co-composting of green wastes [55], the composting of agricultural waste mixtures with and without FPS [28], organic fertilizer produced from sludge in combination with RS or WH [31], and market crop wastes [47]. However, our organic fertilizer was higher in TN, TP, and phosphate compared to compost from mixed agricultural wastes and PPS [28,31,54]. Moreover, the TN, ammonium, and nitrate concentrations in our organic fertilizer were higher than in the compost based on market crop wastes [40] and co-composting of fecal sludge and organic solid waste from agriculture [54].

The initial C/N ratio depends on the quality of the residues and affects the composting process and compost quality, while the final C/N depends on the degree of decomposition [56]. The final C/N ratios of our organic fertilizers ranged between 9.52–17.24 for organic fertilizer based on rice straw, and

14.19–14.82 in fertilizer based on water hyacinth (Table 3). A C/N ratio of around 16 is recommended for compost used in agriculture [54].

4.3. Organic Fertilizer Benefits to Soil and Plants

The indirect integration of aquaculture with agriculture through the reuse of FPS as organic fertilizer for green fodder, vegetables, and rice production has significant potential to contribute to sustainable intensification and nutrition security goals, reducing local environmental impacts associated with sediment disposal, and increasing agricultural production [13,15,17,52]. We hypothesized that organic fertilizer produced from PPS and locally sourced plant residues (RS, or WH) can offer an avenue for sustainable agricultural development in the Mekong Delta region and Southeast Asia. Our experimental results confirmed this expectation, showing higher OM, TN, TP, and available phosphorus, ammonium, and nitrate concentrations in soils at the end of experiment two compared to the initial soil plots (Table 1). However, these results should be treated with caution, since soil samples were pooled before chemical analysis, so we cannot quantify uncertainty around these average values. Similar improvements have been reported when fish pond sediments were used as fertilizer for fodder grass production and in rice fields in Bangladesh [13], China [57], and Palestine [58].

The trends in plant traits between each treatment and between growing seasons at 10 and 20 days are presented in Figures 2 and 3, respectively. The measured parameters did not differ between treatments, except at high organic fertilizer application rates (Tables S1 and S2). In general, cucumber plant indices in the dry season were larger than in the wet season, possibly because of higher solar radiation in combination with abundant water from nearby canals in the dry season. These results thus suggest that organic amendments can promote the vegetative growth of cucumber plants in both wet and dry seasons.

4.4. Organic Fertilizer Benefits to Crop Yields

The highest fruit yield and fruit number were found when applying 50% of the maximum doses of inorganic and organic fertilizers for the crops both during the dry and wet seasons, whilst the lowest values were obtained when growing cucumbers with only organic fertilizer (Table 5). Therefore, the fertilizer combination in this treatment provided enough nutrients to satisfy the requirements of the cucumber plants and improved yields. The best performing treatment combination (T3) resulted in a per hectare equivalent yield in an integrated fish–cucumber system of 28.7 and 20.2 tons ha^{-1} for the wet season and dry season, respectively, using RS. These yields are approximately half of the yields commonly reported in Hau Giang Province (based on a survey of local cucumber production, results not shown), but approximately half of the experimental area was dedicated to fish farming and thus did not contribute to vegetable production. Therefore, considering only the effective growing area, yields were comparable to those found within the province when standard practices were used. However, caution is needed in assessing the benefit of RS over WH as an organic addition. While RS organic amendments performed better than WH amendments, T1 plots within the RS growing area also performed marginally better than T1 plots in the WH area. As these areas are fertilized with an identical amount of chemical fertilizer, this result suggests an inherent (albeit minor) benefit to plant growth within the RS production area, which occurred due to a lack of a fully randomized design.

The other half of the system was dedicated to fish production. The fish yield we obtained (387 kg) equated to approximately 2 tons of fish if the system was scaled up to one hectare. The fish provide a valuable second farm income, an additional protein source, and also have the potential to increase farmer resilience through diversified production (Figure 1).

5. Conclusions

We have demonstrated that the use of organic fertilizers can either replace or supplement chemical inputs and have an overall positive effect on yields. This can also be achieved in combination with fish production. Further work is needed to demonstrate the economic benefits to farmers, given the trade-offs between fish production and reduced area available for vegetable production, and between savings on chemical fertilizers and increased labor costs for the preparation of the organic amendments. However, the results demonstrate a system that may be economically beneficial for farmers over traditional cucumber production systems.

The study demonstrates that the nutrients in organic fertilizer from striped catfish pond sediments combined with rice straw or water hyacinth residues can replace 25%–50%, or even up to 75% of inorganic fertilizers as a nutrient source for cucumber plants. The organic amendments satisfied the nutritional requirements of the cucumber plants and increased yields compared to using only inorganic fertilizers. Moreover, we showed that organic amendments can be combined with integrated fish–vegetable farming to provide a more diversified production system with tangible environmental benefits and potentially improved farm income.

Supplementary Materials: The following are available online at http://www.mdpi.com/2073-4395/10/7/1025/s1, Table S1: Mean growth performance and the indices of cucumber vegetable plants at 10 days after sowing, for all organic fertilizer treatments in both the wet season and dry season (length in cm). Means with different letters within rows are significantly different ($p < 0.01$). Table S2: Mean growth performance and the indices of cucumber vegetable plants at 20 days after sowing, for all organic fertilizer treatments in both the wet season and dry season (length in cm). Means with different letters within rows are significantly different ($p < 0.01$).

Author Contributions: Conceptualization, C.T.D., P.A.T., and V.T.T.; Methodology, C.T.D., P.A.T., and V.T.T.; Formal analysis, C.T.D., P.A.T., J.L., and V.T.T.; Writing—original draft preparation, C.T.D., P.A.T., and V.T.T.; Writing—review and editing, C.T.D., P.A.T., V.T.T., H.B., S.M., and J.L. All authors have read and agreed to the published version of the manuscript.

Funding: This research was partially funded by the Swedish Research Council (Vetenskapsrådet), Formas, and Sida through the joint call "Sustainability and resilience—Tackling climate and environmental changes" (VR 2016-06313).

Acknowledgments: The authors wish to thank the farmers, staff, and students at the Crop Science Department of the Faculty of Agriculture and Natural Resources, An Giang University, and Laboratory of Can Tho University for their support and field and lab assistance. Two anonymous reviewers provided useful comments to the original manuscript.

Conflicts of Interest: The authors declare no conflict of interest.

References

1. FAO. *The State of World Fisheries and Aquaculture 2012*; FAO—Food and Agriculture Organization of the United Nation: Rome, Italy, 2012; 230p.
2. Rahman, M.M.; Yakupitiyage, A.; Ranamukhaarachchi, S.L. Agricultural use of fishpond sediment for environmental amelioration. *Thammasat Inter. J. Sci. Tech.* **2004**, *9*, 1–10.
3. World Bank. *Aquaculture Pollution: An Overview of Issues with a Focus on China, Vietnam, and the Philippines*; The World Bank's Agriculture and Environment and Natural Resources Global Practices; World Bank Regional Agricultural Pollution Study; Working Paper; World Bank: Washington, DC, USA, 2017; pp. 1–15.
4. Vietnam Association of Seafood Exporters and Producers (VASEP). *Vietnam's Fisheries Industry Overview 2018 of Vietnam Association of Seafood Exporters and Producers*; Ministry of Agriculture and Rural Development: Hanoi, Vietnam, 2019; Available online: http://vasep.com.vn/1192/OneContent/tong-quan-nganh.htm (accessed on 9 October 2019).
5. The Ministry of Agriculture and Rural Development (MARD). *Annual Reports of the Ministry of Agriculture and Rural Development*; The Ministry of Agriculture and Rural Development (MARD): Hanoi, Vietnam, 2018. (In Vietnamese)
6. General Statistics Office Vietnam (GSO). *Production of Agriculture, Forestry and Fishing of Vietnam*; Statistical Documentation and Service Centre, General Statistics Office of Vietnam: Hanoi, Vietnam, 2019. Available online: https://www.gso.gov.vn/default_en.aspx?tabid=778 (accessed on 18 February 2020).
7. Halls, A.; Johns, M. *Assessment of the Vulnerability of the Mekong Delta Pangasius Catfish Industry to Development and Climate Change in the Lower Mekong Basin*; Report Prepared for the Sustainable Fisheries Partnership; Johns Associates Limited: Bath, UK, 2013; Available online: www.johnsassociates.co.uk (accessed on 20 November 2019).

8. Tovar, A.C.; Moreno, M.P.; Manuel-Vez, M. Garcia-Vargas. Environmental impacts of intensive aquaculture in marine waters. *Water. Res.* **2000**, *34*, 334–342. [CrossRef]
9. Lin, C.K.; Yi, Y. Minimizing environmental impacts of freshwater aquaculture and reuse of pond effluents and mud. *Aquaculture* **2003**, *226*, 57–68. [CrossRef]
10. Crab, R.; Avnimelech, Y.; Defoirdt, T.; Bossier, P.; Verstraete, W. Nitrogen removal techniques in aquaculture for a sustainable production. *Aquaculture* **2007**, *270*, 1–14. [CrossRef]
11. Anh, P.T.; Kroeze, C.; Bush, S.R.; Mol, A.P.J. Water pollution by *Pangasius* production in the Mekong Delta, Vietnam: Causes and options for control. *Aqua. Res.* **2010**, *42*, 108–128. [CrossRef]
12. Feng, J.; Zhou, F.; Li, X.; Xu, C.; Fang, F. Nutrient removal ability and economical benefit of a rice-fish co-culture system in aquaculture pond. *Ecol. Eng.* **2016**, *94*, 315–319. [CrossRef]
13. Haque, M.M.; Belton, B.; Alam, M.M.; Ahmed, A.G.; Alam, M.R. Reuse of fish pond sediments as fertilizer for fodder grass production in Bangladesh: Potential for sustainable intensification and improved nutrition. *Agric. Ecosyst. Environ.* **2016**, *216*, 226–236. [CrossRef]
14. Oláh, J.; Pekár, F.; Szabó, P. Nitrogen cycling and retention in fish-cum-livestock ponds. *J. Appl. Ichthyol.* **1994**, *10*, 341–348. [CrossRef]
15. Rahman, M.; Yakupitiyage, A. Use of fishpond sediment for sustainable aquaculture—Agriculture farming. *Int. J. Sustain. Dev. Plan.* **2006**, *1*, 192–202. [CrossRef]
16. Muendo, P.N.; Verdegem, M.C.J.; Stoorvogel, J.J.; Milstein, A.; Gamal, E.; Duc, P.M.; Verreth, J.A.J. Sediment accumulation in fish ponds: Its potential for agricultural use. *Int. J. Fisher. Aquat. Stud.* **2014**, *1*, 228–241.
17. Da, C.T.; Phuoc, L.H.; Duc, H.N.; Troell, M.; Berg, H. Use of wastewater from striped catfish (*Pangasianodon hypophthalmus*) pond culture for integrated rice–fish–vegetable farming systems in the Mekong Delta, Vietnam. *Agroecol. Sustain. Food Syst.* **2015**, *39*, 580–597. [CrossRef]
18. Boyd, C.E. *Bottom Soils, Sediment, and Pond Aquaculture*; Chapman and Hall: New York, NY, USA, 1995; 348p.
19. Phu, T.Q.; Tinh, T.K. Chemical compositions of sludge from intensive striped catfish (*Pangasianodon hypophthalmus*) culture pond. *J. Sci. Can Tho Univ.* **2012**, *22*, 290–299. (In Vietnamese)
20. Berg, H. Rice monoculture and integrated rice-fish farming in the Mekong Delta, Vietnam—Economic and ecological considerations. *Ecol. Econ.* **2002**, *41*, 95–107. [CrossRef]
21. Berg, H.; Nguyen, T.T. Integrated rice-fish farming: Safeguarding biodiversity and ecosystem services for sustainable food production in the Mekong Delta. *J. Sustain. Agric.* **2012**, *36*, 859–872. [CrossRef]
22. Lemaire, G.; Franzluebbers, A.; Carvalho, P.C.D.F.; Dedieu, B. Integrated crop–livestock systems: Strategies to achieve synergy between agricultural production and environmental quality. *Agric. Ecosyst. Environ.* **2014**, *190*, 4–8. [CrossRef]
23. Nhan, D.K.; Verdegem, M.C.J.; Milstein, A.J.; Verreth, A.V. Water and nutrient budgets of ponds in integrated agriculture–aquaculture systems in the Mekong Delta, Vietnam. *Aqua. Res.* **2008**, *39*, 1216–1228. [CrossRef]
24. Snow, A.M.; Ghaly, A.E.; Snow, A. A comparative assessment of hydroponically grown cereal crops for the purification of aquaculture wastewater and the production of fish feed. *Am. J. Agric. Biol. Sci.* **2008**, *3*, 364–378. [CrossRef]
25. Graber, A.; Junge, R. Aquaponic systems: Nutrient recycling from fish wastewater by vegetable production. *Desalination* **2009**, *246*, 147–156. [CrossRef]
26. Quynh, H.T.; Kazuto, S. Organic fertilizers in Vietnam's markets: Nutrient composition and efficacy of their application. *Sustainability* **2018**, *10*, 2437. [CrossRef]
27. Li, X.; Zhang, R.; Pang, Y. Characteristics of dairy manure composting with rice straw. *Bioresour. Technol.* **2008**, *99*, 359–367. [CrossRef]
28. Karak, T.; Bhattacharyya, P.; Paul, R.K.; Das, T.; Saha, S.K. Evaluation of composts from agricultural wastes with fish pond sediment as bulking agent to improve compost quality. *CLEAN Soil Air Water* **2013**, *41*, 711–723. [CrossRef]
29. Pouil, S.; Samsudin, R.; Slembrouck, J.; Sihabuddin, A.; Sundari, G.; Khazaidan, K.; Kristanto, A.H.; Pantjara, B.; Caruso, D. Nutrient budgets in a small-scale freshwater fish pond system in Indonesia. *Aquaculture* **2019**, *504*, 267–274. [CrossRef]
30. Tham, H.T. Water Hyacinth (*Eichhornia Crassipes*) Biomass Production, Ensilability and Feeding Value to Growing Cattle. Ph.D. Thesis, Swedish University of Agricultural Sciences, Uppsala, Sweden, 2012.
31. Thanh, X.B.; Hien, V.T.M.; Cong, T.T.; Da, C.T.; Berg, H. Reuse of sediment from catfish pond through composting with water hyacinth and rice straw. *Sustain. Environ. Res.* **2015**, *25*, 1–5.

32. Saldarriaga, J.F.; Gallego, J.L.; López, J.E.; Aguado, R.; Olazar, M. Selecting monitoring variables in the manual composting of municipal solid waste based on principal component analysis. *Waste Biomass Valoriz.* **2019**, *10*, 1811–1819. [CrossRef]
33. Hien, N.T. *Organic Fertilizer: Biofertilizer and Compost Fertilizer*; Institute for Research and Universalization for Encyclopedic Knowledge (IREUK): Hanoi, Vietnam, 2003.
34. Dung, P.T.; Huong, D.T. *Effect of Compost and Micro-Organic Fertilizers on Growth Performances and Yield of Cucumber in Organic Farming System in Gia Lam—Hanoi, Vietnam*; Vietnam National University of Agriculture: Hanoi, Vietnam, 2012.
35. McLean, E.O. Soil pH and lime requirement. In *Methods of Soil Analysis. Part 2. Chemical and Microbiological Properties*; Page, A.L., Miller, R.H., Keeney, D.R., Eds.; American Society of Agricultural Engineers: Madison, WI, USA, 1982; pp. 199–224.
36. Cochrane, K.; De Young, C.; Soto, D.; Bahri, T. *Climate change implications for fisheries and aquaculture*; FAO of the United Nations: Rome, Italy, 2009.
37. Molle, F.; Foran, T.; Käkönen, M. *Contested waterscapes in the Mekong region: Hydropower, livelihoods and governance*; Earthscan: Sterling, VA, USA, 2009.
38. Hanjra, M.A.; Qureshi, M.E. Global water crisis and future food security in an era of climate change. *Food Policy* **2010**, *35*, 365–377. [CrossRef]
39. Stirling, H.P. *Chemical and Biological Methods of Water Analysis for Aquaculturists*; Institute of Aquaculture, University of Stirling: Stirling, NJ, USA, 1985; 117p.
40. Tirado, M.C.; Clarke, R.L.; Jaykus, A.; McQuatters-Gollop, A.; Frank, J.M. Climate change and food safety: A review. *Food Res. Int.* **2010**, *43*, 1745–1765. [CrossRef]
41. Edwards, P. Environmental issues in integrated agriculture—Aquaculture in wastewater-fed fish culture systems. In *Environment and Aquaculture in Developing Countries*; Pullin, R.S.V., Rosenthal, H., Maclean, J.L., Eds.; International Center for Living Aquatic Resources Management: Makati, Philippines, 1993; Volume 31, pp. 139–170.
42. Prein, M. Integration of aquaculture into crop–animal systems in Asia. *Agric. Syst.* **2002**, *71*, 127–146. [CrossRef]
43. Roca-Pérez, L.; Martínez, C.; Marcilla, P.; Boluda, R. Composting rice straw with sewage sludge and compost effects on the soil–plant system. *Chemosphere* **2009**, *75*, 781–787. [CrossRef]
44. Zayed, G.; Abdel-Motaal, H. Bio-active composts from rice straw enriched with rock phosphate and their effect on the phosphorous nutrition and microbial community in rhizosphere of cowpea. *Bioresour. Technol.* **2005**, *96*, 929–935. [CrossRef]
45. Zhu, N.; Deng, C.; Xiong, Y.; Qian, H.Q. Performance characteristics of three aeration systems in the swine manure composting. *Bioresour. Technol.* **2004**, *95*, 319–326. [CrossRef]
46. Abdelhamid, M.T.; Horiuchi, T.; Oba, S. Composting of rice straw with oilseed rape cake and poultry manure and its effects on Faba bean (*Vicia Faba* L.) growth and soil properties. *Bioresour. Technol.* **2004**, *93*, 183–189. [CrossRef]
47. Tumuhairwe, J.B.; Tenywa, J.S.; Otabbong, E.; Ledin, S. Comparison of four low-technology composting methods for market crop wastes. *Waste Manag.* **2009**, *29*, 2274–2281. [CrossRef]
48. Thunjai, T.; Boyd, C.E.; Boonyaratpalin, M. Bottom soil quality in tilapia ponds of different age in Thailand. *Aqua. Res.* **2004**, *35*, 698–705. [CrossRef]
49. Karak, T. Heavy metal accumulation in soil amended with roadside pond sediment and uptake by rice (*Oryza sativa* L.). *Commun. Soil Sci. Plant Anal.* **2010**, *41*, 2577–2594. [CrossRef]
50. Boyd, B.C.E.; Rajts, F.; Firth, J. Sludge management at *Pangasius* farm cuts discharges. Environmental and Social Responsibility. Available online: https://www.aquaculturealliance.org/advocate/sludge-management-pangasius-farm-cuts-discharges (accessed on 18 February 2020).
51. Phung, V.C.; Nguyen, B.P.; Hoang, T.K.; Bell, R.W. Recycling of fishpond waste from rice cultivation in Cuu Long Delta, Vietnam. In *Technologies and Management for Sustainable Biosystems*; Nair, J., Furedy, C., Hoysala, C., Doelle, H., Eds.; Nova Science Publishers: New York, NY, USA, 2009; pp. 85–97.
52. Phu, T.Q.; Tinh, T.K.; Giang, H.T. Reuse ability of bottom sediment from intensive catfish (*Pangasianodon hypophthalmus*) ponds for rice cultivation. *J. Sci. Can Tho Univ.* **2012**, *24*, 135–143. (In Vietnamese)

53. Nguyen, P.Q.; Be, N.V.; Cong, N.V. Quantifying and qualifying sediment load from intensive catfish (*Pangasianodon hypophthalmus*) ponds and sediment application for vegetable-cultured (in Vietnamese). *J. Sci. Can Tho Univ.* **2014**, *35*, 78–89.
54. Cofie, O.; Kone, D.; Rothenberger, S.; Moser, D.; Zubruegg, C. Co-composting of faecal sludge and organic solid waste for agriculture: Process dynamics. *Water. Res.* **2009**, *43*, 4665–4675. [CrossRef]
55. Sun, X.; Wang, S.; Wang, J.; Lu, W.; Wang, H. Co-composting of night soil and green wastes. *Comp. Sci. Util.* **2012**, *20*, 254–259. [CrossRef]
56. Zhu, N. Effect of low initial C/N ratio on aerobic composting of swine manure with rice straw. *Biotechnology* **2007**, *98*, 9–13. [CrossRef]
57. NACA. *Integrated Fish Farming in China*; NACA Technical Manual 7; A World Food Day Publication of the Network of Aquaculture Centres in Asia and the Pacific: Bangkok, Thailand, 1989; 278p, Available online: www.idl-bnc-idrc.dspacedirect.org (accessed on 15 October 2019).
58. Ghasem, S.; Morteza, A.S.; Maryam, T. Effect of organic fertilizers on cucumber (*Cucumis sativus*) yield. *Int. J. Agric. Crop Sci.* **2014**, *7*, 808–814.

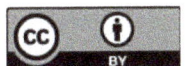

© 2020 by the authors. Licensee MDPI, Basel, Switzerland. This article is an open access article distributed under the terms and conditions of the Creative Commons Attribution (CC BY) license (http://creativecommons.org/licenses/by/4.0/).

MDPI
St. Alban-Anlage 66
4052 Basel
Switzerland
Tel. +41 61 683 77 34
Fax +41 61 302 89 18
www.mdpi.com

Agronomy Editorial Office
E-mail: agronomy@mdpi.com
www.mdpi.com/journal/agronomy

www.ingramcontent.com/pod-product-compliance
Lightning Source LLC
LaVergne TN
LVHW070701100526
838202LV00013B/1007